CT and MR Angiography of the Peripheral Circulation

Dedication

To my parents for their infinite patience, love, and understanding, and who continue to be my source of inspiration, and to my wonderful wife, Suchandra, for her love and support.

Debabrata Mukherjee

I dedicate this book to all the physicists, technicians and physician colleagues in the CT/MR and vascular community from whom I have imbibed what I know in this area. I also dedicate this book to my wife Kyle for her unstinting support through this project.

Sanjay Rajagopalan

CT and MR Angiography of the Peripheral Circulation

Practical Approach with Clinical Protocols

Edited by

Debabrata Mukherjee MD

Gill Foundation Professor of Interventional Cardiology
Director, Cardiac Catheterization Laboratories
University of Kentucky
Lexington, KY
USA

Sanjay Rajagopalan MD FACC

Wolfe Professor of Medicine and Radiology
Director Vascular Medicine and Co-Director of MR/CT Imaging
The Ohio State University
Columbus, OH
USA

Sub editors

Santo Dellegrottaglie MD PhD
Javier Sanz MD

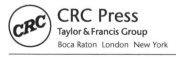

CRC Press
Taylor & Francis Group
Boca Raton London New York

CRC Press is an imprint of the
Taylor & Francis Group, an **informa** business

CRC Press
Taylor & Francis Group
6000 Broken Sound Parkway NW, Suite 300
Boca Raton, FL 33487-2742

First issued in paperback 2019

© 2007 by Taylor & Francis Group, LLC
CRC Press is an imprint of Taylor & Francis Group, an Informa business

No claim to original U.S. Government works

ISBN-13: 978-1-84184-606-4 (hbk)
ISBN-13: 978-0-367-38906-2 (pbk)

Visit the Taylor & Francis Web site at
http://www.taylorandfrancis.com

and the CRC Press Web site at
http://www.crcpress.com

Contents

Contributors

Prachi P Agarwal MD
Assistant Professor
Department of Radiology, Division of Cardiothoracic
    Radiology
University of Michigan
Ann Arbor, MI
USA

Marja Berg MD, PhD
Radiologist
Department of Clinical Radiology
Kuopio University Hospital
Kuopio, Finland

Emil I Cohen MD
Assistant Professor
Department of Radiology
Mount Sinai School of Medicine
New York, NY
USA

Santo Dellegrottaglie MD, PhD
Adjunct Instructor of Medicine (Cardiology)
Mount Sinai School of Medicine
New York, NY
USA

Amish Doshi MD
Mount Sinai School of Medicine
New York, USA

Robert R Edelman MD
Evanston Northwestern Healthcare
Evanston, IL
USA

Andrew J Einstein MD, PhD
Assistant Professor
Department of Medicine, Division of Cardiology
Columbia University College of Physicians and Surgeons
New York, USA

Hale Ersoy MD
Instructor
Department of Radiology
Harvard Medical School
Boston, MA
USA

Claudia Fellner PhD
Institute of Diagnostic Radiology
University Hospital of Regensburg
Regensburg, Germany

Franz A Fellner MD
Institute of Radiology
AK2 Linz
Linz, Austria

Thomas Flohr PhD
Siemens Medical Solutions
Forchheim, Germany

Corey Goldman MD, PhD
Ochsner Clinic Foundation
New Orleans, Louisiana
USA

Michael Grass
Philips Reseach Europe-Hamburg Sector Medical
    Imaging Systems
Hamburg, Germany

John D Grizzard MD
Assistant Professor
Department of Radiology
VCU Medical Center
Section Chief Non-invasive Cardiovascular Imaging
Virginia Commonwealth University
Richmond, VA
USA

James J Jang MD
Kaiser Permanente
Santa Teresa Medical Center
San Jose, CA
USA

Robert M Judd PhD
Duke University Medical Center
Durham, NC
USA

Young S Kang MD, PhD
Santa Clara Valley Medical Center
San Jose, CA
USA

Marko Kangasniemi MD, PhD
Neuroradiologist
Hus-Töölö Hospital
Helsinki University Hospital
Helsinki, Finland

Ella A Kazerooni MD, MS
Professor and Director of Cardiothoracic Radiology
University of Michigan Medical School
Michigan, MI
USA

Raymond J Kim MD, FACC
Associate Professor of Medicine
Co-Director, Duke Cardiovascular Magnetic
    Resonance Center
Duke University Medical Center
Durham, NC
USA

Igor Klem MD
Duke Cardiovascular Magnetic Resonance Center
Duke University
Durham, NC
USA

Robert A Lookstein MD
Assistant Professor
Department of Radiology, Division of Interventional
    Radiology
Mount Sinai School of Medicine
New York, USA

Hannu Manninen MD, PhD
Professor of Interventional Radiology
Department of Clinical Radiology
Kuopio University Hospital
Kuopio, Finland

Robert M Manzke PhD
Senior Member Research Staff
Clinical Sites Research Program
Philips Reseach North America
Massachusetts General Hospital
New York, NY
USA

Diego Martin MD, PhD
Emory University School of Medicine
Atlanta, GA
USA

Debabrata Mukherjee MD
Gill Foundation Professor of
    Interventional Cardiology
Director, Cardiac Catheterization Laboratories
University of Kentucky
Lexington, KY
USA

Chanh D Nguyen MD
Santa Clara Valley Medical Center
San Jose, CA
USA

Bernd Ohnesorge PhD
Siemens Medical Solutions
Forchheim, Germany

Mahesh R Patel MD
Santa Clara Valley Medical Center
San Jose, CA
USA

Martin R Prince MD, PhD
Professor of Radiology
Weill Medical College of Cornell University
Columbia College of Physicians and Surgeons
New York, NY
USA

Sanjay Rajagopalan MD, FACC
Wolfe Professor of Medicine and Radiology
Director Vascular Medicine and Co-Director of
    MR/CT Imaging
The Ohio State University
Columbus, OH
USA

Vasco Gama Ribeiro
Centro Hospitalar V.N.
Gaia
Portugal

Javier Sanz MD
Assistant Professor of Medicine/Cardiology
Mount Sinai School of Medicine
New York, NY
USA

Dipan J Shah MD
Nashville Cardiovascular MRI Institute
Brentwood, TN
USA

Gopi KR Sirineni MD
Emory University School of Medicine
Atlanta, GA
USA

Marc Sirol MD, PhD
Assistant Professor of Medicine
Assistance Publique Hôpitaux de Paris
Hôpital Lariboisière
Paris, France

Mushabbar A Syed MD, FACC
Associate Professor of Medicine/Director of
    Cardiovascular CT & MR Imaging
Gill Heart Institute
University of Kentucky
Lexington, KY
USA

Ritva L Vanninen MD, PhD
Professor (temp.)
Department of Clinical Radiology
Kuopio University Hospital
Kuopio, Finland

Honglei Zhang MD
Research Fellow
Department of Radiology
Weill Medical College of Cornell University
New York, NY
USA

Foreword

The advent of multislice computed tomographic angiography (CTA) and magnetic resonance angiography (MRA) has had a dramatic impact on practice patterns in cardiovascular medicine with a significant proportion of catheter-based diagnostic angiography giving way to these new modalities.

This text represents a comprehensive treatise on CTA and MRA for the diagnosis of peripheral vascular disease and represents a consolidated attempt at bridging the ever-widening gap between innovation in these areas and the knowledge of the general and cardiovascular clinician. A large number of high-quality illustrations make this textbook particularly attractive to the general clinician. Abundant tables and scanning protocols are included in each chapter wherever applicable.

In the first half of the book dedicated to CTA, the introductory chapters address technical principles, image reconstruction, radiation dosimetry, and principles of CT contrast agents and their administration. Subsequently, clinical application of CTA in each major vascular territory is dealt with thoroughly, with clear description of the examination and scanning technique for assessing each specific territory. The section on MRA provides a state of the art overview of this methodology in the peripheral circulation. MR physics relevant to the clinician is succinctly articulated with specific chapters dedicated to pulse sequences commonly used in peripheral angiography and MR contrast agents. Individual chapters on each major vascular territory including the extracranial and intracranial circulation, the pulmonary circulation, the thoracic and the abdominal aorta, the renal, and mesenteric circulation, the lower and upper extremity circulation enable the reader to appreciate the intricacies of MRA techniques for the evaluation of these territories.

In summary, Doctors Debabrata Mukherjee, Sanjay Rajagopalan, Informa Healthcare and colleagues have put together a very didactic and practical book. I believe the information will serve to stimulate the interest not only of the cardiovascular specialist ready to become familiarized with this important technological development of CT and MRI as applied to patients with peripheral vascular disease, but also of a broad range of professionals and students of cardiovascular medicine.

This book is a valuable resource and should help the efforts to incorporate CT and MR in mainstream cardiovascular practice.

Valentin Fuster MD PhD
Professor of Medicine
Director, Mount Sinai Heart
Mount Sinai Medical Center
New York City, NY

1

Fundamentals of multi-slice CT scanning and its application to the periphery

Thomas Flohr and Bernd Ohnesorge

INTRODUCTION

With the introduction of spiral computed tomography (CT) in the early 1990s, volume data could be acquired without the danger of mis-registration or double-registration of anatomic details. Images could be reconstructed at any position along the patient axis (longitudinal axis, z-axis), and overlapping image reconstruction could be used to improve longitudinal resolution. Volumetric data acquisition enabled the development of applications such as CT angiography (CTA). CTA imaging of the lower-extremity arteries had already been attempted with single-slice CT, even though it was limited by either insufficient volume coverage or missing spatial resolution in the z-axis.

Adequate imaging of the peripheral vascular system during a single acquisition and a single injection of contrast medium requires larger volume coverage using shorter scan times and improved longitudinal resolution. This became feasible with the introduction of 4-slice CT systems with 0.5 s gantry rotation by all major CT manufacturers in 1998. The increased performance allowed the optimization of a variety of clinical protocols. Examination times for standard protocols could be significantly reduced or, alternatively, scan ranges could be significantly extended, which is essential for CTA of the lower extremities. Alternatively, a given anatomic volume could be scanned within a time window with substantially reduced slice width and improved longitudinal resolution. This way, for many clinical applications, the goal of isotropic resolution was within reach with 4-slice CT systems. Multi-detector row CT (MDCT) also dramatically expanded

into areas previously considered beyond the scope of third generation CT scanners based on the mechanical rotation of X-ray tube and detector, such as cardiac imaging with the addition of electrocardiographic (EKG) gating capability.

Despite all these promising advances, clinical challenges and limitations remained for 4-slice CT systems. True isotropic resolution had not yet been achieved for many routine applications, such as CTA of the lower extremities, since 2.5 mm collimated slices had to be chosen to complete the scan within a reasonable time frame. For EKG-gated coronary CTA, stents or severely calcified arteries constituted a diagnostic dilemma, mainly due to partial volume artifacts as a consequence of insufficient longitudinal resolution, and reliable imaging of patients with higher heart rates was not possible due to limited temporal resolution. The introduction of an 8-slice CT system in 2000 enabled shorter scan times, but did not yet provide improved longitudinal resolution (thinnest collimation 8×1.25 mm). The latter was achieved with the introduction of 16-slice CT, which made it possible to routinely acquire substantial anatomic volumes with isotropic submillimeter spatial resolution. CT angiographic scans of the peripheral vasculature could now routinely be acquired with 16×0.625 mm or 16×0.75 mm collimation. EKG-gated cardiac scanning benefited from both improved temporal resolution (achieved by gantry rotation times down to 0.375 s) and improved spatial resolution due to near isotropic spatial resolution.

The new generation of 64-slice CT systems introduced in 2004 represents the latest step in the on-going race for more slices. Two different scanner concepts were introduced by the different vendors: the 'volume concept' pursued by GE, Philips, and Toshiba aims at a further increase in volume coverage speed by using 64 detector rows instead of 16 without changing the physical parameters of the scanner compared to the 16-slice version. The 'resolution concept' pursued by Siemens uses 32 physical detector rows in combination with double z-sampling, a refined z-sampling technique enabled by a periodic motion of the focal spot in the z-direction, to simultaneously acquire 64 overlapping slices with the goal of pitch-independent increase of longitudinal resolution and reduction of spiral artifacts. With the most recent generation of CT systems, CT angiographic examinations with submillimeter resolution in the pure arterial phase become feasible even for extended anatomic ranges. The improved temporal resolution due to reductions in gantry rotation times to 0.33 s has the potential of improving the performance of EKG-gated scanning at higher heart rates, thereby significantly reducing the number of patients requiring heart rate control and facilitating the successful integration of CT coronary angiography into routine clinical algorithms.

Figure 1.1 shows the number of slices of new CT systems at the time of their market introduction. Interestingly, analogous to Moore's law, it follows an exponential law, approximately doubling every 2 years. Very useful up-to-date information regarding MDCT is readily available on the Internet, for example at the UK MDCT website www.medical-devices.gov.uk or at www.ctisus.org. An overview of MDCT systems and image reconstruction techniques may be found in other sources as well.

BASIC CT PARAMETERS

CT scale

CT measures the local X-ray attenuation coefficients of the tissue volume elements, or voxels, in an axial slice of the patient's anatomy. The attenuation coefficients are translated into the gray-scale values (CT value) of the corresponding picture elements (pixels) in the displayed two-dimensional image of the slice. The numeric value I_{ij} assigned to a pixel (i,j) corresponds to the average X-ray attenuation $\mu(x_i, y_j)$ within its associated voxel (x_i, y_j), after normalization to the attenuation properties of water

$$I_{ij} = 1000 \frac{\mu(x_i, y_j) - \mu_{water}}{\mu_{water}} [HU]$$

where μ_{water} is the attenuation coefficient of water, typically $\mu_{water} \approx 0.192/cm$. I_{ij} is measured in 'Hounsfield Units' (HU). Pixel values are stored as integers, in the range -1024 to 3071 HU, corresponding to 4096 different values. By definition, $I_{ij} = 0$ HU for water, and $I_{ij} = -1000$ HU for air, independent of the X-ray spectrum. The CT values of human tissue, however, depend on the X-ray spectrum. In general, lung and fat have negative CT values, muscle has positive I_{ij}, and bone has rather large CT values up to 2000 HU. The CT values of different tissues at a typical setting of 120 kV are shown in Figure 1.2.

Administration of iodine contrast agent increases the CT value, with contrast-filled vessels typically having CT values in the range 200 to 600 HU. In most cases they can be easily differentiated from the surrounding tissue which does not exceed a CT value of 100 HU, with the exception of bone. This easy, threshold-based differentiation is the basis for CTA and related image post-processing techniques.

Windowing

CT images are stored with 4096 different gray values; the human eye, however, can distinguish only 30 to 40 gray values at best. To improve visualization, only a user-selectable subset of the 4096 possible gray values is used to display a CT image on the monitor or on film. This subset is called 'window'. It is centered at a CT value called the 'window center', and its width is called the 'window width'. All CT values larger than the maximum CT value in the subset are displayed as white pixels, all CT values smaller than the minimum CT value are displayed as black pixels. Window center and window width have to be selected according to the needs of the clinical application. A 'body' window, for example, is optimized to display the different abdominal tissue types with CT values ranging from −50 HU to 100 HU. It is therefore centered at about 50 HU, with a typical width of 350 to 500 HU. A 'bone' window is intended for best possible visualization of bony details; its width will be much

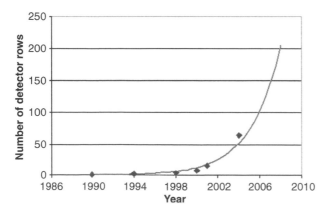

Figure 1.1   The number of detector rows of new CT scanners at the time of market introduction.

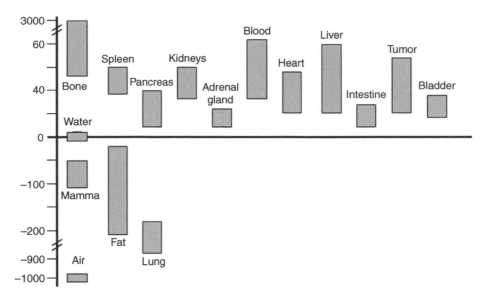

Figure 1.2 CT values (in Hounsfield units, HU) of different tissues at a typical setting of 120 kV. By definition, the CT value is 0 HU for water and −1000 HU for air. Mamma, female breast.

wider and can range from 2000 to 4000 HU. A 'lung' window is usually centered at about −600 HU, with a width of 1200 to 1600 HU.

For CT angiographic examinations of the peripheral vasculature, special attention has to be paid to proper selection of the display window width and center. Choosing a display window that is too narrow can increase the 'blooming' effect of arterial wall calcifications, make them appear larger than they really are, and lead to an overestimation of the degree of stenoses (Figure 1.3). When dealing with heavily calcified arteries, a viewing window width of at least 1500 HU may be required.

MDCT SYSTEM DESIGN

MDCT design has evolved through successive iterations and comprises numerous components outlined below. Besides the inherent challenges involved in designing hardware components for modern CT scanners including gantry design, X-ray sources, and a detector capable of measuring several thousand channels at a time, the acquired data need to be transferred to an image reconstruction system with appropriate post-processing algorithms.

Gantry

Third-generation CT scanners employ the so-called 'rotate/rotate' geometry, in which both X-ray tube and

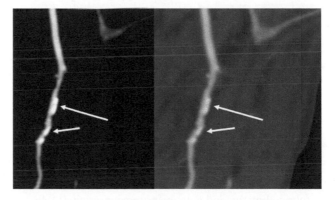

Figure 1.3 Curved multi-planar reformat (MPR) of the peroneal artery in a patient with severe atherosclerotic disease. Left: display window 700 HU. Calcifications (arrows) suffer from increased blooming due to the narrow window setting. They appear much larger than they are and simulate severe stenoses. Right: display window 1500 HU. Blooming is significantly reduced. When dealing with heavily calcified arteries, a viewing window width of at least 1500 HU may be required.

detector are mounted onto a rotating gantry and rotate around the patient (Figure 1.4). In an MDCT system, the detector comprises several rows of 700 or more detector elements which cover a scan field-of-view (SFOV) of usually 50 cm. The X-ray attenuation of the object is measured by the individual detector elements. All measurement values acquired at the same angular position of the measurement system are called a 'projection' or 'view'. Typically 1000 projections are measured during each 360° rotation. Key requirement for the mechanical design of the gantry is the

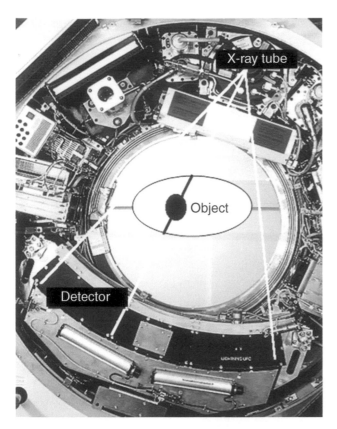

Figure 1.4 Basic system components of a modern 'third generation' CT system.

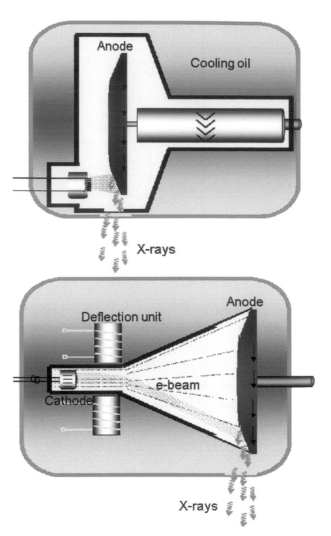

Figure 1.5 Schematic drawings of a conventional X-ray tube (top) and a rotating envelope tube (bottom). The electrons emitted by the cathode are represented by green lines, the X-rays generated in the anode are depicted as purple arrows. In a conventional X-ray tube the anode plate rotates in a vacuum housing. Heat is mainly dissipated via thermal radiation. In a rotating envelope tube, the anode plate constitutes an outer wall of the tube housing and is in direct contact with the cooling oil. Heat is more efficiently dissipated via thermal conduction, and the cooling rate is significantly increased. Rotating envelope tubes have no moving parts and no bearings in the vacuum.

stability of both focal spot and detector position during rotation, in particular with regard to the rapidly increasing rotational speeds of modern CT systems (from 0.75 s in 1994 to 0.33 s in 2003). Hence, the mechanical support for the X-ray tube, tube collimator, and data measurement system (DMS) has to be designed such as to withstand the high gravitational forces associated with fast gantry rotation (~17 **g** for 0.42 s rotation time, ~28 **g** for 0.33 s rotation time). Rotation times of less than 0.25 s (mechanical forces >45 **g**) appear to be beyond today's mechanical limits.

X-ray tube and generator

State-of-the-art X-ray tube/generator combinations provide a peak power of 60–100 kW, usually at various, user-selectable voltages, e.g. 80 kV, 100 kV, 120 kV, and 140 kV. Different clinical applications require different X-ray spectra and hence different kV settings for optimum image quality and/or best possible signal-to-noise ratio at lowest dose. As an example, CT angiographic examinations generally benefit from lower tube voltage. In a conventional tube design, an anode plate of typically 160–220 mm diameter rotates in a vacuum housing (Figure 1.5). The heat storage capacity of

the anode plate and tube housing – measured in mega heat units (MHU) – determines the performance level: the bigger the anode plate is, the larger is the heat storage capacity, and the more scan seconds can be delivered until the anode plate reaches its temperature limit. Typically, a conventional state-of-the-art X-ray tube has a heat storage capacity of 5 to 9 MHU, realized by thick graphite layers attached to the back of the anode plate. An alternative design is the so-called rotating envelope tube (STRATON, Siemens, Forchheim, Germany). The anode plate constitutes an outer wall of the rotating tube housing; it is therefore in direct contact with the cooling oil and can be efficiently cooled via thermal conduction (Figure 1.5). This way, a very high heat dissipation rate of 5 MHU/min is achieved, eliminating the need for heat storage in the anode which consequently has a heat storage capacity close to zero. Owing to the fast anode cooling, rotating envelope tubes can perform high power scans in rapid succession. Due to the central rotating cathode permanent electromagnetic deflection of the electron beam is needed to position and shape the focal spot on the anode (see below and also Figure 1.5). The versatile electromagnetic deflection is a prerequisite for the double z-sampling technology used in a 64-slice CT system.

Tube collimator (prepatient collimator)

In the X-ray tube of a CT scanner a small area on the anode plate, the focal spot, emits X-rays that penetrate the patient and are registered by the detector. A collimator between the X-ray tube and the patient, the tube (prepatient) collimator, is used to shape the beam in the longitudinal (z) direction and to establish the dose profile. For this purpose, a set of collimator blades made of highly absorbing materials such as tungsten or molybdenum is positioned behind the tube entrance window (see Figure 1.6). The opening of these blades is adjusted according to the selected collimated slice width and the size and position of the focal spot. In general, the collimated dose profile is a trapezoid in the longitudinal direction. Usually, additional pre-filters such as bowtie filters can be moved into the X-ray beam to modify its intensity distribution in the scan plane (in the fan angle direction) and to reduce the radiation intensity with increasing distance from the isocenter.

MDCT detector design and slice collimation

Modern CT systems generally use solid state detectors. Each detector element consists of a radiation-sensitive solid state material (such as cadmium tungstate, gadolinium oxide, or gadolinium oxisulfide with suitable dopings), which converts the absorbed X-rays into visible light. The light is then detected by a silicon photodiode. The resulting electrical current is amplified and converted into a digital signal. Key requirements for a suitable detector material are good detection efficiency, i.e. high atomic number, and very short afterglow time to enable the fast gantry rotation speeds that are essential for EKG-gated cardiac imaging. Afterglow is signal decay of the detector following an X-ray irradiation pulse. Ideally, there should be no afterglow – as soon as X-ray irradiation stops, the detector signal should go to zero.

A CT detector must provide different slice widths to adjust the optimum scan speed, longitudinal resolution, and image noise for each application. With a single-slice CT detector, different collimated slice widths are obtained by prepatient collimation of the X-ray beam (see Figure 1.6). For a very elementary model of a 2-slice CT detector consisting of M (number of simultaneously acquired slices) = 2 detector rows, different slice widths can be obtained by prepatient collimation if the detector is separated midway along the z-extent of the X-ray beam.

For $M>2$ this simple design principle must be replaced by more flexible concepts requiring more than M detector rows to simultaneously acquire M slices. Different manufacturers of MDCT scanners have introduced different detector designs. In order to be able to select different slice widths, all scanners combine several detector rows electronically to a smaller

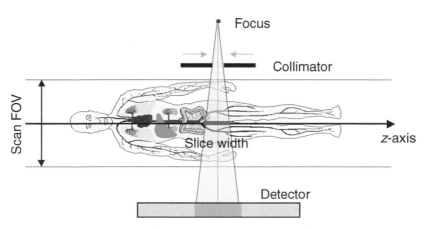

Figure 1.6 Illustration of prepatient collimation of the X-ray beam to obtain different collimated slice widths with a single-slice CT detector.

number of slices according to the selected beam collimation and the desired slice width.

The fixed array detector consists of detector elements with equal sizes in the longitudinal direction. A representative example for this scanner type, the GE Lightspeed scanner, has 16 detector rows, each of them defining a 1.25 mm collimated slice width in the center of rotation. The total coverage in the longitudinal direction is 20 mm at the isocenter; due to geometric magnification the actual detector is about twice as wide. In order to select different slice widths, several detector rows can be electronically combined to a smaller number of slices according to the selected beam collimation and the desired slice width. The following slice widths (measured at the isocenter) are realized: 4×1.25 mm, 4×2.5 mm, 4×3.75 mm, 4×5 mm (see Figure 1.7, top left). The same detector design is used for the 8-slice version of this system, providing 8×1.25 mm and 8×2.5 mm collimated slice width.

A different approach uses an adaptive array detector design, which comprises detector rows with different sizes in the longitudinal direction. Scanners of this type, the Philips M$\times$8000 4-slice scanner and the Siemens SOMATOM Sensation 4 scanner, have 8 detector rows. Their widths in the longitudinal direction range from 1 to 5 mm (at the isocenter) and allow for the following collimated slice widths: 2×0.5 mm, 4×1 mm, 4×2.5 mm, 4×5 mm, 2×8 mm, and 2×10 mm (see Figure 1.7, top center).

Sixteen-slice CT systems have adaptive array detectors in general. A representative example for this scanner type, the Siemens SOMATOM Sensation 16 scanner, uses 24 detector rows (see Figure 1.7, top right). By appropriate combination of the signals of the individual detector rows, either 12 or 16 slices with 0.75 mm or 1.5 mm collimated slice width can be acquired. The GE Lightspeed 16 scanner uses a similar design, which provides 16 slices with either 0.625 mm or 1.25 mm collimated slice width. Yet another design, which is implemented in the Toshiba Aquilion scanner, allows the use of 16 slices with either 0.5 mm, 1 mm, or 2 mm collimated slice width, with a total coverage of 32 mm at the isocenter.

The Siemens SOMATOM Sensation 64 scanner has an adaptive array detector with 40 detector rows. The 32 central rows define a 0.6 mm collimated slice width at the isocenter, the 4 outer rows on both sides define a 1.2 mm collimated slice width (see Figure 1.7, bottom left). The total coverage in the longitudinal direction is 28.8 mm. Using a periodic motion of the focal spot in the z-direction (z-flying focal spot), 64 overlapping 0.6 mm slices per rotation are acquired (see Double z-sampling, below). Alternatively, 24 slices with a 1.2 mm slice width can be obtained. Toshiba, Philips, and GE use fixed array detectors for their systems. The Toshiba Aquilion scanner has 64 detector rows with a collimated slice width of 0.5 mm. The total z-coverage at the isocenter is 32 mm. Both the GE VCT scanner and the Philips Brilliance 64 have 64 detector rows with a collimated slice width of 0.625 mm, enabling the simultaneous read-out of 64 slices (see Figure 1.7, bottom right) with a total coverage of 40 mm in the longitudinal direction.

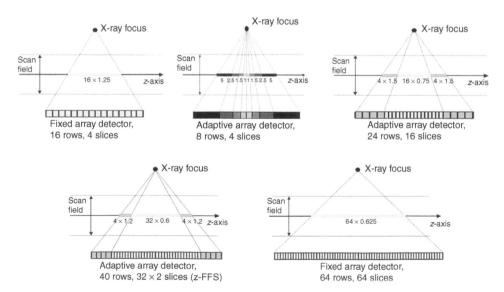

Figure 1.7 Examples of fixed array detectors and adaptive array detectors used in commercially available MDCT systems.

MDCT SPIRAL/HELICAL SCANNING

The two basic modes of MDCT data acquisition are axial and spiral (also called helical) scanning. Using axial scanning, the scan volume is covered by subsequent axial scans in a 'step-and-shoot' technique. The number of images per scan corresponds to the number of active detector rows. In between the individual axial scans the table moves to the next z-position. With the advent of multi-slice CT, axial 'step-and-shoot' scanning has been used in clinical practice for only few applications, such as head scanning or high-resolution lung scanning. It does not play a role in CTA applications, which are exclusively performed in the spiral/helical mode. Spiral/helical scanning is characterized by continuous gantry rotation and continuous data acquisition while the patient table is moving at constant speed (see Figure 1.8).

Pitch

An important parameter to characterize a spiral/helical scan is the pitch p. According to IEC (International Electrotechnical Commission 2002) specifications, p is given by

p = table feed per rotation/total width of the
    collimated beam

This definition holds for single-slice CT as well as for MDCT. It shows whether data acquisition occurs with gaps ($p>1$) or with overlap ($p<1$) in the longitudinal direction.

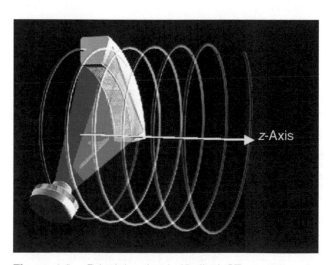

Figure 1.8   Principle of spiral/helical CT scanning: the patient table is continuously translated while multiple rotations of scan data are acquired. The path of the X-ray tube and detector relative to the patient is a helix.

With 4×1 mm collimation and a table-feed of 6 mm/rotation, the pitch is $p=6/(4\times1)=6/4=1.5$. With 16×0.75 mm collimation and a table feed of 18 mm/rotation, the pitch is also $p=18/(16\times0.75)=18/12=1.5$. In the early days of 4-slice CT, the term *volume pitch* had been additionally introduced, which was derived by using the width of one single slice in the denominator. For the sake of clarity and uniformity, the volume pitch should no longer be used. For general radiology applications, clinically useful pitch values range from 0.5 to 2. For the special case of EKG-gated cardiac scanning, very low pitch values of 0.2 to 0.4 are usually applied to ensure gapless volume coverage of the heart during each phase of the cardiac cycle.

Collimated and effective slice width

Both single-slice and multi-slice spiral CT require an interpolation of the acquired measurement data in the longitudinal direction to estimate a complete CT data set at the desired plane of reconstruction. As a consequence of this interpolation the slice profile changes from the trapezoidal, sometimes almost rectangular shape known from axial scanning to a more bell-shaped curve (see Figure 1.9). z-Axis resolution is no longer only determined by the collimated beam width s_{coll} as in axial scanning, but by the effective slice width s which is established in the spiral interpolation process. Usually, s is defined as the full width at half maximum (FWHM) of the slice sensitivity profile (SSP). The wider s gets for a given collimated beam width s_{coll}, the more the longitudinal resolution degrades. In single-slice spiral CT, s increases with increasing pitch (Figure 1.10). This is a consequence of the increasing longitudinal distance of the projections used for spiral interpolation. The SSP is not only characterized by its FWHM, but the entire shape has to be taken into account: an SSP that has far-reaching tails degrades longitudinal resolution more than a well-defined, close to rectangular SSP – even if both have the same FWHM and hence the same effective slice width.

Multi-slice linear interpolation and z-filtering

Multi-slice linear interpolation is characterized by a projection-wise linear interpolation between two rays on either side of the image plane to establish a CT data set at the desired image z-position. In general, scanners relying on this technique

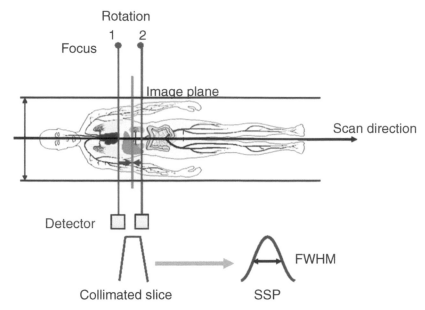

Figure 1.9 Principle of single-slice spiral/helical interpolation. For each view angle, an interpolation of the acquired measurement data (schematically shown as red lines) has to be performed in the z-direction to estimate a complete CT data set at the desired image position (green). As a result of this interpolation (indicated by the two blue arrows), z-axis resolution is no longer determined by the collimated slice width as in axial scanning, but by the effective slice width which is defined as the full width at half maximum (FWHM) of the slice sensitivity profile (SSP).

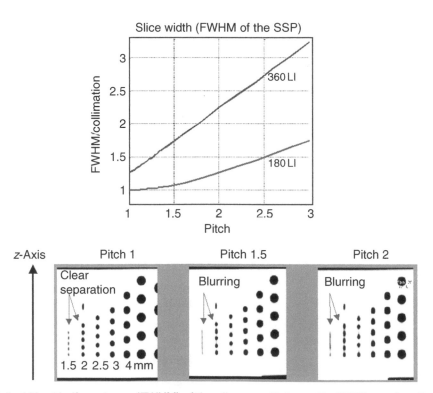

Figure 1.10 Top: full width at half maximum (FWHM) of the slice sensitivity profile (SSP) as a function of the pitch for the two most commonly used single-slice spiral interpolation approaches, 180° linear interpolation (180 LI) and 360° linear interpolation (360 LI). For both, the slice significantly widens with increasing pitch as a result of the increasing distance of the interpolation partners. Bottom: multi-planar reformats (MPRs) of a spiral z-resolution phantom scanned with 2 mm collimation (180 LI) show increased blurring of the 1.5 mm and 2 mm cylinders with increasing pitch as a consequence of the increasing effective slice width.

provide selected discrete pitch values to the user, such as 0.75 and 1.5 for 4-slice scanning or 0.5625, 0.9375, 1.375, and 1.75 for 16-slice scanning. The user has to be aware of pitch-dependent effective slice widths. For low-pitch scanning (at $p=0.75$ using 4 slices and at $p=0.5625$ or 0.9375 using 16 slices), $s \sim s_{coll}$ and for a collimated 1.25 mm slice the resulting effective slice width stays at 1.25 mm. The narrow SSP, however, is achieved by conjugate interpolation at the price of increased image noise. For high-pitch scanning (at $p=1.5$ using 4 slices and at $p=1.375$ or 1.75 using 16 slices), $s \sim 1.27 s_{coll}$ and a collimated 1.25 mm slice results in an effective 1.5–1.6 mm slice. To obtain the same image noise as in an axial scan with the same collimated slice width, 0.73–1.68 times the dose depending on the spiral pitch is required, with the lowest dose at the highest pitch. Thus, as a 'take home point', when selecting the scan protocol for a particular application, scanning at low pitch optimizes image quality and longitudinal resolution at a given collimation, yet at the expense of increased patient dose. To reduce patient dose, either mA settings should be reduced at low pitch or high pitch values should be chosen.

In a z-filter multi-slice spiral reconstruction, the spiral interpolation for each projection angle is no longer restricted to the two rays in closest proximity to the image plane. Instead, all direct and complementary rays within a selectable distance from the image plane contribute to the image. A representative example for a z-filter approach is the adaptive axial interpolation implemented in Siemens CT scanners. Another example is the MUSCOT algorithm used by Toshiba. z-Filtering allows the system to trade off z-axis resolution (SSP) with image noise (which directly correlates with required dose). From the same CT raw data, images with different slice widths can be retrospectively reconstructed. Only slice widths equal to or larger than the sub-beam collimation can be obtained. With the adaptive axial interpolation the effective slice width is kept constant for all pitch values between 0.5 and 1.5. Therefore, longitudinal resolution is independent of the pitch (see Figure 1.11). As a consequence of the pitch-independent spiral slice width, the image noise for a fixed 'effective' mAs (that is mAs divided by the pitch p, see also Radiation dose in MDCT, below) is nearly independent of the spiral pitch. For a 1.25 mm effective slice width reconstructed from 4×1 mm collimation, 0.61–0.69 times the dose is required to maintain the image noise of an axial scan at the same collimation. Radiation dose is also independent of the pitch and equals the dose of an axial scan at the same mAs. Thus, as a 'take-home point', using higher pitch does not result in dose saving, which is an important practical consideration with CT systems relying on adaptive axial interpolation and the 'effective' mAs concept.

With regard to image quality, narrow collimation is preferable to wide collimation, due to better suppression of partial volume artifacts and a more rectangular SSP, even if

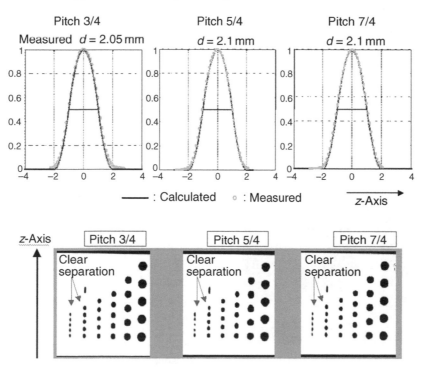

Figure 1.11 Adaptive axial interpolation for a 4-slice CT system: slice sensitivity profile of the 2 mm slice (for 4×1 mm collimation) at selected pitch values. The functional form of the SSP and hence the effective slice width (d in the figure) are independent of the pitch. Consequently, multi-planar reformats of a spiral z-resolution phantom scanned with 2 mm slice width show clear separation of the 1.5 mm and 2 mm cylinders for all pitch values.

the pitch has to be increased for equivalent volume coverage (see Figure 1.12). Similar to single-slice spiral CT, narrow collimation scanning is the key to reduce artifacts and improve image quality. The best suppression of spiral artifacts is achieved by both using narrow collimation relative to the desired slice width and reducing the spiral pitch.

Three-dimensional back-projection and adaptive multiple plane reconstruction

For CT scanners with 16 and more slices, modified reconstruction approaches accounting for the cone beam geometry of the measurement rays have to be considered: the measurement rays in MDCT are tilted by the so-called cone angle with respect to a plane perpendicular to the z-axis. The cone angle is largest for the slices at the outer edges of the detector and it increases with increasing number of detector rows if their width is kept constant. Some manufacturers (Toshiba, Philips) use a three-dimensional (3D) filtered back-projection reconstruction. With this approach, the measurement rays are back-projected into a 3D volume along the lines of measurement, this way accounting for their cone beam geometry. Other manufacturers use algorithms which split the 3D reconstruction task into a series of conventional 2D reconstructions on tilted intermediate image planes. A representative example is the adaptive multiple plane reconstruction (AMPR) used by Siemens. Multi-slice spiral scanning using AMPR in combination with the 'effective' mAs concept is characterized by the same key properties as adaptive axial interpolation. Thus, all recommendations regarding selection of collimation and pitch that have been discussed there also apply to

AMPR. In particular, changing the pitch does not change the radiation exposure to the patient, and using higher pitch does not result in dose saving. Narrow collimation scanning should be performed whenever possible.

Double z-sampling

The double z-sampling concept for multi-slice spiral scanning makes use of a periodic motion of the focal spot in the longitudinal direction to improve data sampling along the z-axis. By continuous electromagnetic deflection of the electron beam in a rotating envelope X-ray tube, the focal spot is wobbled between two different positions on the anode plate. The amplitude of the periodic z-motion is adjusted in a way that two subsequent readings are shifted by half a collimated slice width in the patient's longitudinal direction (Figure 1.13). Therefore, the measurement rays of two subsequent readings with a collimated slice-width s_{coll} interleave in the z-direction, and every two M-slice readings are combined to one 2M-slice projection with a sampling distance of $s_{coll}/2$. In the Siemens SOMATOM Sensation 64, as an example of an MDCT system relying on double z-sampling, two subsequent 32-slice readings are combined to one 64-slice projection with a sampling distance of 0.3 mm at the isocenter. As a consequence, spatial resolution in the longitudinal direction is increased, and objects <0.4 mm in diameter can

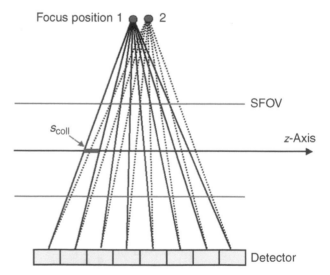

Figure 1.13 Principle of improved z-sampling with the z-flying focal spot technique. Due to a periodic motion of the focal spot in the z-direction two subsequent M-slice readings are shifted by half a collimated slice width $s_{coll}/2$ at the isocenter and can be interleaved to one 2M-slice projection. The simultaneous radial motion of the focal spot in an actual X-ray tube has been omitted to simplify the drawing. SFOV: scan field of view. M, counts the number of simultaneously acquired slices.

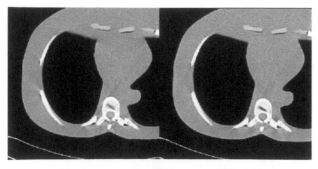

Figure 1.12 Images of a thorax phantom with a 3 mm slice width obtained from 4×2.5 mm collimation at pitch 0.75 (left) and 4×1 mm collimation at pitch 1.75 (right). Despite the higher pitch, the images acquired with 4×1 mm collimation show fewer artifacts at the ribs.

be routinely resolved at any pitch. Another benefit of double z-sampling is the suppression of spiral 'windmill' artifacts at any pitch (Figure 1.14).

VOLUME COVERAGE IN SPIRAL/HELICAL MDCT WITH SPECIAL EMPHASIS ON PERIPHERAL CT ANGIOGRAPHY

In MDCT spiral scans, the volume coverage speed can be increased by choosing wider collimated slice widths, by reducing the gantry rotation time t_{rot}, by increasing the pitch p, and, of course, by increasing the number M of simultaneously acquired slices. A simple equation relates the volume coverage speed v to these parameters:

$$v = \frac{M s_{coll} P}{t_{rot}}$$

A scanner with $M=64$ collimated detector rows, $s_{coll}=0.625$ mm, $p=1.375$, and $t_{rot}=0.5$ s can be as fast as 110 mm/s. However, these high volume coverage speeds are not necessarily useful for CTA of the peripheral vessels, since there is a considerable danger of 'outrunning' the bolus when the table moves faster than the contrast medium bolus. Any stenosis, occlusion, or aneurysm may delay downstream vascular opacification, and both legs may have different circulation times. It has been shown that consistently good results in peripheral CTA can be achieved if a maximum volume

coverage speed $v=30$ mm/s is not exceeded. Assuming a scan range of 1200 mm from the renal artery origins through the feet, this corresponds to a scan time of about 40 s, which is usually well tolerated since breath holding is only required at the beginning of scan data acquisition in the abdominal and pelvic region.

A 4-slice scanner with a beam collimation of 4×2.5 mm, a pitch of 1.5, and 0.5 s gantry rotation time would provide a volume coverage speed of 30 mm/s. The thinnest possible reconstruction slice width is about 3 mm. These data sets are adequate for the visualization of larger arteries such as the aorta, the iliac, or the femoral arteries. They may be of limited value, when visualization of smaller arterial branches is required. With a 16-slice scanner, 16×0.625 mm or 16×0.75 mm collimation (depending on the manufacturer) can be selected. Using 0.5 s gantry rotation time and pitch 1.375 (with 16×0.625 mm collimation) a volume coverage speed of 27.5 mm/s is achieved. Using 0.5 s gantry rotation time and pitch 1.2 (with 16×0.75 mm collimation) the table travels as fast as 28.8 mm/s. Longitudinal resolution in peripheral CTA can be considerably improved with 16-slice systems compared to 4-slice scanners, which immediately translates into diagnostic benefit: Schertler et al compared 16-slice CTA data with different slice widths and reconstruction increments (2.0 mm and 1.0 mm, 1.0 mm and 0.5 mm, 0.75 mm and 0.4 mm, respectively) for 17 patients with occlusive peripheral artery disease and found that specificity was significantly improved for the thin slice data, while sensitivity did not differ. Accuracy of stenosis detection was 88.2%, 90.8%, and 96.1% for the three slice width/reconstruction increment combinations, respectively. Sixty-four-slice systems can be routinely operated at 64×0.6 mm/64×0.625 mm collimation for best possible longitudinal resolution – ideally better than 0.4 mm, e.g. with the use of double z-sampling. In this case, the scanner has to be deliberately slowed down by choosing longer rotation times or reducing the pitch to values below 1. A suitable protocol for a 64-slice CT scanner with 0.6 mm collimation and double z-sampling is 0.5 s gantry rotation time and pitch 0.8 for a volume coverage speed of 30.7 mm/s. A system with 64×0.625 mm collimation has to be operated at a slower gantry rotation time of 0.7 s and pitch 0.5625 to achieve a volume coverage speed of 32 mm/s.

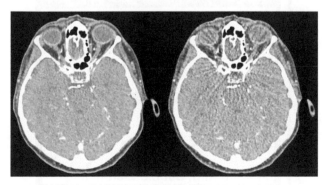

Figure 1.14 Reduction of spiral artifacts with double z-sampling. Left: neck scan acquired with 32×0.6 collimation in a 64-slice acquisition mode with the z-flying focal spot at pitch 1.5. Right: same scan, using only one focus position of the z-flying focal spot for image reconstruction. Due to the improved longitudinal sampling with z-flying focal spot (left) spiral interpolation artifacts (windmill structures on high contrast objects) are suppressed without degradation of z-axis resolution.

SPATIAL RESOLUTION IN MDCT

The matrix size for axial images in CT is generally 512×512 picture elements (pixels). Considered as a part of a 3D image volume an axial image is a layer of 512×512 voxels within that volume. The voxel size in the image plane (in the x–y direction), also called in-plane voxel size, is determined by the reconstruction field-of-view (FOV). The voxel size perpendicular to the image plane (in the z-direction), also called through-plane voxel size, is given by the reconstruction slice width. Calculating FOV/matrix size yields the in-plane voxel size. The reconstruction FOV is selected as an image reconstruction parameter. The larger the FOV, the larger the in-plane voxel size is. A FOV of 250 mm, for example, results in 0.5 mm in-plane voxel size. The in-plane voxel size is often mistaken as the in-plane resolution of a CT image. In most cases, however, the image resolution is mainly determined by the convolution kernel (filter) chosen for image reconstruction and not by the in-plane voxel size. Typical convolution kernels used for abdominal imaging or for CT angiographic studies of the peripheral vasculature provide a resolution of 8–10 line pairs/cm, corresponding to 0.5–0.6 mm object size in the scan plane that can be resolved. All relevant information will be displayed as soon as the image voxel size is smaller than the minimum object size that can be resolved with the selected convolution kernel. For peripheral CTAs, this is usually achieved when the FOV for image reconstruction is not larger than 250–300 mm. Further reducing the FOV will reduce the in-plane voxel size, but will not increase image resolution. Only in special cases, such as high-resolution thorax imaging with a large FOV of 350–400 mm, will the in-plane voxel size be the limiting factor for in-plane resolution.

Sometimes, the reconstruction increment in the z-direction is mistaken for the through-plane voxel size or the longitudinal (z-axis) resolution of the images. Longitudinal resolution, however, is mainly determined by the reconstruction slice width. In a spiral/helical mode, the effective slice width – the FWHM of the spiral SSP – is adjusted in the spiral interpolation process during image reconstruction. In general, slice widths equal to or larger than the collimated slice width can be reconstructed. When scan data have been acquired with, for example, 4×1 mm collimation, the thinnest possible slice is 1 mm. Reconstructing images with an overlap results in improved longitudinal resolution, but no better longitudinal resolution than about 0.7 times the reconstruction slice width, even if the reconstruction increment chosen is incrementally small. Clinical practice suggests a reconstruction increment of 0.5–0.8 times the reconstruction slice width if the corresponding axial images are to be used for 3D post-processing.

While in-plane spatial resolution did not significantly change from 4-slice to 64-slice CT, longitudinal resolution has considerably improved. The progress in longitudinal resolution from 4-slice to 64-slice CT can best be demonstrated with a z-resolution phantom, which consists of a lucite plate with rows of cylindrical holes with different diameters aligned in the z-direction (see Figure 1.15). The 4-slice CT scanner with 4×1 mm collimation can resolve 0.8 mm objects. With 16×0.75 mm collimation, 0.6 mm objects can be delineated. The 64-slice CT scanner with 64×0.6 mm collimation and double z-sampling can routinely resolve 0.4 mm objects. In-plane spatial resolution for routine examinations of chest and abdomen or CT angiographic studies is about 0.4 to 0.6 mm, depending on the selected convolution kernel. Isotropic resolution of 0.4–0.6 mm for routine applications, that is equal spatial resolution in all three dimensions, has been achieved with the latest generation of 64-slice CT systems. For special applications such as inner ear or wrist imaging, both in-plane and longitudinal spatial resolution can be increased up to 0.25 mm with some 64-slice CT systems (Figure 1.16). This resolution level is comparable to the resolution achieved with flat-panel detector technology used in some preclinical prototype CT systems. Increased spatial resolution, however, goes hand in hand with increased pixel noise in the

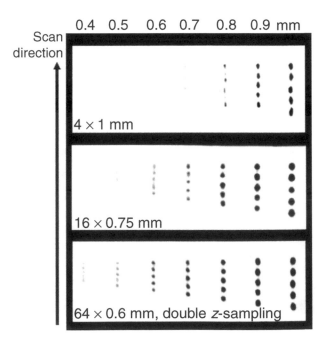

Figure 1.15 Progress in longitudinal resolution from 4-slice to 64-slice CT. The 4-slice CT scanner with 4×1 mm collimation (top) can resolve 0.8 mm objects. With 16× 0.75 mm collimation, 0.6 mm objects can be delineated (center). The 64-slice CT scanner with 64×0.6 mm collimation and double z-sampling can routinely resolve 0.4 mm objects (bottom). The z-resolution phantom was scanned at a pitch of 1.5 for all three scanner types.

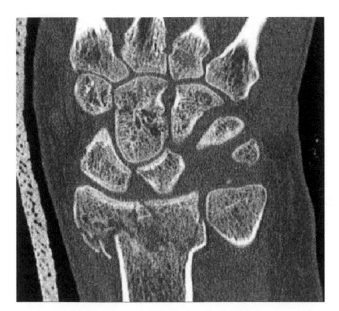

Figure 1.16 Multi-planar reformat (MPR) of a wrist fracture acquired with 0.25 mm isotropic resolution (SOMATOM Sensation 64). The image demonstrates a level of resolution previously known only from research CT systems with flat-panel detectors (image courtesy of Dr C Becker, Klinikum Großhadern, Munich, Germany).

images. Consequently, to maintain a given signal-to-noise ratio, one has to increase the applied radiation dose. If spatial resolution is to be doubled in all three dimensions without increasing the pixel noise, e.g. to perform routine examinations at 0.25 mm isotropic resolution instead of 0.5 mm, the dose needs to be increased 16-fold. It is not expected that the radiation dose to the patient can be increased this much for routine applications. Dose reference values and limitations are now being introduced in many countries. Therefore ultrahigh-resolution imaging will be limited to special applications where high noise levels can be tolerated because of high object contrast, e.g. in lung or bone imaging.

RADIATION DOSE AND RADIATION DOSE REDUCTION

Radiation exposure of the patient by CT and the resulting potential radiation hazard has recently gained considerable attention both in the public and in the scientific literature. Typical values for the effective patient dose of selected CT protocols are 1–2 mSv for a head examination, 5–7 mSv for a chest CT, and 8–11 mSv for CT of the abdomen and pelvis. This radiation exposure must be appreciated in the context of the average annual background radiation, which is 2–5 mSv (3.6 mSv in the US).

Radiation dose in MDCT

The principles of radiation dosimetry are discussed in Chapter 3. To represent the dose in a spiral scan, both single-slice and multi-slice, it is essential to account for gaps or overlaps between the radiation dose profiles from consecutive rotations of the X-ray source. For this purpose $CTDI_{vol}$, the volume $CTDI_w$, has been introduced:

$$CTD_{vol} = 1/p \times CTDI_w = 1/p \times mAs \times (CTDI_w)_n$$
$$= mA \times 1/p \times (CTDI_w)_n$$

where t_{rot}, rotation time; p, pitch; mA, X-ray tube current; CTDI, computerized tomographic dose index; $CTDI_w$, weighted computerized tomographic dose index; $(CTDI_w)_n$, weighted CTDI normalized per mAs. The factor $1/p$ accounts for the increasing dose accumulation with decreasing spiral pitch due to the increasing spiral overlap. In principle, this equation holds for single-slice CT as well as for MDCT. Some manufacturers such as Siemens have introduced an 'effective' mAs concept for spiral/helical scanning which includes the factor $1/p$ into the mAs definition:

$$(mAs)_{eff} = mA \times t_{tot} \times 1/p = mAs \times 1/p$$

For spiral/helical scans, $(mAs)_{eff}$ is indicated on the user interface. The dose of a multi-detector row spiral/helical scan is simply given by:

$$CTDI_{vol} = (mAs)_{eff} \times (CTDI_w)_n.$$

Some other manufacturers, such as Toshiba and GE, stay with the conventional mAs definition, and the user has to perform the $1/p$ correction himself. When comparing the scan parameters for CT systems of different manufacturers, the underlying mAs definition has to be taken into account. This is of particular importance for scan protocols relying on very low pitch settings such as in EKG-gated cardiac CT. If the scanner is operated at a pitch of 0.25 – a typical value for EKG-gated examinations of the heart – 150 mAs, for example, correspond to 600 effective mAs.

$CTDI_w$ is a physical dose measure; it does not provide full information on the radiation risk associated with a CT examination. For this purpose the concept of 'effective dose' has been introduced by the ICRP (International Commission on Radiation Protection). The effective dose is given in mSv and is discussed in detail in Chapter 3 on radiation dosimetry.

Despite its undisputed clinical benefits, multi-slice scanning is often considered to require an increased patient dose compared with single-slice CT. And indeed, a certain increase in radiation dose is unavoidable due to the underlying physical principles.

In general, the collimated dose profile is a trapezoid in the longitudinal direction. In the umbral region, that is the plateau region of the trapezoid, X-rays emitted from the entire area of the focal spot illuminate the detector. In the penumbra regions, only a part of the focal spot illuminates the detector, while the prepatient collimator blocks off other parts. With single-slice CT, the entire trapezoidal dose profile can contribute to the detector signal and the collimated slice width is determined as the FWHM of this trapezoid. The relative dose utilization of a single-slice CT system can therefore be close to 100%. With MDCT, in most cases only the plateau region of the dose profile is used to ensure equal signal level for all detector elements. The penumbra region is then discarded, either by a post-patient collimator or by the intrinsic self-collimation of the multi-slice detector, and represents 'wasted' dose. The relative contribution of the penumbra region increases with decreasing slice width, and it decreases with increasing number of simultaneously acquired slices. This is demonstrated in Figure 1.17, which compares the 'minimum width' dose profiles for a 4-slice CT system and a corresponding 16-slice CT system with an equal collimated width of one detector slice. Correspondingly, the relative dose utilization at 4×1 mm collimation with 4-slice CT is 70% or less, depending on the scanner type. With 16-slice CT systems and submillimeter collimation, dose utilization can be improved up to 84%, again depending on scanner type. Some MDCT systems offer special implementations of even more dose-efficient modes which use a portion of the penumbral region. As a 'take-home point', routine submillimeter scanning is possible with CT systems equipped with 16 and more slices without the penalty of limited dose efficiency and thus increased radiation dose to the patient.

Radiation dose reduction

Approaches for radiation exposure reduction are discussed in detail in Chapter 3. The most important factor is an adaptation of the dose to patient size and weight. This is of particular importance in pediatric imaging. Dose reduction in CT angiography can be obtained by lower kV settings (Figure 1.18).

Another approach for dose reduction which finds increased implementation in clinical practice is anatomic tube current modulation. With this technique the tube output is adapted to the patient geometry during each rotation of the scanner to compensate for strongly varying X-ray attenuations in asymmetric body regions such as the shoulders and pelvis. In studies with cardiac synchronization, dose exposure can be minimized with the use of EKG-controlled tube output modulation (EKG-pulsing).

EKG-TRIGGERED AND EKG-GATED CARDIOVASCULAR CT

Principles of EKG triggering and EKG gating

For EKG-synchronized examinations of the cardiothoracic anatomy, either EKG-triggered axial scanning or EKG-gated spiral scanning can be used. A technical overview on EKG-controlled CT scanning may be found in other sources (see Further reading).

In EKG-triggered axial scanning, the heart volume is covered by subsequent axial scans in a 'step-and-shoot' technique. The number of images per scan corresponds to the number of active detector slices. In between the individual axial scans, the table moves to the next z-position. Due to the

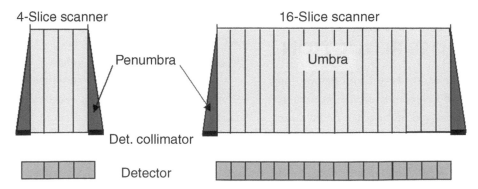

Figure 1.17 Dose profiles for a 4-slice CT system and a 16-slice CT system with an identical collimated width of one detector slice. The relative contribution of the penumbra region, which represents wasted dose, decreases with increasing number of simultaneously acquired slices. Det. collimator, detector collimator (post-patient collimator).

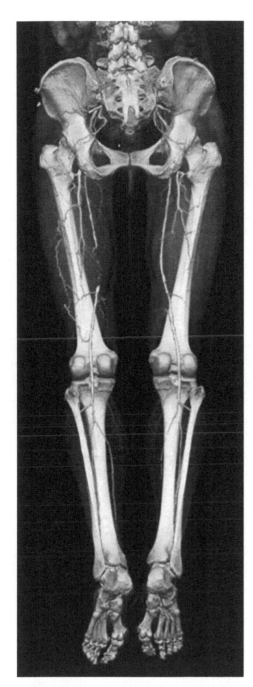

Figure 1.18 Peripheral run-off acquired on a 16-slice scanner at 100 kV, 150 eff mAs. Effective patient dose for this scan was 3.4 mSv, 25% less than for the standard 120 kV protocol (courtesy of Dr C Becker, Klinikum Großhadern, Munich, Germany).

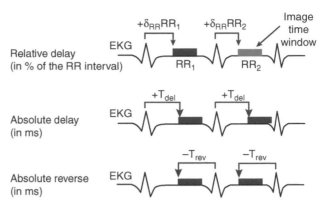

Figure 1.19 Schematic illustration of absolute and relative phase setting for EKG-controlled CT examinations of the cardiothoracic anatomy.

certain percentage of the RR interval time) or absolute (given in ms) and either forward or reverse (Figure 1.19).

Since the table is stationary for each individual scan and moves only in between scans, no multi-detector row spiral interpolation is necessary. To improve temporal resolution, modified reconstruction approaches for partial scan data have been proposed, which provide a temporal resolution up to half the gantry rotation time per image in a sufficiently centered region of interest. Some of the recently introduced 16-slice and 64-slice CT systems offer gantry rotation times shorter than 0.5 s, such as 0.4 s, 0.37 s, or even 0.33 s. In this case, temporal resolution can be as good as 200 ms, 185 ms, or 165 ms.

With retrospective EKG gating, the heart volume is covered continuously by a spiral scan. The patient's EKG signal is recorded simultaneously to data acquisition to allow for a retrospective selection of the data segments used for image reconstruction. Only scan data acquired in a predefined cardiac phase, usually the diastolic phase, are used for image reconstruction. The data segments contributing to an image start with a user-defined offset relative to the onset of the R-waves, similar to EKG-triggered axial scanning (Figure 1.20).

Image reconstruction generally consists of two parts: multi-detector row spiral interpolation to compensate for the continuous table movement and to obtain scan data at the desired image z-position, followed by a partial scan reconstruction of the axial data segments (Figure 1.20). Image reconstruction during different heart phases is feasible by shifting the start points of the data segments used for image reconstruction relative to the R-waves. For a given start position, a stack of images at different z-positions covering a small subvolume of the heart can be reconstructed thanks to the multi-slice data acquisition.

time necessary for table motion, only every second heart beat can be used for data acquisition, which limits the minimum slice width to 2.5 mm with 4-slice or 1.25 mm with 8-slice CT systems if the whole heart volume has to be covered within one breath-hold period. Scan data are acquired with a predefined temporal offset relative to the R-waves of the patient's EKG signal which can be either relative (given as a

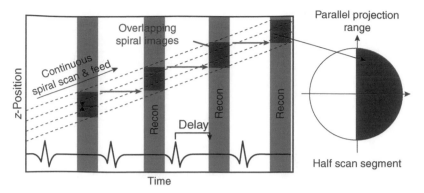

Figure 1.20 Principle of retrospectively EKG-gated spiral scanning with single-segment reconstruction. The patient's EKG signal is indicated as a function of time on the horizontal axis, and the position of the detector slices relative to the patient is shown on the vertical axis (in this example for a 4-slice CT system). The table moves continuously, and continuous spiral scan data of the heart volume are acquired. Only scan data acquired in a predefined cardiac phase, usually the diastolic phase, are used for image reconstruction (indicated as red boxes). The spiral interpolation is illustrated for some representative projection angles.

EKG-gated single-segment and multi-segment reconstruction

In a single-segment reconstruction, each image is reconstructed by using data from one heart cycle only, which are acquired at a predetermined period within the RR interval. There is no mixture of data from different heart cycles in an image (see Figure 1.20). At low heart rates, a single-segment reconstruction yields the best compromise between sufficient temporal resolution on the one hand and adequate volume coverage with thin slices on the other.

The temporal resolution of an image can be improved up to $t_{rot}/(2N)$ by using scan data of N subsequent heart cycles for image formation in a so-called multi-segment reconstruction. With increased N, better temporal resolution is achieved, but at the expense of slower volume coverage: every z-position of the heart has to be seen by a detector slice at every time during the N heart cycles. As a consequence, the larger N and the lower the patient's heart rate is, the more the spiral pitch has to be reduced. With this technique, the patient's heart rate and the gantry rotation time of the scanner have to be properly desynchronized to allow for improved temporal resolution. Depending on the relationship between the rotation time and the patient heart rate, the temporal resolution is generally not constant, but varies between one half and $1/(2N)$ times the gantry rotation time in an N-segment reconstruction. There are 'sweet spots', heart rates with optimum temporal resolution, and heart rates where temporal resolution cannot be improved beyond half the gantry rotation time. Multi-segment approaches rely on a complete periodicity of the heart motion, and they encounter their limitations for patients with arrhythmia or patients with changing heart rates during examination. They may improve image quality in selected cases, but the reliability of obtaining good-quality images with N-segment reconstruction goes down with increasing N. In general, clinical practice suggests the use of 1 segment at lower heart rates and $N \geq 2$ segments at higher heart rates. In some CT scanners (Siemens), the partial scan data segment is automatically divided into 1 or 2 subsegments depending on the patient's heart rate during examination (adaptive cardio volume (ACV) algorithm). In some other CT scanners (GE), the single-segment partial scan images are reconstructed prospectively as base-line images, followed by a 2-segment reconstruction retrospectively for a potential gain of temporal resolution for higher heart rates.

EKG-controlled dose modulation

Prospective EKG triggering combined with 'step and shoot' acquisition of axial slices has the benefit of smaller patient dose than EKG-gated spiral scanning, since scan data are acquired in the previously specified heart phases only. However, it does not provide continuous volume coverage with overlapping slices and increases the likelihood of misregistration of anatomic details. Furthermore, reconstruction of images in different phases of the cardiac cycle for functional evaluation is not possible. Since EKG-triggered axial scanning depends on a reliable prediction of the patient's next RR interval by using the mean of the preceding RR intervals, the method encounters its limitations for patients with severe arrhythmia. To maintain the benefits of EKG-gated spiral CT but obviate the resulting increments in dose,

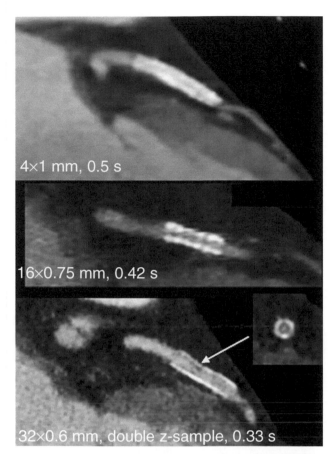

4×1 mm, 0.5 s

16×0.75 mm, 0.42 s

32×0.6 mm, double z-sample, 0.33 s

Figure 1.21 Patient examples depicting a similar clinical situation (a stent in the proximal LAD) for the 4-slice system, the 16-slice system, and the 64-slice system with double z-sampling, demonstrating the improvement in longitudinal resolution from one MDCT scanner generation to the next. With the 64-slice system, an in-stent restenosis (arrow) can be evaluated. Four-slice case courtesy of Hopital de Coracao, Sao Paulo, Brasil; 16-slice case courtesy of Dr A Küttner, Tübingen University, Germany, and 64-slice case courtesy of Dr CM Wong, Hong Kong, China.

EKG-controlled dose modulation has been developed. During the spiral scan, the output of the X-ray tube is modulated according to the patient's EKG. It is kept at its nominal value during a user-defined phase of the cardiac cycle, in general the mid- to end-diastolic phase. During the rest of the cardiac cycle, the tube output is typically reduced to 20% of its nominal value, although not switched off entirely to allow for image reconstruction throughout the entire cardiac cycle. Depending on the heart rate, dose reduction of 30–50% has been demonstrated in clinical studies.

SUMMARY AND CONCLUSIONS

The major improvements of 16-slice CT compared with established 4-slice scanners include improved temporal resolution due to shorter gantry rotation times, better spatial resolution owing to submillimeter collimation, and considerably reduced examination times. Sixty-four-slice CT with further improvements in spatial resolution by techniques such as double z-sampling, and further improvements in temporal resolution is expected to further improve clinical performance, in particular for EKG-gated applications (Figure 1.21).

MDCT evaluation of the peripheral vasculature has revolutionized diagnostic evaluation of peripheral vascular disease. These techniques currently play a dominant role in the management of these patients and in concert with magnetic resonance angiographic techniques will likely represent the standard of care for these patients.

FURTHER READING

Fleischmann D, Hallett RL, Rubin GD. CT angiography of peripheral arterial disease. J Vasc Interv Radiol 2006; 17: 3–26.

Flohr T, Stierstorfer K, Raupach R, Ulzheimer S, Bruder H. Performance evaluation of a 64-slice CT system with z-flying focal spot. Rofo 2004; 176: 1803–10.

Flohr TG, Schoepf UJ, Kuettner A et al. Advances in cardiac imaging with 16-section CT systems. Acad Radiol 2003; 10: 386–401.

Flohr TG, Schaller S, Stierstorfer K et al. Multi-detector row CT systems and image-reconstruction techniques. Radiology 2005; 235: 756–73.

Fraioli F, Catalano C, Napoli A et al. Low-dose multidetector-row CT angiography of the infra-renal aorta and lower extremity vessels: image quality and diagnostic accuracy in comparison with standard DSA. Eur Radiol 2006; 16: 137–46.

Hu H, He HD, Foley WD, Fox SH. Four multidetector-row helical CT: image quality and volume coverage speed. Radiology 2000; 215: 55–62.

International Electrotechnical Commission 60601–2–44. Amendment 1: Medical electrical equipment, Part 2–44: Particular requirements for the safety of X-ray equipment for computed tomography. Geneva, Switzerland: International Electrotechnical Commission, 2002.

McCollough CH. Patient dose in cardiac computed tomography. Herz 2003; 28: 1–6.

Morin RL, Gerber TC, McCollough CH. Radiation dose in computed tomography of the heart. Circulation 2003; 107: 917–22.

Ohnesorge B, Flohr T, Becker C et al. Cardiac imaging by means of electrocardiographically gated multisection spiral CT: initial experience. Radiology 2000; 217: 564–71.

Rubin GD, Schmidt AJ, Logan LJ, Sofilos MC. Multi-detector row CT angiography of lower extremity arterial inflow and runoff: initial experience. Radiology 2001; 221: 146–58.

Schertler T, Wildermuth S, Alkadhi H, Kruppa M, Marincek B, Boehm T. Sixteen-detector row CT angiography for lower-leg arterial occlusive disease: analysis of section width. Radiology 2005; 237: 649–56.

Schoepf UJ, Becker CR, Hofmann LK et al. Multislice CT angiography. Eur Radiol 2003; 13: 1946–61.

Wintersperger B, Jakobs T, Herzog P et al. Aorto-iliac multidetector-row CT angiography with low kV settings: improved vessel enhancement and simultaneous reduction of radiation dose. Eur Radiol 2005; 15: 334–41.

2

Image reconstruction with multi-slice CT

R Manzke and Michael Grass

INTRODUCTION

The history of modern computed tomography (CT) pre-dates the introduction of the first CT scanner in 1968 by Godfrey Hounsfield. In 1917, the Czech mathematician Johann Radon formulated the basic mathematic theory for reconstruction methods used in today's CT systems (Radon transform). The first clinical CT scanner was installed in 1971 at Atkinson Morley Hospital, UK, while the first commercial scanners became available in 1974 (head only scanners) and 1976 (single-slice whole body scanners). Dual-slice scanners became available in 1992, quad slice (4-slice) in 1998 followed, in a few years, by the introduction of 16- and 64-detector scanners. Together with hardware developments, efficient image reconstruction algorithms have played a very important role in the evolution of the current generation of CT scanners. With the availability of multi-detector scanners, reconstruction challenges have shifted from single-slice two-dimensional (2D) reconstruction, mainly through filtered back projection (FBP) algorithms, to three-dimensional (3D) volume reconstruction strategies. See Table 2.1 for the nomenclature used in this chapter.

MULTI-SLICE CT PHYSICS AND INSTRUMENTATION

For additional details on this section, the reader is referred to Chapter 1.

X-ray absorption physics and terminology

The X-ray source produces photon beams that, on passing through the object, are subject to two physical effects, namely absorption (photon effect) and scattering (Compton and Rayleigh scattering). In an ideal case scenario, only attenuated rays, passing through the object, should be measured at the detector. However, the real measurement comprises both attenuated rays and scattered photons. Usage of a fairly narrow X-ray spectrum, and anti-scatter grids at the detector and collimators at the source, restrict the beam to the utilizable space on the detector and prevent detection of scattered rays to a large extent. The attenuation of X-rays can be expressed with an absorption function $\mu(x, y, z)$. The absorption of photons is energy dependent, which causes effects such as beam hardening. The attenuation of the X-rays along a line through a 3D object can be described by equation (1), which is equivalent to the Lambert–Beer law of spectrophotometry:

$$I_{out} = I_0 \exp\left(-\int_{line} \mu(x, y, z) \mathrm{d}l\right) \tag{1}$$

where I_{out} is the intensity measured at the detector, I_0 is the intensity of the X-ray at the source, $\mu(x, y, z)$ are the absorption coefficients of the object, and $\mathrm{d}l$ is an infinitesimal small element along the line. Consequently, the intensity value at the detector corresponds to the integral of absorption

Table 2.1 Nomenclature

I_0	X-ray source intensity
I_{out}	X-ray intensity after absorption in object
exp( )	Euler exponential function
$\mu(x, y, z)$	Object function
dl	Infinitesimal line element
ln( )	Natural logarithm
π	Slice pitch
TF	Table feed (mm/revolution)
h_D	Detector collimation (mm)
I_{tube}	Tube current (mA)
U_{tube}	Tube voltage (kV)
K_{tube}	Tube constant
D	Dose
T_{rot}	Gantry rotation time (s/revolution)
T_{scan}	Scan time
$P_{line}(x)$	Projection along line, 2D Radon transform, line-integral
$P_{line}{}^{\pi}(x)$	All projections over an angular interval of π
FT_1	One-dimensional Fourier transform
FT_2^{-1}	Inverse two-dimensional Fourier transform
$Rf_{plane}(z)$	3D Radon transform, plane-integral
r, κ	Cone angle parameters, angle and magnitude, polar coordinates
ϕ	Gantry rotation angle in parallel-beam geometry
β	Gantry rotation angle in fan-beam geometry
γ	Fan angle
ξ	Detector coordinate in parallel-beam geometry
$\overline{SO}$	Distance source to origin
$p^F()$	Fan beam projection
$p^P()$	Parallel-beam projection
$\phi_{f, l}(x, y, z)$	First/last projection angle of voxel illumination
$\psi_{all}()$	Normalized weighting function
$\psi_c()$	Cardiac weighting function
$\psi_{il}()$	Illumination weighting function

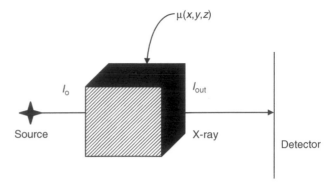

Figure 2.1 The measurements of X-rays is the measurement of line integrals. The figure shows the absorption process during CT projection measurement.

Table 2.2 Typical Hounsfield unit (HU) values for selected tissue types

Tissue type	HU range
Water	0
Air	−1000
Bone	50 to 3000
Milt	30 to 50
Fat	−10 down to −800
Lung	−180 down to −900
Pancreas	10 to 40
Kidney	35 to 50
Blood	35 to 80
Heart	30 to 55
Liver	35 to 70
Gut	10 to 40
Tumor	35 to 55
Bladder	30 to 40

coefficients through the object function (Figure 2.1) after the logarithmic transformation:

$$\ln(I_0/I_{out}) = \left(\int_{line} \mu(x, y, z) \mathrm{d}l\right) \tag{2}$$

The challenge with CT image reconstruction is to compute the object function and hence the absorption coefficients μ (x, y, z).

CT images are usually presented in Hounsfield units (HU) rather than in the units of the pure absorption coefficients. Hounsfield units are calculated according to the following formula:

$$\text{Hounsfield unit} = \frac{\mu - \mu_{water}}{\mu_{water}} 1000 (HU) \tag{3}$$

Typical Hounsfield units for body tissue are shown in Table 2.2 and Figure 2.2. CT data sets are optimally visualized by adjusting the so-called level and window of the Hounsfield interval on the workstation.

Scanner design

CT systems consist of several components: (1) the gantry, composed by stator and rotor, (2) the X-ray source including the high-voltage generator, (3) the beam collimator, (4) the anti-scatter grid, (5) the detector and data acquisition system (DAS), and (6) the reconstruction and back-end visualization unit.

In the late 1980s, the power supply for the X-ray tube and data connections were achieved by hooking a set of long cables to the gantry. This restricted the rotation time and, indeed, the continuous rotation angle allowing for current helical scanning modes. At the beginning of the 1990s the so-called 'slip ring technique' was introduced and has developed since. The power supply for the X-ray tube as well as the data connections are provided by the slip ring allowing for continuous rotation. Scanners nowadays mostly use mechanical slip rings for the power distribution and optical slip rings for the data path. Mechanical issues such as the bearing of the gantry and the weight distribution on the gantry are still an enormous engineering challenge, particularly when aiming for faster rotation times. Next to other technical developments being described in the following sections, the capability to perform continuous rotations was key to enable new applications for CT, including imaging the peripheral circulation and e.g. cardiac CT imaging in a single breath hold.

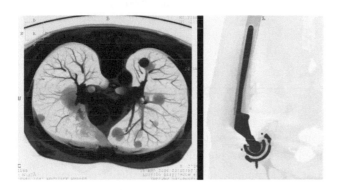

Figure 2.2 Left image shows Hounsfield level window settings for soft-tissue lung nodule detection (wide window, low level settings). Right image shows typical Hounsfield scaling for bone imaging depicting an orthopedic implant (narrow window, high level settings).

Source and detector design

X-ray source and focal spot

An X-ray source used for CT typically consists of a fixed cathode from which electrons are emitted onto a rotating anode (rotation due to better heat distribution) (Figure 2.3). The size of the focal spot on the anode determines the sharpness of the projection and hence influences the spatial resolution of the image reconstruction. X-rays are emitted through a window, typically consisting of a filter material (metal) absorbing X-ray photons of low energies, which assures a narrow energy spectrum of the beam. Some manufacturers use tubes, which allow for a dynamic deflection of the electron beam leading to a so-called 'flying focal spot'. With this technique the data sampling is improved, leading to a better spatial resolution. This approach can be used to improve the sampling either within the slice plane or along the patient axis (focal spot in the z-direction).

Detector design

The detector consists of several elements, grouped together into a matrix. Each detector element consists of a scintillator crystal, which converts the X-ray photons into light impulses, and a photodiode, which converts the light impulse into an electrical signal (Figure 2.4). The electrical signals corresponding to projections and intensity values are then read out at a specific sampling rate (about 2300 frames/rotation) and transferred via the slip ring to the image reconstruction unit. The slice thickness of the detector rows (element height) typically varies from 1.25 mm down to 0.6 mm. The volume coverage of multi-slice scanners varies depending on the slice collimation and the number of available slices. For example, a high-end 64-slice system provides a detector volume coverage

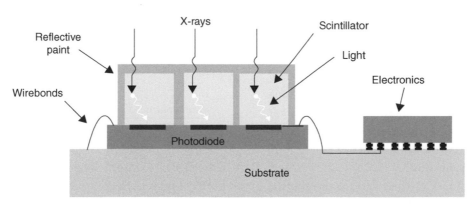

Figure 2.3 Schematic representation of a detector element with a front illuminated photodiode.

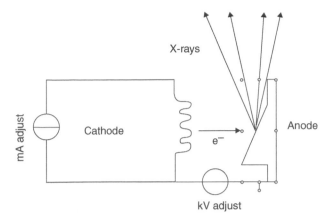

Figure 2.4 Simplified plot of the electric circuits within an X-ray tube. Current is adjustable for the coil heating circuit. Voltage is adjustable for the electron emission circuit. X-rays are produced when electrons (e⁻) impinge on the anode.

Table 2.3 Typical parameter settings for cardiac CT scanning (40- and 64-slice scanners)	
Tube energy	120–140 kVp
Current	100–300 mAs
Detector configuration	40 × 0.625 mm and 64 × 0.625 mm
Volume of coverage	12–14 cm
Rotation time	0.33–0.4 s
Acquisition time	10–12 s (for 12–14 cm, 40-slice scanner) 6–8 s (for 12–14 cm, 64-slice scanner)
Reconstructed slice thickness	0.67–0.9 mm
Reconstruction filters	Standard
Contrast volume	60–100 cc
Contrast density	320–375
Injection rate	4–5 ml/s
Saline chaser volume	20–30 ml
Injection rate (saline)	4–5 ml/s
Targeted phases for reconstruction (for coronary imaging)	Low heart rate: physiologic phases 70–80 (diastasis) (High heart rate: physiologic phases 40–50 (isovolumetric relaxation time) and 70–80 (diastasis)

of about 4 cm at a collimation of 64 × 0.625 mm. The spatial resolution of the reconstructed image depends on various parameters such as the focal spot size, the distance between the focal spot and the detectors, the detector element size, the data sampling strategy (flying focal spot, quarter detector offset, etc.) and the reconstruction algorithm properties. Usually it is measured using so-called slice sensitivity profiles (SSPs), which are discussed later in this chapter.

Scan parameter considerations

Acquisition parameter

While performing a CT scan, several parameters have to be chosen according to the actual application (Table 2.3). These parameters, which influences the spatial and the temporal resolution and the volume coverage, include: the gantry rotation time T_{rot} (s/revolution), the detector collimation (detector height) h_D (mm) and the pitch. With multi-slice CT, the definition of pitch is given by the ratio between table travel per gantry rotation (in mm) and the nominal slice width (in mm).

The I_{tube} or tube current (expressed as mA) may be defined as the number of photons emanating from the focal spot and is a major determinant of signal-to-noise ratio (Figure 2.4). Thus a high I_{tube} improves image quality but also increases radiation dose (see below). Often an effective tube current (I_{eff} or effective mAs) is given by $I_{eff} = I_{tube} \cdot T$, where T is the illumination time.

The tube voltage U_{tube} (kV) determines the energy of the X-ray beam or the hardness of the X-ray. A high kV results

in a smaller fraction of the X-ray beam being absorbed (reduced attenuation) but will result in improvements in contrast. The amount of X-ray dose delivered may be expressed by the equation:

$$D \approx k_{tube} \cdot I_{tube} \cdot U_{tube}^3 \cdot T \tag{4}$$

Depending on whether a step and shoot approach or a continuous feed is used, different source trajectories may result (Figure 2.5). For a step and shoot (i.e. no table feed [TF]), the source moves on a circular orbit. Otherwise, if a table feed is chosen (TF > 0), the source moves on a helical orbit around the patient leading to helical (or spiral) CT.

The scan time can be calculated by:

$$T_{scan} = \frac{\text{Scan volume} \cdot T_{rot}}{\text{TF}} = \frac{\text{Scan volume} \cdot T_{rot}}{\prod \cdot h_D} \tag{5}$$

A collimation of 40×0.625 mm, pitch of 1.175 and rotation time of 0.75 s yields a table speed of 39.2 mm/s. Thus a 1200 mm scan can be performed in 30.6 s.

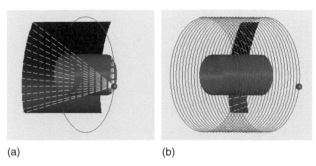

(a)   (b)

Figure 2.5 Different acquisition paths. (a) Cone beam acquisition on a circular source trajectory. (b) Moving source on a helical orbit.

Spatial resolution and signal-to-noise ratio

In CT, the spatial resolution is often determined using so-called SSPs or by estimating the modulation transfer function (MTF). Both depend on several parameters such as the characteristics of the X-ray source (focal spot size), the detector characteristics (detector element size), and the reconstruction algorithm (filter kernel). The MTF can be estimated by analytic observations taking into account the properties of the reconstruction algorithm and the physical acquisition set-up. It can also be estimated by phantom experiments where line pairs of different resolution are imaged and evaluated. The SSP of a CT system can be determined approximately using relatively simple experiments. Phantoms made of thin absorbing disks (for instance, 20 mm diameter in the x–y plane and 0.2 mm thickness along the patient axis) are scanned. The dispersion of the disks along the patient axis is evaluated in the CT image, leading to SSPs specific to the scanner and the chosen scan and reconstruction protocol. In this way the spatial resolution along the z-axis can be determined.

Similar to the spatial resolution, the signal-to-noise ratio (SNR) depends on several parameters such as detector element distance, the amount of measured projections, the amount of X-ray photons measured per detector element, the reconstruction algorithm, and the filter kernel. In general, the pixel noise is small when a small detector element distance (distance between detector elements) is chosen, a large number of projections is calculated, and a high number of photons is measured (increased dose). It can be further adjusted by using an adequate filter kernel and choosing either an edge-enhancing filter (better spatial resolution, more noise) or a smoothing filter (reduced spatial resolution, less noise).

Depending on the application, the optimal parameter settings must be chosen. Usually, current CT systems offer templates for different applications. Full body scans, for example, are performed using a large collimation in order to use the full detector coverage at an intermediate rotation time, resulting in an adequate number of projections which enables medium spatial resolution reconstructions. If high-resolution reconstructions of specific body regions are required, a low pitch is chosen combined with a smaller detector collimation. If high-contrast resolution is required, for example for lung imaging, a higher tube voltage and current are chosen in order to increase the SNR.

CT IMAGE RECONSTRUCTION

In the following sections, CT image reconstruction will be discussed starting with the introduction of the Radon transform and the Fourier slice theorem leading to 2D FBP reconstruction algorithms. Following this, the shift from reconstruction approaches from single-slice systems to multi-slice systems (fan beam to cone beam acquisition) and the linked problem with exact cone beam reconstruction will be discussed. Some practical 2D FBP reconstruction approaches for helical scanning such as the 180 LI, 360 LI (LI = linear interpolation) and an adaptive method, ASSR (advanced single-slice rebinning and the related AMPR (adaptive multiple plane reconstruction) method), will be introduced. Techniques such as rebinning and Parker weighting will be explained. The limitations of 2D techniques will be outlined leading to practical 3D cone beam FBP approaches, such as the Feldkamp (FDK) method (circular scanning) and the extended wedge method (helical scanning). The determination of the spatial resolution by means of an SSP and the parameters influencing the SNR will be outlined too.

2D Radon transform and Fourier slice theorem

In 2D, the Radon transform is linked to X-ray imaging by the fact that both describe line integrals (Figure 2.6):

$$p_{\text{line}}(x) = \int \mu(x, y) \mathrm{d}y \tag{6}$$

Where $p_{\text{line}}(x)$ represents the Radon transform of the object, which corresponds to a measured X-ray on the detector (a projection).

With the Fourier slice theorem it can be shown that the one-dimensional (1D) Fourier transform of the Radon transform of the object corresponds to the 2D Fourier

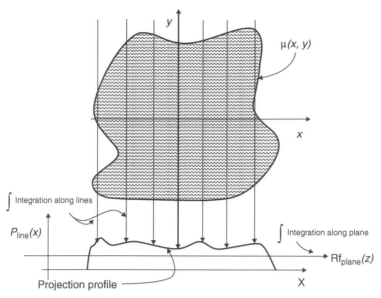

Figure 2.6 The 2D and 3D Radon transform. In the 2D case, the Radon values correspond to line integrals, whereas in the 3D case they correspond to plane integrals.

transform of the object. With this knowledge an object reconstruction approach can be formulated:

$$\mu(x,y) = \mathrm{FT}_2^{-1}(\mathrm{FT}_1(p_{\mathrm{line}}{}^{\pi}(x))), \tag{7}$$

where $p_{\mathrm{line}}{}^{\pi}(x)$ corresponds to all projections over an angular interval of π, FT_1 corresponds to the 1D Fourier tansform and $\mathrm{FT}^{-1}{}_2$ stands for the inverse 2D Fourier transform. This means that the object can be reconstructed by performing a 1D Fourier transform of the projection data followed by an inverse 2D Fourier transform. In practice, this approach is not widely used, since resampling in the Fourier domain is crucial. Furthermore, the object reconstruction cannot be carried out in parallel with the data acquisition. Another technique, known as the FBP, can be implemented more efficiently and is therefore widely used. The above reconstruction formulation based on the Fourier transforms can be reformulated obtaining the following expression:

$$\mu(x,y) = \text{Back projection (Ramp filter}(p_{\mathrm{line}}{}^{\pi}(x))). \tag{8}$$

One step of the FBP approach is a filtering along the row direction of the projection with a ramp filter (high-pass). In practice, different filter kernels are used according to the clinical application in order to get either better edge enhancement or a better SNR ratio. During the back projection process, all filtered projections acquired over an angular range of π must be back projected over the imaging grid in order to reconstruct the object (Figure 2.7). (FBP = smearing out the filtered projections over the image grid.)

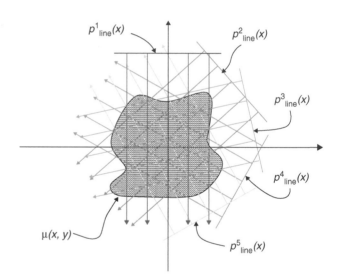

Figure 2.7 Back projection process. Projections over an angular range of p^1 through p^5 are back projected (smeared out along the original paths of the rays over the imaging grid) in order to reconstruct the object.

3D object reconstruction

In 3D, the Fourier slice theorem also holds true and respective inversion formulae can be derived. The 3D Radon transform $Rf_{\mathrm{plane}}(z)$ corresponds to plane integrals rather than line integrals (Figure 2.6):

$$\mathrm{Rf}_{\mathrm{plane}}(z) = \int p_{\mathrm{line}}(x,z)\mathrm{d}x = \iint \mu(x,y,z)\mathrm{d}x\mathrm{d}y, \tag{9}$$

meaning that the line integrals obtained from the X-ray projections taken from the system have to be integrated along the x-axis in order to obtain plane integrals and, hence, 3D

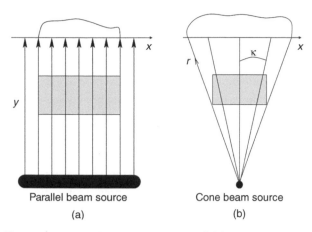
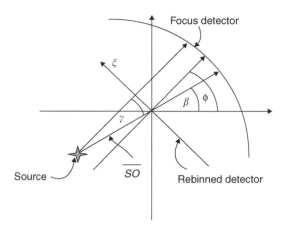

Figure 2.8   Parallel beam geometry (a) is non-existent in the reality due to the fact that the X-ray source emits an X-ray cone (b).

Figure 2.9   Principles of the rebinning approach.

Radon values. This, however, is a problem due to the ray divergence of the real X-ray source, which produces a cone beam and not a set of parallel beams (Figure 2.8). The 3D Radon transform can be expressed in a cone beam co-ordinate system by:

$$\mathrm{Rf}_{\mathrm{plane}}(z) = \iint \mu(x,y,z)\mathrm{d}x\mathrm{d}y = \iint \mu(r,\kappa,z)r\mathrm{d}r\mathrm{d}\kappa, \qquad (10)$$

which obviously differs from the cone beam CT data represented by:

$$\mathrm{Rf}_{\mathrm{plane}}(z) \neq \int p_{\mathrm{line}}(\kappa,z)\mathrm{d}\kappa = \iint \mu(r,\kappa,z)\mathrm{d}r\mathrm{d}\kappa \qquad (11)$$

by the absence of the proportion factor . In practice, this leads to the problem known as 'exact cone beam reconstruction'. In addition, a sufficiency condition with regard to the trajectory must be fulfilled in order to allow for exact object reconstruction, known as the Tuy–Smith condition: 'if on every plane that intersects the object, there exists at least one cone beam source point, then one can reconstruct the object'. This obviously means that only approximate reconstructions can be performed with multi-slice CT when circular and step and shoot acquisition modes are chosen (Figure 2.5). In contrast, a helical trajectory fulfills the condition. In current CT systems, predominantly approximate reconstruction algorithms are used for the image reconstruction, since they can be implemented very efficiently, offering a reasonable accuracy.

Practical 2D reconstruction methods

Back in the time when only single-slice CT systems were available, simple 2D approaches based on FBP were used. They can be applied in a straightforward manner in the case that a circular trajectory is chosen and are able to deliver an exact reconstruction of the 2D slice. In order to allow for object reconstruction, projections over an angular coverage of at least π plus fan angle must be acquired. In reality, the

source produces an X-ray cone, which irradiates the patient. If the detector consists of a single row, one can speak about fan-beam CT since projection data are taken from a fan beam irradiating the patient. The physically acquired fan-beam data can be rebinned into a parallel-beam geometry (Figure 2.9), which enables the use of parallel-beam reconstruction formulae. Given that:

$$\phi = \beta + \gamma \text{ and } \beta = \gamma - \phi, \gamma = \arcsin\left(\frac{\xi}{\overline{SO}}\right) \qquad (12)$$

where ϕ, β, and γ describe, respectively, the rotation angle of the parallel-beam geometry, the rotation angle of the fan-beam geometry, and the fan angle, ξ is the coordinate along the detector row and $\overline{SO}$ is the distance from the source to the rotation center. Parallel beam projections $p^{\mathrm{P}}(\phi, \xi)$ can be obtained from the fan-beam projections $p^{\mathrm{F}}(\beta, \gamma)$ according to:

$$p^{\mathrm{P}}(\phi,\xi) = p^{\mathrm{F}}\left(\phi - \arcsin\left(\frac{\xi}{\overline{SO}}\right), \arcsin\left(\frac{\xi}{\overline{SO}}\right)\right) \qquad (13)$$

A simple parallel-beam reconstruction algorithm would look as follows:

(1) Rebinning of the fan-beam data to parallel-beam data (equation (13))

(2) Filtering of the rebinned data along the detector row with a ramp filter

(3) Back projection over the parallel-beam grid.

If full rotation acquisitions are performed, fan-beam projection data over an angular interval of 2π are acquired. This is more than theoretically required. In order to make optimal use of the data redundancy the so-called Parker weighting can be applied.

As previously mentioned, helical scanning was introduced at the beginning of the 1990s. In this case, a constant gantry rotation is performed while the table is moved with a constant velocity. From the image reconstruction perspective, new approaches were required for the object reconstruction. The 180 LI and the 360 LI approach are two well-known techniques for single-slice helical image reconstruction. When using the 180 LI algorithm, projection data are obtained at a given z-slice by means of linear interpolation between acquired projections, which are closest to the z-slice and π apart. The 360 LI algorithm, instead, uses projections, which are 2π apart for obtaining the projection data at an arbitrary z-slice position, again using linear interpolation. The actual image reconstruction can be performed using the FBP techniques mentioned above. However, these algorithms cannot be applied in the case of multi-slice detectors due to the increased cone angle and would, hence, result in image artifacts.

For a small number of detector rows, adaptive methods can be used for image reconstruction, where the reconstruction plane is tilted according to the slope of the helix at a given slice position. One such approach is the ASSR algorithm. In this approach, the plane is tilted in such a way that it optimally fits a π segment of the helix. The optimal tilt angle is derived from the supposition that the plane is to be centered around the reconstruction position such that the deviation of the focus is minimal if moving a fraction of half a rotation from the reconstruction position. After the optimal angle is found, the multi-slice CT data are rebinned and interpolated to fit that tilted slice. The tilted slice can be reconstructed using standard 2D algorithms such as FBP methods discussed above. The reconstructed image planes must be interpolated to an isotropic Cartesian volume, since the reconstruction delivers tilted image planes. The AMPR approach (Siemens) is an extension of the ASSR method.

Practical 3D reconstruction methods

Cone-beam CT systems were already used for non-destructive imaging in the automotive industry as far back as 1984. For such purposes, a well-known approximate 3D reconstruction technique referred to as FDK had been developed. This approximate 3D reconstruction algorithm is based on a circular source trajectory (Figure 2.10). It employs a weighted 3D back projection (back projection over an image volume rather than an image slice). This is taken into account approximately with the application of a specific preweighting function to the measured data. The FDK method has been the basis for different enhancements and modifications. The basic idea may be considered as the foundation for all approximate reconstruction algorithms based on filtered 3D back projection.

In 2000, Tuy proposed a 3D cone-beam reconstruction method for helical trajectories referred to as the 'wedge method'. This approximate method is based on 3D filtered back projection, similar to the before mentioned FDK technique, but can be applied to helical trajectories. Compared with the FDK approach, a different virtual detector geometry is used (Figure 2.11) which is obtained by the parallel rebinning known from 2D reconstruction approaches. The wedge method uses an illumination weighting function in order to handle redundant data, which are acquired when small helical pitches are chosen (Figure 2.12). The illumination interval is the angular projection interval in which the voxel is irradiated by the X-rays and projections of it are taken. The wedge algorithm can be used for multi-slice CT with a large number of detector rows. It is able to reconstruct CT volumes for helical acquisitions with arbitrary, non-discrete pitches.

For volume CT applications when, for example, flat X-ray detectors are mounted on CT gantries or when the number of detector rows is significantly larger than 64

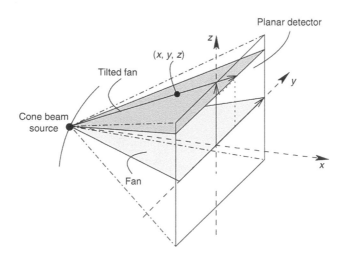

Figure 2.10   Geometry used in the Feldkamp (FDK) reconstruction approach.

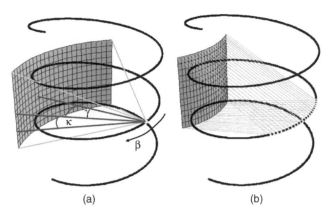

Figure 2.11 Part (a) shows the standard cone-beam geometry of a real CT system. Part (b) shows the rebinned virtual geometry used by the wedge and extended cardiac reconstruction (ECR) method.

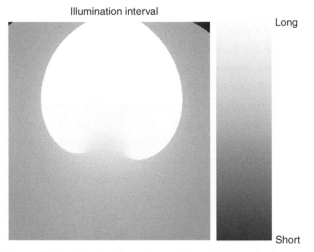

Figure 2.12 Illumination interval for a CT slice in the x–y plane, perpendicular to the patient axis. Some voxels have a longer illumination interval (they are seen by the X-ray source for a longer time) whilst others remain in the X-rays for a shorter time (shorter illumination interval).

(standard flat X-ray detectors have an element matrix of about 1k times 1k detector elements), FDK-based methods are likely to fail to deliver the best possible image quality due to their approximate character. In this case, exact or iterative reconstruction approaches promise to deliver better results. Iterative reconstruction approaches have the further advantage to incorporate, for example, noise models in order to improve the SNR of the reconstruction.

Phase-correlated cardiac CT

The advent of faster gantry speeds and multi-row detectors with volume coverage has made imaging in specific phases of the cardiac cycle possible. Current generation scanners offer a gantry rotation time of <0.4 s. Theoretically, this implies a temporal resolution of <200 ms. Therefore, it is necessary to select appropriate phases throughout one or multiple cardiac cycles for volume reconstruction. The most favorable points in time are those in which the heart is least subject to motion. Acquisition can be related or gated to a synchronously recorded electrocardiogram (EKG) or pulse detector. Prospective triggering or gating (step and shoot) implies that X-rays are switched on and off related to a specific phase or interval related to an event (usually the R-wave). Retrospective triggering or gating means that the X-ray source illuminates constantly and acquisition occurs continuously in time, but with the possibility to be related retrospectively to an event (usually R-wave or a percentage of the RR interval). The prospective gating approach is widely used in EBCT (electron beam CT) and results in significant dose reduction. On the other hand the retrospective gating approach results in higher

levels of radiation exposure (which can be tackled by tube current modulation), but also allows one to reconstruct data at multiple phases of the cardiac cycle.

Single- and multi-slice reconstruction approaches

With the advent of gantries with rotation times of <0.5 s, there is renewed interest in cardiac CT. In 1998, an EKG gating approach was introduced for subsecond helical scanning. This approach basically uses a special z-interpolation technique derived from the known 180 LI and makes use of the information provided by a synchronously recorded EKG, resulting in two new algorithms: the 180 CI (cardio interpolation) and the 180 CD (cardio delta). As previously mentioned, the 180 LI algorithm employs linear interpolation to obtain the projection data of a slice at a given position along the rotation axis (Figure 2.13). The linear interpolation takes place between two opposed projections. With the 180 CI algorithm, the slices, which can be used for interpolation, are tagged as good or bad with regard to the recorded EKG. The algorithm performs a linear interpolation between projections labeled good that are π apart to obtain the projection data for the required slice, at the projection angle. Of course, a low pitch must be used for data acquisition since the maximum distance of the used projections from the required slice is restricted in order to maintain an acceptable narrow slice sensitivity profile. For example, several projections at the same angle or the opposed angle within the maximum distance must be available to ensure that data are present for different gating windows. The 180 CD is a short-scan reconstruction algorithm (projection data from the minimal interval of π) which aims to reduce the effective scan time. No z-interpolation is performed, instead the projection next to the required z-position (nearest neighbor), which is tagged as good, is used for reconstructing the image. With the advent of the first multi-row detector scanners, modifications to multi-row reconstruction algorithms for small cone angles were introduced, resulting in a significant improvement in cardiac imaging results due to the faster acquisition of larger volumes. Two new interpolation algorithms, called the multi-slice cardio delta (MCD) and the multi-slice cardio interpolation (MCI), which are generalizations to the single-slice algorithms CD and CI, were introduced. In the case of 180 MCI the basic idea remains the same as in CI. The cone divergence is neglected. Only data within gated phases of the cardiac cycle are accepted and used for the interpolation of the slice's projection data (Figure 2.13). An appropriate weighting kernel is used for interpolation of the slice data at a required z-position and a required position in the cardiac cycle. For the interpolation, the weighted selection out of the redundant data is used, which may cover multiple cardiac cycles. Data are acquired at arbitrary but small pitches leading to an overlap of the detector rows and, therefore, the acquisition of redundant data. The redundancy definition does not

account for the cone angle. The temporal resolution of a slice depends on the data combination and, hence, on parameters such as the rotation time, heart rate, and pitch. Care must be taken while setting the rotation time of the gantry and the pitch to decorrelate the acquisition from the heart rate in order to achieve a good temporal resolution. The interpolation itself is a combination of two weighting functions, one for the distance weighting along the z-direction and one for the weighting according to the cardiac gating. The 180 MCD algorithm is a short-scan algorithm, similar to the 180 CD. This differs from the 180 MCI, which gathers data from several rotations. The aim of the MCD is, again, to reduce the effective scan time by doing a partial scan reconstruction. With both algorithms, the image is reconstructed after the interpolation of the projection data at a given z-position and a given heart phase by applying a rebinning-based 2D FBP algorithm. Depending on the number of cardiac cycles used for the reconstruction, single- or multi-segment reconstruction is performed (where single- and multi-segment corresponds to single- and multi-cycle). Another approach to cardiac CT image reconstruction is the multi-section cardiac volume (MSCV) technique, which employs a multi-slice helical weighting approach. Related to this approach is a reconstruction approach called the adaptive cardio volume (ACV) reconstruction (Siemens). The ACV approach is an extension of the MSCV approach employing short-scan reconstruction with multi-slice helical weighting too. Both approaches disregard the cone geometry. The short-scan data interval is composed, depending on the heart rate, by data segments of up to three subsequent cardiac cycles (three segment reconstruction), leading to multi segment (or multi-cycle) reconstruction. The temporal resolution depends on the number of data segments from subsequent cardiac cycles used to compose the data interval.

Advanced multi-slice cone beam CT reconstruction

As mentioned in the section on CT reconstruction techniques, an increased cone angle introduced by wider detectors in cardiac CT demands dedicated cone beam reconstruction algorithms to prevent artifacts. One approach for heart-rate-adaptive cone beam cardiac CT reconstruction is referred to as extended cardiac reconstruction (ECR) (Philips). With the ECR framework, the heart-rate-adaptive helical cardiac cone beam reconstruction is achievable. This approach is based on 3D FBP, integrating retrospective cardiac gating based on, for example, EKG information. Neglecting the cardiac

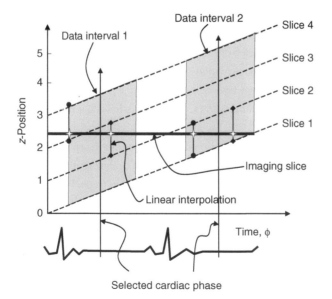

Figure 2.13 Principle of multi-slice cardiac CT reconstruction. For a given imaging slice, the data for the 2D reconstruction approach are interpolated from the different slices according to a preselected cardiac phase. In this case, two cardiac cycles contribute data for the reconstruction.

gating, the reconstruction technique relates to the wedge method described before. In the following the ECR framework is outlined.

The source moves along a helical path around the object. Cone beam projections $p(\beta, \gamma, \kappa)$ are acquired at the projection angle β, where γ denotes the angle in the fan direction and κ is the angle in the cone direction (Figure 2.11). Subsequently, the following steps are performed for the object reconstruction:

(1) The cone beam projections undergo parallel rebinning (equation 13) leading to projections $p(\phi, \xi, \kappa)$ in the wedge geometry, where ξ denotes the position along the detector row.

(2) The rebinned projections are weighted with the cosine of the cone angle, resulting in $p'(\phi, \xi, \kappa)$.

(3) The preweighted projections are filtered along each detector row with the ramp filter kernel resulting in projections $p''(\phi, \xi, \kappa)$.

(4) Cardiac phase-correlated 3D FBP according to:

$$\mu(x,y,z)=\int_{\phi_f(x,y,z)}^{\phi_l(x,y,z)}\psi_{all}(\phi,x,y,z)\bullet p''(\phi,\xi,\kappa)d\phi \qquad (14)$$

delivers the object reconstruction, where $\phi_{f,l}(x, y, z)$ describe the first/last projection angle illuminating the voxel, hence defining the illumination interval (also referred to as the sunrise/sunset projection angle). $\phi_{all}(\phi, x, y, z)$ denotes the voxel-specific weighting function which takes into account potential data redundancy (refer to the wedge method) and the cardiac gating.

The voxel-specific weighting term $\psi_{all}(\phi, x, y, z)$ consists of two weighting functions, one, the illumination weighting $\psi_{il}(\phi, x, y, z)$ known from the wedge method and, two, the cardiac weighting $\psi_c(\phi)$, which facilitates the phase correlated reconstruction. These two weightings are combined using a normalizing approach:

$$\psi_{all}(\phi,x,y,z)=\frac{\psi_c(\phi)\times\psi_{il}(\phi,x,y,z)}{\displaystyle\sum_{j=-\infty}^{\infty}\psi_c(\phi+j\pi)\times\psi_{il}(\phi+j\pi,x,y,z)} \qquad (15)$$

Both the illumination weighting and the cardiac weighting are normalized for all redundant projections, which are π apart (π-partners) (Figure 2.14). The illumination weighting is a voxel-dependent function. It is introduced to minimize discontinuities between the normalized weighted projections in order to suppress bending and streak artifacts. The cardiac weighting is used to select projections from a

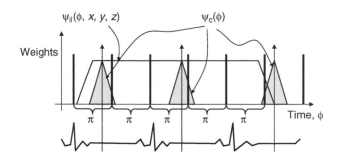

Figure 2.14 Normalizing approach of the extended cardiac reconstruction (ECR) algorithm. All so-called π-partners are normalized according to their weights from the illumination and cardiac weighting function. In this case, three cardiac cycles contribute data for the reconstruction.

pre-selected cardiac phase, enabling retrospective gating. Its width determines the amount of projection data used from each cardiac cycle and primarily determines the temporal resolution. Note that with ECR every voxel obtains a different contribution of projection data and, hence, the temporal resolution varies for each voxel throughout the volume depending on the heart rate, rotation time, and pitch.

Parameter considerations for phase-correlated CT

In cardiac CT, parameters such as the gating interval width and the gating interval position have a strong influence on the image quality. The gating interval width influences the temporal resolution. In the case of single-cycle reconstruction, projection data over an interval of at least π are used for the reconstruction, which results in a temporal resolution of $T_{rot}/2$. If multi-cycle reconstruction is chosen, the temporal resolution can be reduced depending on the number of cardiac cycles used. With the ECR framework, the number of cardiac cycles used for the reconstruction is determined automatically depending on the chosen pitch, the rotation time, and the heart rate, which varies over time (hence, adaptive multi-cycle reconstruction). The cardiac weighting function can be optimized such that the minimal amount of data is used in order to achieve the best temporal resolution. A π interval of data may be composed by data of distinct subintervals from multiple cardiac cycles. The temporal resolution varies depending on the heart rate throughout the scan and is specific for every voxel (Figure 2.15). The rotation time should be chosen according to the heart rate of the patient, in order to avoid resonance effects, where the temporal resolution is suboptimal. The smaller the pitch chosen, the more redundant projection

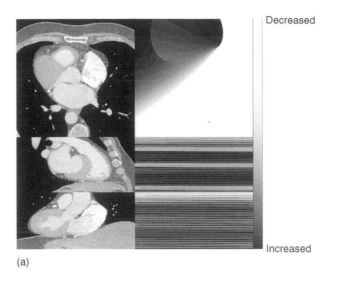

(a)

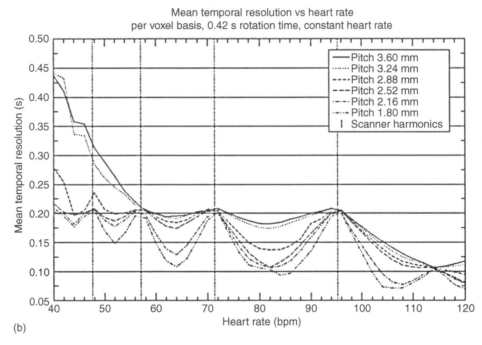

(b)

Figure 2.15 Voxel-dependent temporal resolution variation for different slices (a). Brighter areas correspond to decreased temporal resolution whilst darker areas correspond to increased temporal resolution. The variation is caused by different illumination intervals and heart rate variations during the scan. Temporal resolution variation depending on the heart rate and the pitch (b). At scanner harmonics, the temporal resolution is reduced. Therefore, the rotation time should be chosen according to the patient's heart rate.

data are available and the better the temporal resolution becomes, however at the cost of an increased dose given to the patient. With current systems, using adaptive multi-cycle reconstruction approaches temporal resolutions between 125 ms and 225 ms are feasible depending on the clinical situation. A significant reduction in temporal resolution can be achieved by further reductions in pitch, which in turn is limited by increased scan time and the dose given to the subject. A reduction of rotation time, which is limited physically by the mechanical construction of the gantry or the integration of

multiple tube-detector systems on a single gantry (dual source CT), which adds additional X-ray cross scatter to the image would also be a way.

CONCLUSIONS

Multi-slice CT has evolved dramatically during the past years. Extended volume coverage using detectors with a large number of rows has enabled peripheral imaging applications with

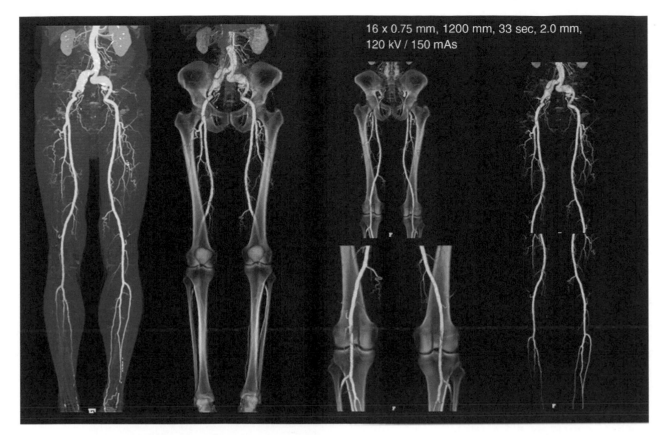

16 x 0.75 mm, 1200 mm, 33 sec, 2.0 mm, 120 kV / 150 mAs

Figure 2.16   Several CT image results of peripheral scans.

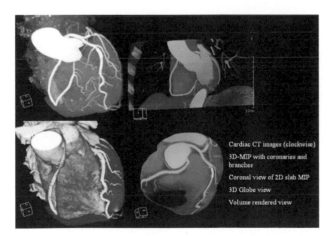

Cardiac CT images (clockwise)

3D-MIP with coronaries and branches

Coronal view of 2D slab MIP

3D Globe view

Volume rendered view

Figure 2.17   Several cardiac reconstructions using different visualization techniques.

extended volume coverage (Figure 2.16). This along with improvements in gantry rotation speed has made multi-slice CT a promising modality for cardiovascular imaging with high spatial and temporal resolution (Figure 2.17). In the future, new CT systems with even larger detectors or higher rotation speeds may result in further improvements in both cardiac CT and peripheral applications.

ACKNOWLEDGEMENTS

The authors would like to thank Mani Vembar and Peter Johnson from Philips Medical Systems in Cleveland, Ohio, USA for kindly providing CT images and practical scan parameters.

FURTHER READING

Dössel O. Bildgebende Verfahren in der Medizin. Berlin: Springer, 1999.

Feldkamp LA, Davis LC, Kress JW. Practical cone-beam algorithm. J Opt Soc Am 1984 ; A6: 612–19.

Flohr T, Ohnesorge B. Heart rate adaptive optimization of spatial and temporal resolution for EKG gated multislice spiral CT of the heart. J Comp Assist Tomogr 2001; 25(6): 907–23.

Grangeat P. Mathematical Methods in Tomography. Berlin: Springer, 1991: 66–97.

Grass M, Manzke R, Nielsen T et al. Helical cardiac cone beam reconstruction using retrospective EKG gating. Phys Med Biol 2003; 48(18): 3069–84.

Hoffmann MHK, Shi H, Schmitz BL et al. Noninvasive coronary angiography with multislice computed tomography. JAMA 25(293): 2471–78.

Kachelrieß M, Fuchs T, Schaller S et al. Advanced single-slice rebinning in cone beam spiral CT. Med Phy 2000; 27(4): 754–72.

Kachelrieß M, Kalender WA. Electrocardiogram-correlated image reconstruction from subsecond spiral computed tomography scans of the heart. Med Phy 1998; 25(12): 2417–31.

Kachelrieß M, Ulzheimer S, Kalender WA. EKG-correlated image reconstruction from subsecond multi-slice spiral CT scans of the heart. Med Phys 2000; 27(8): 1881–1902.

Kak AC, Slaney M. Principles of Computerized Tomography. New York: IEEE Press, 1987.

Kalender WA. Computed Tomography: Fundamentals, System Technology, Image Quality, Application. Munich, Publics MCD Verlag, 2000.

Lackner K, Thurn P. Computed tomography of the heart: EKG-gated and continuous scans. Radiology 1981; 140(2): 413–20.

Manzke R. Cardiac Cone-Beam CT. PhD thesis, University of London, King's College, www.cardiac-ct.net. 2004.

Marchal G, Vogl TJ, Heiken JP et al. Multi-detector-Row Computed Tomography. Italy: Springer Verlag, 2005.

Natterer F. The Mathematics of Computerized Tomography. New York: John Wiley and Sons, 1986 .

Ning R, Tang X, Conover D, Yu R. Flat panel detector-based cone beam computed tomography with a circle-plus-two-arcs data acquisition orbit: preliminary phantom study. Med Phy 30(7): 1694–705.

Ohnesorge B, Flohr T, Becker C et al. Cardiac imaging by means of electrocardiographically gated multisection spiral CT: Initial experience. Radiology 2000; 217(2): 564–71

Parker DL. Optimal short scan convolution reconstruction for, fan-beam CT. Med Phy 1982; 9(2): 254–7.

Radon J. Über die Bestimmung von Funktionen durch ihre Integralwerte längs gewisser Mannigfaltigkeiten. Berichte Sächsische Akademie der Wissenschaft, Mathematik und Physik 1917; 69: 262–7.

Smith BD. Image reconstruction from cone-beam projections: necessary and sufficient conditions and recontruction methods. IEEE Trans Med Imag 1985; 4(1): 14–25.

Taguchi K, Anno H. High temporal resolution for multislice helical computed tomography. Med Phy 2000; 27(5): 861–72.

Tuy HK. 3D image reconstruction for helical partial cone beam scanners using wedge beam transform. US Patent No 6104775, 2000.

Webb S. From the Watching of Shadows. New York: Adam Hilger, 1990.

3

Radiation dosimetric considerations in peripheral CT angiography

Andrew J Einstein and Sanjay Rajagopalan

INTRODUCTION

Performance of any diagnostic test requires a careful assessment of the risks and benefits of the test, and optimization of test protocols to minimize the risk to patients, staff members, and the public. The underlying principle in radiation protection is the as low as reasonably achievable (ALARA) principle. Implicit in ALARA is the assumption that any dose of radiation, however small, may confer biologic risk and thus it is prudent to minimize exposure wherever possible. While the nature of the health effects of low doses of ionizing radiation remains a subject of some controversy, two expert consensus committees, the National Council on Radiation Protection and Measurements' Scientific Committee and the National Research Council's Committee to Assess the Health Risks from Exposure to Low Levels of Ionizing Radiation, have exhaustively reviewed the currently available data and concluded that the risk is best described by a 'linear-no-threshold' risk model. This would therefore imply, at least in theory, that for any type of examination involving radiation, reduction in radiation dose should translate to a reduction in attributable cancer incidence and mortality.

Epidemiologic studies have shown a strong correlation between the frequency of medical X-ray examinations and the attributable risk of cancer. One recent study comparing cancer incidence in 14 countries showed a strong relationship between annual *per capita* X-ray/computed tomography (CT) examination frequency and attributable risk of cancer, as illustrated in Figure 3.1. Radiation doses from multi-detector row CT (MDCT) examinations in general, and those involving the peripheral vascular system in particular, are among the highest of any X-ray study. The United Nations Scientific Committee on the Effects of Atomic Radiation (UNSCEAR) has concluded that while CT constitutes 5% of medical X-ray examinations, it contributes 34% of the resultant collective dose of radiation (Figure 3.2). These figures are higher in developed countries. One report of a single center's experience in the United States found CT to constitute 15% of the exams and 75% of the collective dose. Thus, adherence to the ALARA principle is particularly crucial for peripheral CT examinations.

The first step to minimizing radiation dose from MDCT examinations is to understand how radiation dosimetry is quantified. In this chapter, we shall first discuss the approach to measurement of radiation, both in general and for CT in particular, and then proceed to discuss dosimetry in peripheral CT angiography (CTA) and digital subtraction angiography (DSA).

FUNDAMENTALS OF RADIATION DOSIMETRY

Deterministic and stochastic effects of radiation

Biologic effects of ionizing radiation can be classified as deterministic or stochastic. Deterministic effects such as skin injury

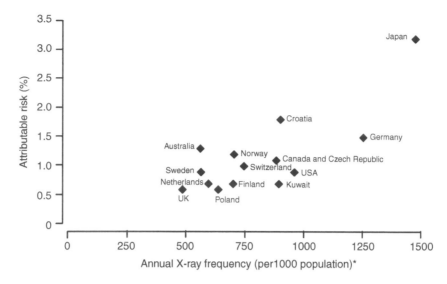

Figure 3.1 Risk of cancer attributable to diagnostic X-ray exposure vs annual X-ray frequency. Reproduced with the permission of Elsevier Health Sciences from Berrington de Gonzalez A, Darby S. Risk of cancer from diagnostic X-rays: estimates for the UK and 14 other countries. Lancet 2004; 363: 345–51.

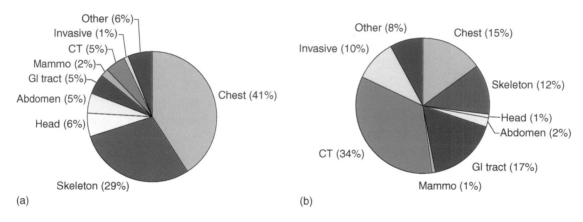

Figure 3.2 Worldwide contributions to frequency (a) and collective dose (b) of medical X-ray examinations. Data from United Nations Scientific Committee on the Effects of Atomic Radiation. UNSCEAR 2000 Report to the General Assembly. New York and Geneva: United Nations Publications, 2000. CT: computed tomography; GI: gastrointestinal.

and cataract formation occur predictably when the dose exceeds a certain threshold, while stochastic effects such as cancer incidence and germ cell mutations occur with a probability which increases with dose. Radiation dose for CT examinations is well below levels where deterministic effects occur, and thus the safety concern is mainly in terms of stochastic effects.

Organizations setting terminology

A number of units and measures are used to quantify radiation. There is some ambiguity in the terminology used in the literature, confounded by multiple sets of units and changing nomenclature between guidelines. The currently used

terminology is a product of the efforts of multiple international organizations, notably the International Commission on Radiation Units and Measurements (ICRU), International Commission on Radiological Protection (ICRP), International Electrotechnical Commission (IEC), and the Conference Gènèrale des Poids et Mesures (CGPM; General Conference on Weights and Measures).

The ICRU (www.icru.org) was founded in 1925 by the International Congress of Radiology, and was initially known as the International X-ray Unit Committee. Its objective is to develop international recommendations on quantities and units of radiation, on procedures for the measurement and application of these quantities, and on physical data required in the application of these procedures. It works closely with the ICRP (www.icrp.org), a daughter organization of the International Society of Radiation, which was founded in 1928 as the International X-ray and Radium Protection Committee. The ICRP's work focuses on all aspects of protection from ionizing radiation, not limited to medical applications, so as to provide an 'appropriate standard of protection for man without unduly limiting the beneficial practices giving rise to radiation exposure.' Towards these ends, the ICRP has issued approximately a hundred reports, each providing specific recommendations in radiologic protection, as well as periodically updated general recommendations, reflecting the state of knowledge on the biologic effects of ionizing radiation. These general recommendations have been offered in 1958, 1964, 1966, 1977 (ICRP Publication 26), and 1991 (ICRP Publication 60). A new update is currently being formulated. It was circulated in draft form in 2005, and succeeded by foundation documents addressing individual aspects of radiologic protection. The IEC was founded in 1906. Its mission is to prepare and publish international standards for electrical, electronic, and related technologies.

The CGPM (www1.bipm.org/en/convention/cgpm/) is one of three linked organizations established by the Convention du Mètre, an international treaty signed in 1875 and now with 51 states as members, as having authority to conduct international activities in standardizing measurement. The CGPM meets every four years. It established the Système International d'Unités (SI) in 1960 and continues to maintain and update it. While the CGPM attempts to keep the SI as parsimonious as possible, special units have been introduced to quantify ionizing radiation, so as to avoid its underestimation and thereby safeguard human health.

Radiation metrics

Exposure measures the total charge of ions of one sign (positive or negative) produced in a unit of dry air by a given amount of X-ray or γ-ray radiation. In SI, exposure is measured in terms of coulombs (C)/kg or amperes (A) · seconds/kg. Exposure is also commonly measured in units of roentgens, where 1 roentgen (R) equals 2.58×10^{-4} C/kg.

Absorbed dose is the mean energy imparted to the matter in a volume by ionizing radiation, divided by the mass of the matter in the volume. The SI unit of absorbed dose, introduced at the 15th CGPM in 1975, is the gray (Gy), where 1 Gy equals 1 Joule/kg. The traditional unit is the rad, short for radiation absorbed dose. One rad equals 1 cGy or 10^{-2} Gy.

While absorbed dose is a useful concept, the biologic effect of a given absorbed dose varies depending on the type

Table 3.1 Radiation weighting factors w_R in ICRP 2005 draft

Particle type	w_R
Photons	1
Electrons, muons	1
Protons	2
Alpha particles, fission fragments, heavy nuclei	20
Incident neutrons	0–20, depending on neutron energy

Adapted from ICRP 2005 Table S3.

and quality of radiation emitted by the radionuclide or external radiation field. Current ICRP terminology uses a dimensionless *radiation weighting factor* (w_R) to normalize for this effect, where the weighting factor ranges from 1 for photons (including X-rays and γ-rays) and electrons to 20 for α particles. Proposed radiation weighting factors in the new ICRP guidelines are summarized in Table 3.1.

Equivalent dose (similar to the ICRP 26 term *dose equivalent* and, currently proposed to be renamed *radiation weighted dose*) in a tissue or organ due to a radiation field is defined as the product of the absorbed dose and the radiation-weighting factor. If the field is composed of different types of radiation with unique radiation weighting factors, then equivalent dose is determined by the sum of the products, based on the constituent radiation types. A special SI unit, the Sievert (Sv), was adopted at the 16th CGPM in 1979 to avoid possible confusion between absorbed dose and equivalent dose, and the resultant underestimation of equivalent dose. One Sv equals 1 Joule/kg. The traditional unit for equivalent dose is the rem, short for roentgen equivalent man. One rem equals 1 cSv, i.e. 10^{-2} Sv. A new name for the unit for radiation weighted dose is currently under consideration, to avoid confusion with the unit for effective dose.

In addition to the absorbed dose and type of radiation, the probability of stochastic effects varies depending on the organ or tissue irradiated. A second weighting factor, the dimensionless *tissue weighting factor* (w_T) is used to normalize for this effect. Equivalent dose multiplied by tissue weighting factor is often termed *weighted equivalent dose*, properly measured in Sv or rem. The sum of the weighted equivalent dose over all organs or tissues in an individual is termed the *effective dose* (E). The older and more cumbersome term *effective dose equivalent*, supplanted by effective dose, is still found in some current literature.

Table 3.2 Tissue-weighting factors in ICRP 2005 Foundation Document, ICRP 60, and ICRP 26

Tissue	ICRP 2005	ICRP 60	ICRP 26
Bladder	0.05	0.05	
Bone	0.01	0.01	0.03
Brain	0.01		
Breast	0.08	0.05	0.15
Colon	0.12		
Liver	0.05	0.05	
Lower large intestine			0.12
Lungs	0.12	0.12	0.12
Esophagus	0.05	0.05	
Ovaries	0.08	0.20	0.25
Red marrow	0.12	0.12	0.12
Remainder tissues	0.12	0.05	0.30
Salivary gland	0.01		
Skin	0.01	0.01	
Stomach	0.12	0.12	
Testes	0.08	0.20	0.25
Thyroid	0.05	0.05	0.03

Tissue-weighting factors are chosen to sum to 1 so that a uniform equivalent dose over the whole body results in an effective dose equal to that equivalent dose. The ICRP has offered recommended tissue weighting factors in ICRP Publication 26 and the subsequent Publication 60. The highest ICRP 60 tissue-weighting factor is that of the gonads (0.2), followed by the bone marrow, colon, lung, and stomach (0.12 each). The 2005 draft and the foundation document on dosimetric quantities introduce a new set of tissue-weighting factors. These weighting factors are summarized in Table 3.2; the major difference is a higher tissue-weighting factor for the female breast and a lower factor for the gonads. Weighting factors for the 'remainder tissues' are determined by complicated rules, which differ in each guideline. When describing the radiation burden to a population, the term *collective dose* is used, referring to the sum of effective doses over all individuals in the population. The unit of collective dose is the man-Sv.

CT-specific terminology

In addition to the general system of nomenclature for radiation dosimetry described above, a particular set of terms has developed for CT. The *dose profile* (D(z)) for a CT scanner is a mathematical description of the dose as a function of position on the z-axis (perpendicular to the tomographic plane). The *CT dose index* (CTDI), measured in units of Gy, is the area under the radiation dose profile for a single rotation and fixed table position along the axial direction of the scanner, divided by the total nominal scan width or beam collimation, i.e.

$$\text{CTDI} = \frac{\int_{2\infty}^{\infty} D(z)dz}{N \times T} \tag{1}$$

where N is the number of tomographic sections produced simultaneously in the rotation of the X-ray tube, and T the section thickness. CTDI is difficult to measure and therefore not commonly reported. Rather, in practice, the CTDI_{100} is determined. CTDI_{100} represents the integrated radiation dose from acquiring a single scan over a length of 100 mm. Exposure is measured using a pencil ionization chamber placed in a cylindrical polymethylmethacrylate phantom (Figure 3.3), and converted to a dose. This is done both at the center of the phantom and at its periphery. Typically, a phantom 16 cm in diameter is used to model the head, and a 32 cm phantom is used to model the body. *Weighted CTDI* (CTDI_w) estimates from CTDI_{100} measurements the average radiation dose to a cross-section of a patient's body. It is determined using the equation

$$\text{CTDI}_w = \frac{2}{3}\text{CTDI}_{100} \text{ at periphery} + \frac{1}{3}\text{CTDI}_{100} \text{ at center} \tag{2}$$

CTDI_w, depends on scanner geometry, slice collimation, and beam prefiltration as well as on X-ray tube voltage, tube current mA, and gantry rotation time t_{rot}. The product of mA and t_{rot} is often referred to as the mAs value of the scan. To obtain a parameter characteristic for the scanner used, it is helpful to eliminate the mAs dependence and to introduce a *normalized* ($_n\text{CTDI}_w$) given in mGy per mAs:

$$\text{CTDI}_w = \text{mA } 3 \, t_{rot} \, 3 \, (\text{CTDI}_w)_n = \text{mAs} \times (\text{CTDI}_w)_n \tag{3}$$

An important CT-specific dosimetry term is the *volume weighted* CTDI, or CTDI_{vol}. This quantity, established by the IEC in 2002, represents the average radiation dose over the volume scanned in a helical or sequential sequence. It is determined from the CTDI_w by the equation

$$\begin{aligned}\text{CTDI}_{vol} &= \text{CTDI}_w/\text{pitch} \\ &= \text{CTDI}_w \times \text{total nominal scan width}/ \\ &\quad \text{distance between scans}\end{aligned} \tag{4}$$

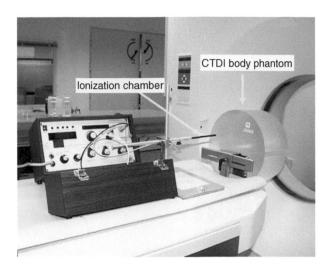

Figure 3.3 Typical equipment used for CT dose index measurements. Courtesy of Thomas Flohr and Berndt Ohnesorge, Siemens, Erlangen, Germany.

$CTDI_{vol}$ can be used in turn to determine the *dose–length product* (DLP). Measured in units of mGy×cm, DLP reflects the integrated radiation dose for a complete CT examination, and is calculated by

$$DLP = CTDI_{vol} \times \text{length irradiated} \qquad (5)$$

Many CT scanner consoles report the $CTDI_{vol}$ and DLP for a study. DLP can be related to E by the formula

$$E = E_{DLP} \times DLP \qquad (6)$$

where E_{DLP}, measured in units of mSv/(mGy×cm), is a body region-specific conversion factor. The most commonly used E_{DLP} values are those of the European Guidelines on Quality Criteria for Computed Tomography (1999), although newer values are reported in the 2004 CT Quality Criteria. These E_{DLP} values are determined using Monte Carlo methods, averaged for multiple scanners. They are summarized in Table 3.3. Thus, for an actual study E can be determined from equations (2) through (6) with knowledge of the $CTDI_{100}$ measurements, total nominal scan width or beam collimation, distance between scans, length irradiated, and region of the body scanned.

METHODS FOR DETERMINING RADIATION DOSE

The actual dose received by a person from a given CT examination can be estimated using one of several methods.

Table 3.3 Relation between DLP and ED: $ED = E_{DLP} \times DLP$

Region of body	E_{DLP} (mSv· mGy^{-1}·cm^{-1}) European Guidelines 1999	E_{DLP} (mSv· mGy^{-1}·cm^{-1}) 2004 CT Quality Criteria, Appendix C
Head	0.0023	0.0021
Neck	0.0054	0.0059
Chest	0.017	0.014
Abdomen	0.015	0.015
Pelvis	0.019	0.015

Dosimetry in CT can be performed using either Monte Carlo simulations or calculations based on CT dose indices measured using an ionization chamber or thermoluminescent dosimeters and applying equations (2) through (6) above. Monte Carlo simulations assume a mathematical patient phantom (Figure 3.4) and model photon transport through this simulated patient. The two most widely used models are those developed by the Gesellschaft für Strahlen- und Umweltforschung (GSF) and the United Kingdom's National Radiological Protection Board (NRPB), now the Health Protection Agency (HPA).

Software is available using data derived from each of these models to estimate patient doses for current scanners using particular scan protocols. These programs include ImpactDose (formerly WinDose, http://www.vamp-gmbh. de/Products/ImpactDose.htm), which uses GSF data, and CTDosimetry.xls (http://www.impactscan.org/ctdosimetry. htm) and CTDose (http://www.nrl.moh.govt.nz/Software. html), which use HPA data. Using these Monte Carlo method-based programs, parameters such as the scanner, tube current, tube voltage, pitch, and scan area in the simulation can be matched to those in an actual examination, enabling realistic simulation of radiation dosimetry in a clinical CT examination. An advantage of Monte Carlo based approaches is that they can determine organ equivalent doses, as well as whole-body E. Current software uses geometric phantoms (Figure 3.4a and b), modeling organs as simple geometric shapes. Newer, more anatomically detailed voxel phantoms (Figure 3.4c) have been developed, and offer the potential of more accurate dosimetry, tailored to body habitus. Regardless of the phantom used for dosimetry, be it geometric, voxel, or a physical phantom, one must be aware that the effective dose accurately estimates the radiation dose to the patient only insofar as the phantom is reflective of the patient's anatomy.

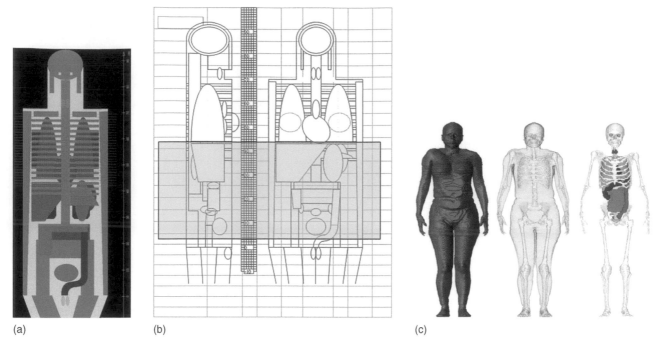

(a)   (b)   (c)

Figure 3.4 Mathematical phantoms used for Monte Carlo simulations of radiation dosimetry. (a) Geometric phantom used in ImpactDose software. (b) Geometric phantom used in CTDosimetry software. (c) Voxel phantom (NAOMI). Reproduced with the permission of the Institute of Physics Publishing. Dimbylow P. Development of the female voxel phantom, NAOMI, and its application to calculations of induced current densities and electric fields from applied low frequency magnetic and electrical fields. Phys Med Biol 2005; 50: 1047–70.

DOSE REDUCTION TECHNIQUES

There are several ways to lower dose delivered to a patient. These methods can be used either alone or together. The appropriate composite dose reduction approach, which provides for ALARA for a number of CTA applications, needs to be developed. The number and energy of photons produced by the X-ray tube are controlled by the tube current, expressed in milliamperes (mA), and the tube voltage, expressed in kilovolts (kV) or peak kilovolts (kVp). The current multiplied by the exposure (rotation time) is known as the tube current-time product (mAs). This can also be divided by the pitch and expressed as effective mAs (eff mAs).

Reduction of tube current

Lowering mAs settings according to the patient's body habitus can lead to decreases in radiation dose. This can be achieved, for example, in peripheral CTA by using protocols with down to 50 effective mAs at 120 kV without compromising diagnostic accuracy.

Reduction of tube voltage

In contrast-enhanced studies, such as CTA, the contrast-to-noise ratio for fixed patient dose increases with decreasing X-ray tube voltage. As a consequence, to obtain the desired contrast-to-noise ratio, patient dose can be reduced by choosing lower kV settings. The potential for dose saving is more significant for smaller patient diameter. Clinical studies have demonstrated a potential for dose reduction of about 50% when using 80 kV instead of 120 kV for performing CTA. This, however, may not be possible in a number of patients as the maximum achievable tube current at 80 kV is generally not sufficient to scan large patients. A recent study recommends 100 kV as the standard mode for aorto-iliac CTA and reports dose savings of 30% without loss of diagnostic information and therefore this may be one potential approach. However, the impact of using lower tube voltage in conjunction with other dose saving modalities such as electrocardiographically (EKG)-controlled dose modulation needs to be investigated.

EKG-controlled dose modulation

The principles of EKG-controlled dose modulation are explained in detail in Chapter 1. Continuous imaging with

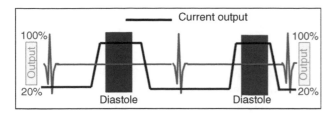

Figure 3.5 EKG-gated tube current modulation. The blue bars represent the acquisition during the nominal value of tube current (mid- to end-diastolic phase in the figure) while, during the rest of the cardiac cycle, the tube output is reduced to 20% of its value to allow for image reconstruction throughout the entire cardiac cycle.

retrospective EKG gating provides continuous volume coverage with overlapping slices, decreases the likelihood of spatial misregistration, and enables reconstruction of specific phases of the cardiac cycle. Since specific phases of the cardiac cycle, typically in diastole, provide minimal coronary motion, it is standard practice in coronary CTA to perform reconstructions in these phases. Typically the output is kept at its nominal value during a user-defined phase (in general the mid- to end-diastolic phase) while during the rest of the cardiac cycle, the tube output is reduced to 20% of its nominal value to allow for image reconstruction throughout the entire cardiac cycle (Figure 3.5). Using this technique, dose reduction of 30–50% has been demonstrated in clinical studies.

Anatomic tube current modulation

In this technique, tube output is adapted to the patient geometry during each rotation of the scanner. The tube output is modulated on the basis of the tissue attenuation characteristics of the localizer scan or determined online by evaluating the signal of a detector row. By employing such a technique, the dose can be reduced by 15–35% without degrading image quality, depending on the body region. A more sophisticated variation of anatomic tube current modulation varies the tube output according to the patient geometry along the longitudinal direction, in order to maintain adequate dose when moving to different body regions, for instance from thorax to abdomen (automatic exposure control). Automatic adaptation of the tube current to patient size prevents, both over- and under-irradiation, considerably simplifies the clinical workflow for the technician, and eliminates the need for look-up tables of patient weight and size for adjusting the mAs settings.

DOSIMETRY IN PERIPHERAL CTA

A number of studies have addressed dosimetry issues in peripheral multi-detector row CTA. These reports have addressed a variety of applications and utilized diverse scanner hardware and imaging protocols.

Thoracic CTA

Three recent studies have addressed non-cardiac thoracic CTA, two focusing on imaging of the pulmonary arteries, and the other on imaging of the thoracic outlet. All three studies used a Siemens 4-slice scanner. Kuiper and colleagues compared dosimetry for 27 consecutive patients undergoing CTA to rule out pulmonary embolism, with 12 patients undergoing (DSA). CT studies were performed with a tube voltage of 120 kV, the effective tube current–time product averaged 124 mAs (range 90–160 mAs), the gantry rotation time was 0.5 s, and collimation was 4×1 mm. Tube current modulation was not employed. The average effective dose in CTA was 4.2 mSv (range 2.2 to 6.0 mSv), while the average effective dose in DSA was 7.1 mSv (range 3.3 to 17.3 mSv).

While concern had been raised about the increased radiation dose to the patient in CT pulmonary angiography, this study demonstrated that 4-slice CTA actually had a lower effective dose than conventional angiography. Tack and colleagues investigated the effect of the tube current–time product on the quality of images and of scan interpretation. Raw data from 21 scans with known pulmonary embolism and filling defects, obtained at 90 mAs, were used to derive simulated scan data at lower tube current–time products ranging from 10 to 60 mAs. Eleven of the 21 patients were women (average body mass index 24.8 kg/m²). The simulated scan data were obtained using a validated method that adds noise to the original raw data such that the magnitude of the noise is proportional to the square root of the X-ray attenuation measured for each detector channel. The raw data sets for both the original 21 scans and the noise-added scans were transferred to a post-processing workstation, where images were reconstructed using 1.25 mm section thickness, 0.8 mm increment, and a soft-tissue kernel. Three readers blinded to the scans, except for knowing that at least one filling defect was present, read each study on two separate occasions. At each reading session, each artery and segment was rated for the presence of a filling defect (absent, present, or inconclusive). In addition, the reader was asked to record the branching order of the most distal artery with a filling defect noted, and to grade the quality of contrast between thrombus and normal vascular content. In this study, the number of inconclusive segments was dependent on the reader, but not on the tube current–time product. The quality score of contrast was noted to be lower at 10 mAs for all readers and at 20 mAs as well for the most experienced reader. Thus, in simulated low-dose pulmonary CTA, lowering the tube current–time product to 40 mAs appeared to result in no significant difference in contrast difference between blood clots and vascular content, in the number of filling defects or inconclusive segments, or in the branching order of the smallest defect noted. This represents a tube current–time product less than half of the minimum value used by Kuiper. Tack's study suggests that it should be routinely possible to perform pulmonary CTA on a 4-slice scanner with an effective dose less than 2 mSv; however, it requires further validation with actual, rather than simulated, images, as well as scans with no filling defects. The study, however, serves as an illustration of how careful optimization of scanning protocols can result in comparable diagnostic performance with significant reduction in dose.

Tube current modulation is an important technique for dose reduction, and can be performed in a variety of ways as outlined above. Mastora et al evaluated the effect of anatomically adapted tube current modulation, using an anatomic dose reduction algorithm (CARE Dose), on image quality in CTA of the thoracic outlet. One hundred patients referred for CTA due to suspicion of thoracic outlet arterial syndrome were studied. The CTA protocol in this evaluation involved performing two acquisitions, one with the patient in neutral position and the other after a postural maneuver, which exacerbates vascular compression at the level of the thoracic outlet. Standard scan protocols were a tube voltage of 140 kV, a tube current time product of 140 mAs (170 mAs when tube current modulation was applied), a collimation of 4×1 mm, and pitch of 1.75. Patients were divided into four equally sized groups, with half of patients receiving dose reduction in the neutral position scan and half in the post-maneuver scan, and half receiving a minimum dose reduction of 20% and the other half receiving a minimum dose reduction of 32%. With the minimum dose reduction set to 20%, the mean dose reduction was 35% (range 27–47%), which was greater when dose reduction was employed after postural maneuver. In these scans, the mean noise level, severity of graininess, and severity of linear streak artifacts did not differ between reference scans and low-dose scans. With the minimum dose reduction set to 32%, the mean dose reduction was only 33% (range 17–38%). Here dose-reduced scans had a greater

severity of graininess but less severity of linear streak artifacts than reference scans, while the mean noise levels did not differ. The presence of artifacts did not compromise the diagnostic value of sagittal reformations or volume-rendered images. Thus, anatomically adapted tube current modulation was effective in reducing radiation dose in CTA of the thoracic outlet by a third, with no effect on image noise, graininess, or streak artifacts, when the minimum reduction was set to 20%. However, the actual reduction did not improve when the reduction was set to a higher value, and was associated with more image graininess, suggesting an upper limit to dose reduction settings for this angiographic application. In addition, the high tube voltage used in this setting suggests the question whether tube current modulation would still be effective if used with lower standard tube voltages, such as 120 kV.

Renal CTA

Kemerink et al assessed dosimetric issues in renal angiography, comparing three different DSA protocols to CTA. The effective dose averaged 22 mSv for the first DSA protocol, 11 mSv for the second, and 9 mSv for the third. CT was performed using a 2-slice scanner, imaging from the celiac artery to the lower pole of the kidneys, an average scan length of 11 cm. Scan parameters were tube voltage 120 kV, tube current 265 mAs, gantry rotation time 1 s, collimation 2.5 mm, and pitch 0.7. The effective dose of CTA averaged 4.9 mSv in men and 5.6 mSv in women. Thus, at least for older scanners, renal CTA is associated with a lower dose than DSA.

Aorto-iliac and lower extremity CTA

It has been suggested that the issue of radiation dosing is less crucial for patients with aorto-iliac and lower extremity arterial disease. These patients are typically older and without long life expectancies. Since the average lag time for the development of a solid tumor from an exposure to low-level radiation is estimated at 14 years, the argument goes that these patients are unlikely to live long enough to develop a malignancy attributable to the CT scan. Even so, current American College of Cardiology and American College of Radiology standards mandate the uniform application of ALARA principles, and these recommendations should be followed for all patients. The initial report of lower extremity multi-detector row CTA was published by Rubin et al.

CTA was performed on 24 patients with suspected lower extremity arterial disease, using a 4-slice scanner. Tube voltage was 120 kV, current was 300 mA, gantry rotation time was 0.8 s, pitch was 6, and slice thickness was 2.5 mm. Effective doses averaged 9.3 mSv, in comparison with 36.2 mSv for DSA.

Three recent studies (one using 4-slice and two using 16-slice scanners) have addressed dosimetric considerations in aorto-iliac and lower extremity CTA. Fraioli et al, using a 4-slice scanner, assessed the performance characteristics and radiation dose from CTA in 75 patients referred for vascular surgery. All scans were performed with a tube voltage of 120 kVp, gantry rotation time of 0.5 s, 4×2.5 mm collimation, 3 mm section thickness, and field of view to fit. Patients were divided into three groups of 25, with tube current–time products of 50 mAs in the first group, 100 mAs in the second, and 130 mAs in the third. The arterial system was divided into 19 anatomic segments, and each segment was evaluated for degree of patency. All patients had DSA performed, which served as the gold standard. CT dosimetry was determined using WinDose, a predecessor to ImpactDose. These authors found the accuracy in the three groups to be 95%, 96%, and 97%, respectively, while the corresponding mean effective doses were 3.7, 8.2, and 13.7 mSv for men and 4.0, 8.9, and 14.8 mSv for women. Sensitivities and specificities were at least 94% in all cases. Thus, low-dose CTA of the infrarenal aorta and lower extremities is both feasible and highly accurate.

Wintersperger et al studied the effect of a reduction in tube voltage from 120 to 100 kVp on noise, image quality, and effective dose in abdominal 16-slice CTA, in 43 patients with abdominal malignancies and 5 with vascular disease. All patients were scanned with an effective tube current–time product of 200 mAs, 16×0.75 mm collimation, 0.5 s gantry rotation time, and a pitch of 1. No significant differences in signal-to-noise (mean 37.0 vs 36.0) or contrast-to-noise (31.1 vs 31.7) ratios were observed between the two protocols. Image quality, assessed on a 5-point scale, was good to excellent, again with no significant differences between the two voltages. Effective dose was determined using both phantom measurements with an ionization chamber and WinDose calculations. The mean effective dose determined using the phantom measurements was 9.6 mSv at 120 kVp and 6.2 mSv at 100 kVp; the corresponding values using WinDose were 12.0 mSv for males and 15.6 mSv for females at 120 kVp, and 6.9 mSv for males and 9.6 mSv for females at 100 kVp. Thus, CTA using the low-voltage 16-slice protocol, at least in these two studies and for these anatomic areas, was associated with a considerably higher effective dose than low-current 4-slice protocols.

Willman et al studied 39 patients with peripheral arterial disease, who underwent both 16-slice CTA and DSA. CTA was performed using the same scanner model as in the study by Wintersperger et al, with the tube voltage being 120 kV. However, a mean tube current of 210 mA was employed, with a gantry rotation time of 0.5 s and a pitch of 1.5, resulting in a mean effective tube current–time product of 70 mAs, a value close to a third of that used by Wintersperger et al. In addition, anatomic tube current modulation was employed to further lower radiation dose. Stenoses were graded using a 4-point scale, and a stenosis >50% was considered significant. There was 96% agreement between CTA and DSA, and excellent agreement between CTA readers (κ=0.84 to 1.0). The effective dose averaged 3.0 mSv in men (range 2.1 to 3.9) and 2.3 mSv in women (range 1.6 to 3.0). Thus, 16-slice aorto-iliac and lower extremity CTA can be performed with high accuracy and low dose.

CONCLUSIONS

Peripheral CTA has emerged as an important diagnostic modality. The potential for high radiation doses necessitates its practitioners to optimize scan protocols in accordance with the ALARA principle. This is predicated on a fundamental understanding of both the principles of CTA as described in Chapter 1 and radiation dosimetry, as well as familiarity with the literature addressing scan protocol optimization. Further studies are needed to address dosimetric considerations using the newer scanners with 64 and more slices and with various dose reduction algorithms.

PRACTICAL PEARLS

- Lowering the pitch increases E (effective dose). (Since $E=E_{DLP}\times DLP$; where E_{DLP} is a body part specific conversion factor; $DLP=CTDI_{vol}\times$length irradiated; and $CTDI_{vol}=CTDI_w/$pitch. Thus $E=E_{DLP}\times$length irradiated$\times CTDI_w/$pitch.)*

- EKG dose modulation should be routinely employed in all cases requiring gating unless there are specific issues related to changing cycle length (e.g. atrial fibrillation, respiratory arrhythmia, or premature beats) where employment of dose modulation may preclude adequate quality reconstruction during phases that correspond to dose lowering.

- Anatomic tube current modulation may allow dose reduction by 15–35%.

- 100 kV rather than 120 kV may be used for lower extremity angiographic applications and may result in dose savings of at least 30% without loss of diagnostic information.

- Using higher pitch may not always result in dose saving as in CT systems relying on adaptive axial interpolation and the 'effective' mAs concept (Chapter 1).

FURTHER READING

Berrington de Gonzalez A, Darby S. Risk of cancer from diagnostic X-rays: estimates for the UK and 14 other countries. Lancet 2004; 363: 345–51.

Committee to Assess Health Risks from Exposure to Low Levels of Ionizing Radiation, Board on Radiation Effects, Research Division on Earth and Life Sciences, National Research Council of the National Academies. Health Risks from Exposure to Low Levels of Ionizing Radiation: BEIR VII, Phase 2. Washington: National Academies Press, 2006.

Dion AM, Berger F, Helie O et al. Dose reduction at abdominal CT imaging: reduced tension (kV) or reduced intensity (mAs)? J Radiol 2004; 85: 375–80.

European Commission. 2004 CT Quality Criteria. Available at: http://www.msct.info/CT_Quality_Criteria.htm. Accessed 28 March, 2006.

European Commission's Study Group on Development of Quality Criteria for Computed Tomography. European Guidelines on Quality Criteria for Computed Tomography. EUR 16262. European Commission, 1999. Available at: http://www.drs.dk/guidelines/ct/quality/mainindex.htm. Accessed 28 March, 2006.

Fleischmann D, Hallett RL, Rubin GD. CT angiography of peripheral arterial disease. J Vasc Interver Radiol 2006; 17: 3–26.

Fraioli F, Catalano C, Napoli A et al. Low-dose multidetector-row CT angiography of the intra-renal aorta and lower extremity vessels: image quality and diagnostic accuracy in comparison with standard DSA. Eur Radiol 2006; 16: 137–46.

Gerber TC, Kuzo RS, Morin RL. Techniques and parameters for estimating radiation exposure and dose in cardiac computed tomography. Int J Cardiovasc Imag 2005; 21: 165–76.

International Commission on Radiological Protection. Recommendations of the International Commission on Radiological Protection (ICRP Publication 26). Ann ICRP 1977; 3: 1–53.

International Commission on Radiological Protection. 1990 Recommendations of the International Commission on Radiological Protection (ICRP Publication 60). Ann ICRP 1991; 21: 1–201.

International Electrotechnical Commission. International Standard IEC 60601-2-44 Edition 2.1. Medical Electrical Equipment – Part 2-44: Particular Requirements for the Safety of X-ray Equipment for Computed Tomography. Geneva: International Electrotechnical Commission, 2002.

Katz DS, Hon M. CT angiography of the lower extremities and aortoiliac system with a mult-detector row helical CT scanner: promise of new opportunities fulfilled. Radiology 2001; 221: 7–10.

Kemerink GJ, Dettaan MW, Vasbinder GBC et al. The effect of equipment set up on patient radiation dose in conventional and CT angiography of the renal arteries. Br J Radiol 2003; 76: 625–30.

Kuiper JW, Geleijns J, Matheijssen NAA, Teeuwisse W, Pattynama PMT. Radiation exposure of multi-row detector spiral computed tomography of the pulmonary arteries: comparison with digital subtraction pulmonary angiography. Eur Radiol 2003; 13: 1496–500.

Limacher MC, Douglas PS, Germano G et al. ACC expert consensus document. Radiation safety in the practice of cardiology. J Am Coll Cardiol 1998; 31: 892–913.

Mastora I, Remy-Jardin M, Delannoy V et al. Multi-detector row spiral CT angiography of the thoracic outlet: dose reduction with anatomically adapted online tube current modulation and preset dose savings. Radiology 2004; 230: 116–24.

McCollough CH. Patient dose in cardiac computed tomography. Herz 2003; 28: 1–6.

Morin RL, Gerber TC, McCollough CH. Radiation dose in computed tomography of the heart. Circulation 2003; 107: 917–22.

Rubin GD, Schmidt AJ, Logan LJ, Sofilos MC. Multi-detector row CT angiography of lower extremity arterial inflow and runoff: initial experience. Radiology 2001; 221: 146–58.

Shrimpton PC. Assessment of Patient Dose in CT. NRPB-PE/1/2004. Chilton: NRPB, 2004. Also published as Appendix C of the 2004 CT Quality Criteria.

Tack D, Demaertelaer V, Petit W et al. Multi-detector row CT pulmonary angiography: comparison of standard-dose and simulated low-dose techniques. Radiology 2005; 236: 318–25.

Upton AC, National Council on Radiation Protection and Measurements Scientific Committee 1–6. The state of the art in the 1990's: NCRP Report No. 136 on the scientific bases for linearity in the dose–response relationship for ionizing radiation. Health Phys 2003; 85: 15–22.

Weinreb JC, Larson PA, Woodard PK et al. American College of Radiology clinical statement on noninvasive cardiac imaging. Radiology 2005; 235: 723–7.

Wiest PW, Locean JA, Heintz PH, Mettler FA. CT scanning: a major source of radiation exposure. Semin Ultrasound CT MRI 2002; 23: 402–10.

Willmann JK, Baumert B, Schertler T et al. Aortoiliac and lower extremity arteries assessed with 16-detector row CT angiography: prospective comparison with digital subtraction angiography. Radiology 2005; 236: 1083–93.

Wintersperger B, Jakobs T, Herzog P et al. Aorta-iliac multidetector-row CT angiography with low KV settings: improved vessel enhancement and simultaneous reduction of radiation dose. Eur Raidol 2005; 15: 334–41.

4

Image post-processing in CT

James J Jang

INTRODUCTION

Modern multi-detector computed tomographic (MDCT) scanners are able to acquire data comprised of volumetric elements called *voxels*. For clinical interpretation, MDCT raw data are reconstructed and reformatted into a diagnostic image. It is important to understand that the terms 'image reconstruction' and 'reformatting' are not interchangeable. While the *reconstruction process* refers to conversion of raw data into an axial image using filtered backprojection algorithms (Chapter 2), *reformatting* manipulates the image orientation and/or the original voxel intensity to highlight specific aspects of the acquired image. Reformatted images can, thus, be displayed in different orientations (i.e., axial, coronal, and sagittal views) (Figure 4.1), or by using different bi-dimensional (2D) formats (such as maximum- and minimum-intensity projections, multiplanar or curved planar reformations) and three-dimensional (3D) formats (such as shaded surface displays or volume rendering). This chapter will discuss in detail various reconstruction and reformatting approaches applicable in evaluating a peripheral angiographic data set. Of note, most of the described reformatting techniques are fully applicable to magnetic resonance (MR) images as well.

SPATIAL RESOLUTION IN MDCT

A general concept in imaging analysis is that the smaller the size of the acquired voxel, the better the ability to spatially discriminate objects (*spatial resolution*). In 3D imaging, the performance of any post-processing method is determined by the voxel size and characteristics. A voxel, by definition, has dimensions in all 3 axes (x-, y-, and z-axis) and it may be isotropic (equally sized in 3 dimensions) or anisotropic (x-y-z dimensions are not identical). Application of post-processing methods to data composed by isotropic voxels results in images that are less distorted.

In-plane spatial resolution

The voxel size in the image plane (typically the x–y direction), also called *in-plane voxel size*, is determined by the ratio between the size of the reconstruction field of view (FOV) and the matrix size (voxel size = FOV/matrix size). The matrix size for axial images in CT is typically 512×512. An FOV of 250 mm, for example, will result in 0.5 mm in-plane voxel size. In general, the wider the selected FOV, the larger will be the obtained in-plane voxel size.

A key concept is that, while in MR imaging the in-plane voxel size is always equal to the in-plane spatial resolution, this is not true with CT imaging. In fact, image resolution is mainly determined in CT imaging by the convolution kernel (filter). In a CT image, all relevant information will be displayed as soon as the image voxel size is smaller than the minimum object size that can be resolved with the selected convolution kernel. Then, further reductions in FOV will reduce the in-plane voxel size, but may not result in improvements in spatial resolution.

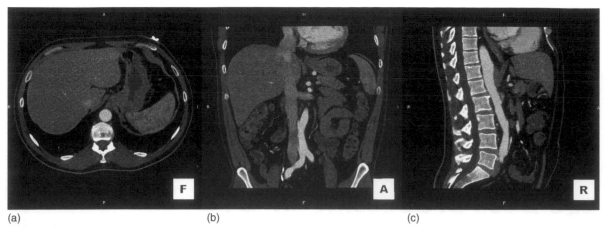

Figure 4.1   Images of abdominal aorta in axial (a), coronal (b), and sagittal (c) orientations. Images are displayed as multiplanar reformations (MPRs).

Through-plane spatial resolution

The voxel size perpendicular to the image plane (in the z-direction), also called *through-plane voxel size*, is given by the reconstruction slice width. The spatial resolution in the longitudinal or the z-plane in MDCT is determined by the slice collimation. In a spiral/helical mode, the *effective slice width* may not be identical to the slice collimation and is actually represented by the full width half maximum (FWHM) of the spiral slice sensitivity profile (SSP) (Chapter 1). A slice width equal to or larger than the collimated slice width can then be reconstructed. The *reconstructed slice width*, especially when wider than the slice collimation, should not be mistaken for the z-axis resolution. Reconstructing images with an overlap results in improved apparent longitudinal resolution, but no better than about 0.7 times the reconstruction slice width. Typically, in clinical practice a reconstruction increment of 0.5–0.8 times the reconstruction slice width is recommended when the corresponding axial images are to be used for 3D post-processing.

POST-PROCESSING TECHNIQUES

Table 4.1 summarizes the most common techniques used for representation of 3D CT data sets. The relative value of the information provided by each of these techniques is summarized in Table 4.2.

Axial images

In MDCT, *axial images* are reconstructions of the source data. Many experts believe that most vascular pathology can be easily identified through review of these axial images. Rapid review of axial images can provide ready information

Table 4.1   Common reconstruction and reformatting techniques used with CT imaging. The relative value in displaying vascular and non-vascular structures for clinical interpretation is summarized

Technique
Axial images
Maximum intensity projection (MIP)
Minimum intensity projection (MinIP)
Multi-planar reconstruction (MPR)
Curved multi-planar reconstruction (cMPR)
Shaded surface display (SSD)
Volume rendering (VR)

on the orientation of the vasculature, identification of anomalies, and evaluation of extravascular structures (Figure 4.2).

Although axial images are easy to scroll through, interpreting peripheral run-off vessels that may comprise 1000–2000 stacked axial images may be difficult and time consuming. Reformatting techniques as described below, allow more efficient means of interpreting peripheral vascular images. The raw data can be reconstructed as thicker slices that allow rapid review of the entire peripheral data set (3 mm or 5 mm thick slices) and present less of an archiving challenge.

Maximum intensity projections and minimum intensity projections

Maximum intensity projection (MIP) and *minimum intensity projection* (MinIP) images are volume data sets obtained by passing parallel rays in a specified direction and displaying only the highest (with MIP) or lowest (with MinIP) attenuation voxels in the selected slab of data (Figure 4.3). As a consequence, with this approach only a limited portion of the original data set is used for image reconstruction while most of it (about 95%) is excluded.

Table 4.2 Differential information provided by multiple reformatting technique

	Reconstruction efficiency	Interpretation efficiency	Luminal, intimal and mural information	Vascular contour	Adjacent nonvascular structures	Stenosis grading accuracy
Axial or MPR	+++	+	+++	+	+++	++
CPR	++	++	+++	++	++	+++
MIP	+ to +++[a]	+++	++	++	+	++
SSD	++	+++	+	+++	+	+
VR	++	+++	++	+++	++	+

Abbreviations: CPR – curved planar reformation; MIP – maximum intensity projections; SSD – shaped surface display; VR – volume rendering.
[a] Depending on degree of prerendering editing of osseous structures.

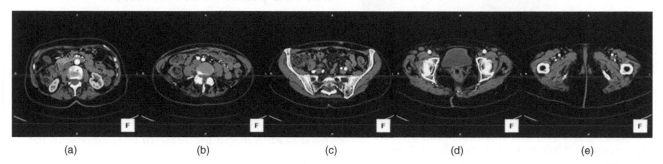

(a)   (b)   (c)   (d)   (e)

Figure 4.2 Volume rendered images (a) provide more depth and improved perspective of coronary arteries against the cardiac background compared to shaded surface display (SSD) (b) and maximum intensity projection (MIP) (c) images.

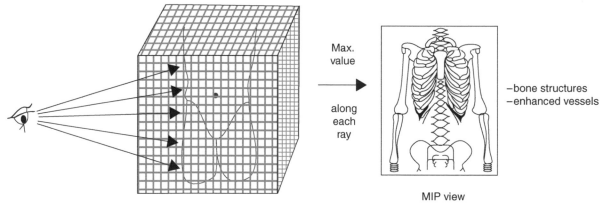

Figure 4.3 Volume rendered image of the abdominal aorta depicting a near total occlusion of the aorta at the level of the superior mesenteric artery with extensive collateral vessels that reconstitute the common iliac arteries on both sides.

MIP displays may provide images similar to that of conventional X-ray angiography and are frequently used for vascular imaging. An important advantage with the MIP post-processing technique is represented by the possibility to adjust the slab thickness on the workstation. In fact, thick (>15–25 mm) MIP slabs can help identify the course of blood vessels that would otherwise not be seen in axial or thin MIP images. However, MIP reformatted images have a tendency to obscure and eliminate low attenuation objects such as thrombi. MIPs in general, and thick slab MIPs in particular, are less sensitive in detecting abnormalities such as thrombi or subtle abnormalities in the vessel wall such as dissection or ulcerations. Sliding thin slab MIPs can follow the course of blood vessels through solid tissue and allow the systematic evaluation of a blood vessel with the ability to evaluate small and tissue-embedded vessels (Figure 4.4).

A major disadvantage with MIP projections is that high-density materials such as bones, endovascular stents, and

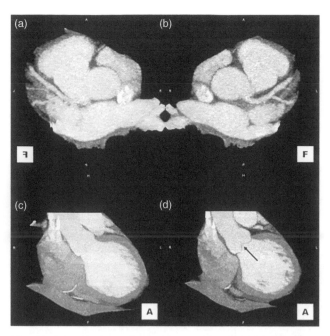

Figure 4.4 Maximum intensity projections (MIPs) displayed with different slab thickness. Although the course of coronary arteries can be well visualized as thick slab MIPs (15 mm) (a), thin slab MIPs (5 mm) offer improved resolution of small caliber vessels (b). Additionally, thick slab MIPs (15 mm) can provide a wide cardiac projection (c), but thin slab MIPs can better visualize the anatomy of thinner cardiac structures such as aortic valves (arrow) (d).

calcification may superimpose on blood vessels and obscure the visualization of important vascular details (Figure 4.5). Manipulation of the window level in conjunction with cropping of the image can be performed in order to exclude highly attenuated structures from the data set.

MinIPs are helpful in evaluating structures with small areas of attenuation. They can be used to detect and analyze abnormalities in the lung such as emphysema, bronchiectasis, and heterogeneous lung attenuation. Since MinIP slabs only project low attenuated voxels, vascular structures will be eliminated and MinIPs are therefore not used in angiography.

Multi-planar reformation

Multi-planar reformation (MPR) images are obtained using a relatively simple post-processing algorithm available on all workstations and represent the reconstructed source data projected in different planes. MPR images display 100% of the information (i.e. there is no loss of information or selective display of information). Thus, MPR images may be used to obtain accurate measurements of the imaged anatomic structures. The MPR technique allows depiction of the object of interest in standard axial, coro-

nal, or sagittal planes (Figure 4.1). The quality of MPR images is dependent on the quality of the source images.

Since MPR images are reformatted source data that lie in a specified single plane, the reader can scroll through stacks of MPR images to appreciate the course of a blood vessel. As discussed previously, on MIP images it is difficult to adequately evaluate the lumen of vessels with calcification or endovascular stents. However, MPR may allow the visualization of luminal contrast material and assessment of patency even in a vessel that is heavily calcified or stented (Figure 4.5).

Curved planar reformation

To better visualize an object that travels in and out of a single 2D plane, *curved planar reformation* (CPR) images can be created to display the entire object in a single axis. Points are assigned to the center of the object of interest along its entire course. Then the midline points along the curved line are connected into a linear projection (Figure 4.6). CPR is similar to MPR in that the displayed image represents the source data and is a single voxel thick projection. Despite the strengths of CPR, there are a number of limitations with this reformatting process. Since 3D volume images are collapsed into a 2D plane, CPR has limited depth resolution. CPR images are created using manual or semi-automated tracings of the vessel centerline. Thus, inaccurate selection of the points along the structure (vessel) of interest can cause spurious pseudostenosis or occlusion.

Shaded surface display image

The *shaded surface display* (SSD) technique is based on the identification of surface voxel intensity on the object of interest. The surface voxels depict a 3D shadow effect by using a threshold criterion, with some regions illuminated and others remaining darker like if they were illuminated by an external light source. Intensity thresholding generates images with a grayscale representation which provides perception of depth. The threshold ranges are based on the Hounsfield units of the displayed voxels. Thresholding is a concept that requires at least four intensity thresholds (t_1–t_4) (Figure 4.7). For intensities that are within t_2–t_3 threshold value the objectiveness or contrast intensity is 1 (100%). Intensities below t_1 and above t_4 are given objectiveness of 0 (0%). However, voxel intensities between t_1–t_2 and t_3–t_4 are given objectiveness values ranging between 0–100%. This range of objectiveness gives the displayed object a perception

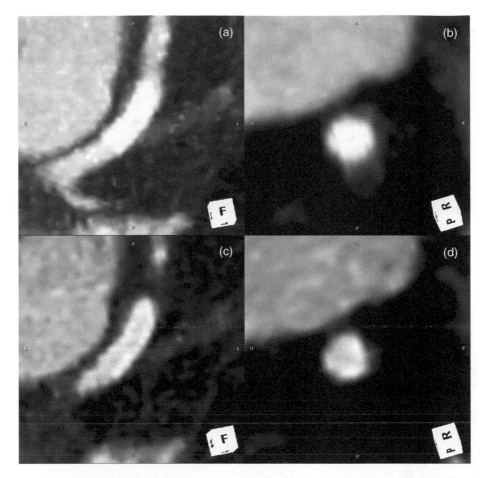

Figure 4.5 Visualization of endovascular stent in the proximal right coronary artery. Using the maximum intensity projection (MIP) technique (5 mm slab thickness), the high-density endovascular stent cast is displayed through the contrast medium inside the vessel. This makes it impossible to evaluate the intrastent patency in a longitudinal view (a) as well as a transverse view (b) of the vessel. The presence of an intrastent stenosis may be better established by displaying multiplanar reformation (MPR) of the same longitudinal (c) and transverse (d) views.

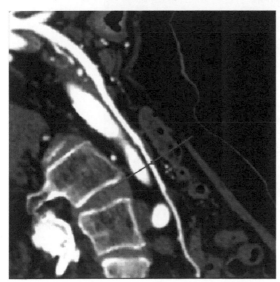

Figure 4.6 Curved planar reformatted (CPR) image allows the visualization of the entire course of the superior mesenteric artery (SMA) to be displayed in one plane. The arrow head notes the position of the aorta, the arrow to the origin of the SMA and the red line denotes the transverse orientation of the aorta and SMA at that level.

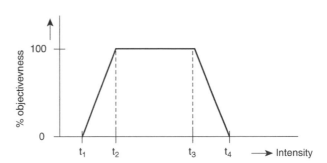

Figure 4.7 The objectiveness of a displayed image is determined by a set of threshold intensity parameters. Intensities within the t_2–t_3 threshold value are given 100% objectiveness. For intensities below t_1 and above t_4, 0% is displayed. Voxel intensities between t_1–t_2 and t_3–t_4 are given objectiveness values ranging between 0–100%.

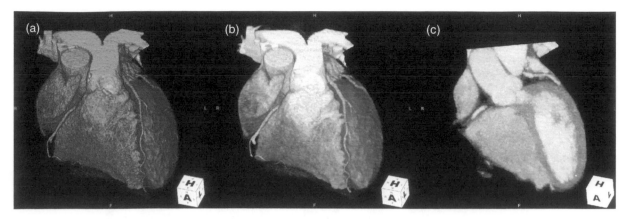

Figure 4.8 Volume rendered images (a) provide more depth and improved perspective of coronary arteries against the cardiac background compared to shaded surface display (SSD) (b) and maximum intensity projection (MIP) (c) images.

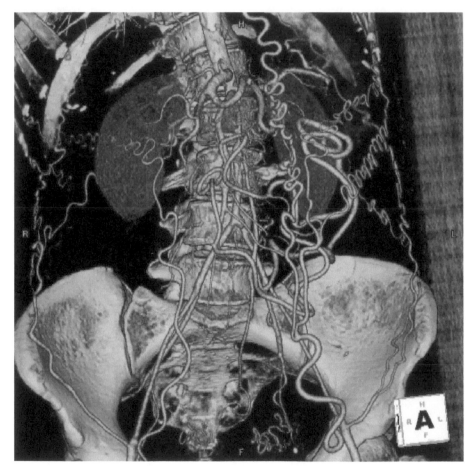

Figure 4.9 Volume rendered image of the abdominal aorta depicting a near total occlusion of the aorta at the level of the superior mesenteric artery with extensive collateral vessels that reconstitute the common iliac arteries on both sides.

of depth. SSD is primarily used to evaluate tubular structures such as airways (i.e. virtual bronchoscopy), colon (i.e. virtual colonoscopy), and blood vessels (virtual angioscopy). This technique is usually faster and requires less data storage because only the points on the surface of the vessel are manipulated rather than every single voxel in the image, as in volume rendering.

Although the final SSD image provides a very appealing visual display, there are several potential pitfalls with the thresholding technique. Since thresholding parameters

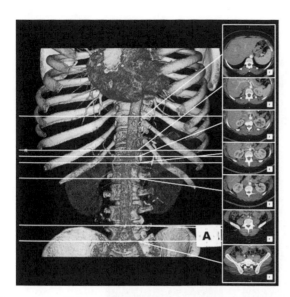

Figure 4.10 Volume rendered image of the abdominal aorta and branching vessels in the anterior-posterior view with corresponding stacked multiplanar reformation (MPR) images.

are arbitrarily set, the true anatomy of the target object may be lost. If the threshold value is set too high, parts of the displayed object may be cut off. This artifact could be misinterpreted as a stenosis. If the threshold value is set too low, surrounding tissue may be rendered as part of the target object owing to partial volume averaging. SSD is a useful tool for giving an overall picture of the course and shape of a (blood) vessel, but it should never be used when accurate measures of luminal dimension are required (Figure 4.8).

3D volume rendering image

Volume rendering (VR) imaging is a technique that uses all the information from the original data set to display a 3D representation of the object of interest (Figures 4.8 and 4.9). Unlike other reformatting techniques such as MIP, there is no loss of data from the conversion of a 3D object into a 2D display.

The advantage of VR imaging is that it gives the true perspective of the object of interest with that of the surrounding tissues. This allows the reader to follow the full course of blood vessels and determine if any external surrounding structure is causing a pseudostenosis. Additionally, the VR images can be rotated and can be helpful in identifying gross anatomic variations in blood vessels, such as anomalous origins and course.

To convey depth perception each voxel in the data set is assigned a degree of opacity based on the value of attenuation. Each voxel contributes 0–100% of opacity to the final image. The final image takes into account image intensities and opacity values for each displayed voxel. As a result of displaying an image with a gradation of attenuation values,

blood vessels can be evaluated in relationship to bones, calcifications, and stents. Since VR imaging is similar to SSD imaging in that an arbitrary scale is used to assign opacity, VR imaging should not be used for diagnostic purposes or to measure anatomic structures.

POST-PROCESSING TECHNIQUES IN PERIPHERAL CT ANGIOGRAPHY

The evaluation of a peripheral angiographic data set usually begins by quickly reviewing the axial source images to detect gross anatomic abnormalities or angiographic variations, to evaluate the quality of acquisition (timing of contrast, signal-to-noise ratio), and to recognize any accompanying artifacts or source of misinterpretation (motion, metal, streaking, poor contrast opacification, calcium, etc.). The same data set is then evaluated by using a MIP format (with a variable thickness depending on the vessel bed) in traditional projections such as anterior–posterior, sagittal, and coronal views as well as in oblique projections. Using the three orientations, the operator attempts to orient the views to the anatomic axis of the vessel or structure of interest. If the workstation allows it, the entire 3D data set can be manipulated in non-conventional views to define stenosis or other abnormalities.

Rapid review of the data set in such a fashion can help rule out abnormalities. If an abnormality is detected, the segment is magnified and viewed as an MPR image to characterize the abnormality and to make measurements. The abnormality should always be viewed in multiple planes, often orthogonal to each other. Scrolling through an MPR data set in a plane along the axis of the lumen will allow one to define the anatomic degree of stenosis and characterize other abnormalities including the performance of measurements (Figures 4.10 and 4.11). Three-dimensional techniques such as VR may be generated either in the beginning or at the end of the evaluation to define anatomic course and to evaluate anatomic variations if needed (Figures 4.10 and 4.11).

CONCLUSIONS

Analysis of CT images requires optimal visualization and resolution of the target object. Much of the image quality is dependent on the image acquisition and, to a lesser extent, on post-processing algorithms. However, post-processing techniques may facilitate accurate interpretation of CT

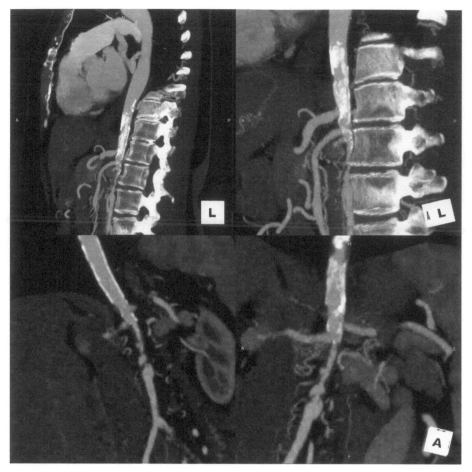

Figure 4.11 Orthogonal projections of the aortic occlusion seen in Figure 4.8, to attempt to visualize the occlusion. It is apparent that the stenosis is high grade and that there is a narrow central channel that reconstitutes the infra-renal aorta (thin caliber) and also the iliac arteries on both sides.

images. It is knowledge and hands-on experience that allow operators to best utilize these post-processing techniques to enhance their ability in image interpretation.

- Measurements should always be made wall-to-wall in the MPR mode after ensuring orientation along the long axis of the vessel.

PRACTICAL PEARLS

- MIP images can allow quick review of angiograms, but often underestimates stenoses and subtle abnormalities.

- Always review source images in the axial orientation and as MPR images.

- Calcified vessels are better visualized in the MPR mode with appropriate windowing and thresholding.

- For assessment of stent lumen patency, especially if the stent involves a small vessel, repeat reconstruction on the scanner console using a sharper kernel (B50f or B45f).

- To assess the anomalous course of vessels a volume rendered image may often be very helpful.

FURTHER READING

Addis KA, Hopper KD, Iyriboz TA. CT angiography: in vitro comparison of five reconstruction methods. Am J Roentgenol 2001 Nov; 177(5) : 1171–6.

Chiang EE, Boiselle PM, Raptopoulos V et al. Detection of pulmonary embolism: comparison of paddle wheel and coronal CT reformations–initial experience. Radiology 2003; 228: 577–82.

Chow LC, Rubin GD. CT angiography of the arterial system. Radiol Clin North Am 2002; 40(4): 729–49.

Cody DD. AAPM/RSNA Physics Tutorial for Residents: Topics in CT Imaging Processing in CT. Radiographics 2002; 22 : 1255–68.

Gruden JF. Thoracic CT performance and interpretation in the multi-detector era. J Thorac Imaging 2005; 20(4): 253–64.

Haaga JR, Lanzieri CF, Gilkeson RC et al. CT and MR Imaging of the Whole Body, Vol 1, 4th edn. St Louis Missouri: Mosby online 2003.

Henschke CI, McCauley DI, Yankelevitz DF. Early lung cancer action project: a summary of the findings on baseline screening. Oncologist 2001; 6(2): 147–52.

Hiatt MD, Fleischmann D, Hellinger JC, Rubin GD. Angiographic imaging of the lower extremities with multidetector CT. Radiol Clin North Am 2005; 43(6): 1119–27.

Kwan SW, Partik BL, Zinck SE et al. Primary interpretation of thoracic MDCT images using coronal reformations. Am J Roentgenol 2005; 185(6): 1500–8.

Napel S, Rubin GD, Jeffrey RB Jr. STS-MIP: a new reconstruction technique for CT of the chest. J Comput Assist Tomogr 1993; 17(5): 832–8.

Ney DR, Fishman EK, Magid D et al. Three-dimensional volumetric display of CT data: effect of scan parameters upon image quality. J Comput Assist Tomogr 1991; 15: 875–85.

Richenberg JL, Hansell DM. Image processing and spiral ST of the thorax. Br J Radiol 1998; 71: 708–16.

Upuda SK. Three-dimensional visualization and analysis methodologies: a current perspective. Radiographics 1999; 19(3): 783–806.

5

X-ray contrast agents and contrast timing considerations

Debabrata Mukherjee and Sanjay Rajagopalan

INTRODUCTION

CT angiography (CTA) may be used to visualize arteries and veins throughout the body and is an attractive alternative to traditional catheter-based angiography in appropriate circumstances. CTA uses contrast agents for the visualization of blood vessels. Many different contrast agents are available today, for CTA. Iodine, the main component of X-ray contrast media, has a high molecular weight which can be combined with larger molecules to form radio-opaque contrast agents. ^{127}I is the only stable isotope and is used in all iodinated contrast media. Iodine has a K-edge at 33.2 keV and therefore X-ray attenuation in blood vessels is enhanced compared to surrounding tissue. Iodinated contrast media may be divided into water-soluble, water-insoluble, and oily contrast media (Figure 5.1).

The two major clinically important attributes of a contrast agent are its iodine dose (concentration X volume) and osmolality. To maintain good radiographic efficacy and safety, contrast agents must balance the somewhat paradoxical relationship between these two properties. Iodine dose refers to the amount of iodine delivered in an injected dose of contrast material. The iodine, delivered by iodinated benzene ring compounds, produces radiographic 'contrast' by blocking X-rays. Visualization is typically improved by increasing the iodine load, a function of the percentage of iodine and the concentration of the compound present upon injection. Increasing the iodine load, however, results in increased osmolality. Osmolality refers to the number of dissolved particles in a solution, or the concentration. Ideally,

contrast agents injected into the vasculature should have an osmolality as close to that of body fluids as possible. Solutions with osmolality greater (hypertonic) or less (hypotonic) than that of body fluids can cause cells to shrink or swell, respectively, contributing to hemodynamic, physiologic, and biologic adverse effects. The body also attempts to quickly dilute and excrete hypertonic solutions to maintain osmotic equilibrium. Therefore, the benefits gained from increasing the iodine load in contrast agents to improve radiographic efficacy may be offset by the adverse effects associated with higher osmolality solutions. The goal should be to use the lowest dose and volume of contrast necessary for adequate CTA.

FUNDAMENTALS

Currently used contrast agents are chemical modifications of a 2,4,6-tri-iodinated benzene ring (Figure 5.2) and are classified on the basis of their physical and chemical characteristics. For clinical purposes, categorization based on osmolality is widely used. Broadly, there are two types of agents, *high-osmolality*, *and low-osmolality* agents, with distinct advantages and disadvantages. *Iso-osmolarity* agents which have traditionally been included within *low-osmolarity* agents are now viewed as a separate class. In general, individuals with prior significant contrast reactions, active asthma, severe heart failure, aortic stenosis, severe pulmonary hypertension, or significant renal dysfunction (serum creatinine >2 mg/dl) should receive either a low-osmolar or preferably an iso-osmolar agent. Iso-osmolal agents have also been shown

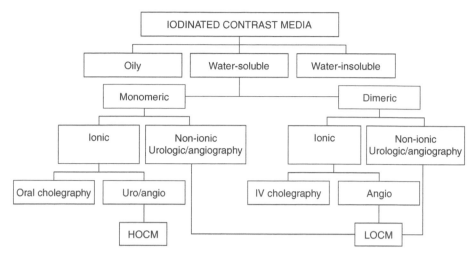

Figure 5.1 Schematic diagram of iodinated X-ray contrast media. HOCM: high-osmolar contrast media, LOCM: low-osmolar contrast media. *Image source*: www.medcyclopaedia.com by GE Healthcare.

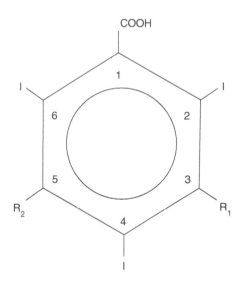

Figure 5.2 The molecular structure of tri-iodinated benzoic acid. In solution, the carboxyl acid group (COOH) will dissociate into its anion (COO⁻) and the appropriate cation (usually either sodium or meglumine). *Image source*: www.medcyclopaedia.com by GE Healthcare.

to cause significantly less discomfort for patients and may also reduce the relative risk of developing contrast media-induced renal failure.

Advances in multi-slice CT technology have resulted in a 4- to 6-fold increase in imaging speed and have enabled both the acquisition of thinner slices and an increase in coverage. These improvements are prompting reconsideration of conventional approaches to the use of contrast media.

Now, along with setting appropriate parameters for pitch, slice thickness, and the number of passes to make during various phases of contrast enhancement, imaging specialists tailor the delivery of iodinated contrast by adjusting volume, concentration, rate, and the timing between injection and scanning.

High-osmolar contrast agents

The osmolality of these *ionic* agents in solution ranges from 600 to 2100 mOsm/kg, versus 290 mOsm/kg for human plasma. Commonly used high-osmolar contrast agents are Renografin™ or Hypaque™ (diatrizoate anion) and Conray (iothalamate anion). The iodine content of diatrizoate is 370 mgI/ml and iothalamate is 400 mgI/ml. When injected for CTA, high-osmolar agents (Hypaque, Conray, Renografin) opacify blood vessels and are then rapidly carried via the bloodstream to the kidneys, where they are excreted unchanged mainly by glomerular filtration, permitting visualization of opacified heart chambers and blood vessels. With these agents, the degree of enhancement is directly related to the amount of iodine administered. Peak iodine blood levels occur immediately following rapid injection of the dose and fall rapidly within 5 to 10 minutes. The exact dose and rate of injection depend on the particular territory of interest, the particular CT scanner, and the number of detectors. It should be noted that very few clinicians currently use *high-osmolarity* contrast agents.

Low-osmolar non-ionic contrast agents

Common examples of low-osmolar and *non-ionic* monomers are iohexol (Omnipaque™) (Figure 5.3), iopamidol (Isovue™), ioversol (Optiray™), and iopromide (Ultravist™). The respective iodine contents are iohexol: 140, 180, 210, 240, 300 and 350 mgI/ml; iopadimol: 200, 250, 300 and 370 mgI/ml; ioversal: 160, 240, 300, 320 and 350 mgI/ml; and iopromide: 150, 240, 300 and 370 mgI/ml. Low-osmolar *non-ionic* contrast agents are used in a broad range of intravascular diagnostic procedures such as peripheral and coronary angiography, spinal cord imaging, and body cavity procedures including shoulder and knee joints. Immediately following intravascular injection, these agents reach peak plasma concentration and are then rapidly distributed throughout the extracellular fluid compartment. Low-osmolar agents do not normally cross the blood brain barrier to any significant extent. It is excreted unchanged by the kidneys, mainly by glomerular filtration and a very small quantity (1 to 2%) is excreted via the bile. Typically these agents are injected intravenously through a 20 gauge antecubital angiocatheter with a power injector. The rate of injection and volume depend on the vascular bed. Low-osmolar agents are the most commonly used contrast agents for CTA.

Iso-osmolar contrast agents

The lower osmolality of iso-osmolar agents such as iodixanol (Visipaque™, GE Healthcare) which is non-ionic isotonic with blood causes fewer and less severe osmolality related disturbances, such as, pain, heat, and a burning sensation, upon injection. Iodixanol has approximately one-third the osmolality of the non-ionic media and one-sixth that of the monomeric ionic media of equi-iodine concentration. Visipaque is the only contrast medium currently available for intravascular to use that is isosmolar to blood at all available iodine concentrations. In other words, it has the same osmolality as blood at the 270 mgI concentration and the 320 mgI concentration. It is used in the same way, for the same examinations as *low-osmolarity* agents but due to its *iso-smolar* property may have benefits as is highlighted in terms of patient comfort and a reduction in rate of contrast-induced nephropathy. Iodixanol 320 mgI/ml (Figure 5.4) is typically injected with a power injector through an 18 to 20 gauge IV cannula in an antecubital vein. A saline chaser bolus is then injected through the second head of the power injector immediately after injection of contrast material has been completed. The rate of injection and volume depend on the vascular bed of interest, but usually 80–100 ml of contrast material is injected followed by a 40–50 ml saline chaser bolus, at an injection rate of 4 ml/s.

Gadolinium

Recently, several groups have reported the use of high-dose gadolinium for CTA of the neck, thorax, abdomen, and pelvis. This may be appropriate for a small percentage of patients who need non-invasive vascular imaging but who have contraindications to both iodinated contrast and MR angiography. On a per-molar basis, gadolinium is a better attenuator of X-rays than iodinated contrast agents, but to achieve this level of enhancement on CTA a much larger volume of gadolinium must be administered than for MRA. With the advent of 64–128 detector CT scanners, in combination with bolus tracking, the overall dose of gadolinium needed for diagnostic CTA examinations will be lower but safety remains a concern. Current guidelines state that the use of gadolinium based contrast media for radiographic

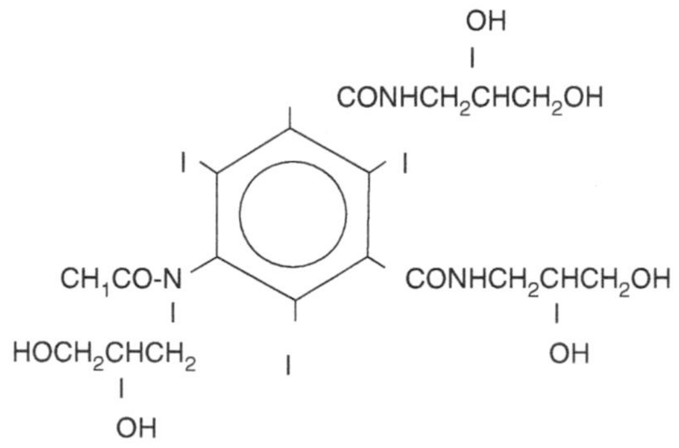

Figure 5.3 The molecular structure of iohexol (Omnipaque), a non-ionic monomer. *Image source*: www.medcyclopaedia.com by GE Healthcare.

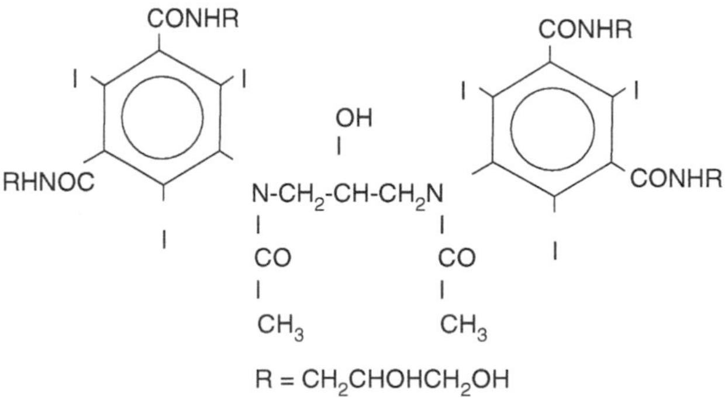

Figure 5.4 The molecular structure of iodixanol (Visipaque), a non-ionic dimer. *Image source*: www.medcyclopaedia.com by GE Healthcare.

examinations is not recommended to avoid nephrotoxicity in patients with renal impairment since they are more nephrotoxic than iodinated contrast media in equivalent X-ray attenuating doses. The use of gadolinium based contrast medium in approved intravenous doses up to 0.3 mmol/kg body weight will not give diagnostic radiographic information in most cases (www.esur.org).

CONTRAST ADMINISTRATION

Contrast material

Non-ionic low osmolar such as iohexol (Omnipaque™), iopamidol (Isovue™, Niopam™), ioversol (Optiray™), iopromide (Ultravist™), ioxaglate (Hexabrix™), or an iso-osmolar agent, iodixanol (Vispaque™) is typically used. The iodine concentrations of these agents are in the range of 300–400 mgI/ml.

Injection site

For most peripheral applications contrast material may be safely administered in one of the forearm superficial veins that drain into the deep venous system of the upper extremity. For most applications involving the arch and thoracic aorta, the right upper extremity is preferred because of the shorter course of the right brachiocephalic vein that results in less 'streaking' artifact. Additionally this allows unimpeded evaluation at the internal mammary artery when indicated. However, this may be irrelevant if the only access site available is the left upper extremity.

Intravenous access

For most applications at least a 20 gauge access is recommended to allow faster injection rates. A smaller gauge iv cannula may require higher iodine-containing contrast agents to allow higher peak attenuation values.

CONTRAST KINETICS

Bolus geometry

The kinetics of contrast arrival and dissipation in an arterial bed is referred to as bolus geometry. For CTA this corresponds to the rate of change of CT attenuation with injection (Figure 5.5). A uniphasic injection protocol is the most common method to administer contrast agents. It involves delivery of the contrast agent at a uniform speed throughout

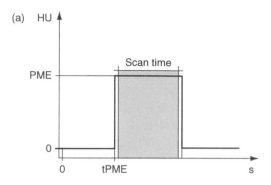

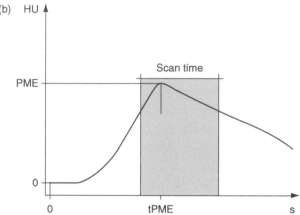

Figure 5.5 Optimal and actual bolus geometry in CT angiography (CTA). (a) Optimal bolus geometry. The abrupt rise and the steady plateau of attenuation characterize the optimal pattern of bolus geometry. Ideally the scan time tightly overlaps with the length of the plateau of enhancement in order to use the entire volume of contrast material (CM) administered for the acquisition. (b) Actual bolus geometry. The pattern of actual bolus geometry is quite different from the ideal one. Before and after the peak of maximum enhancement there are slopes of enhancement. Generally the up slope is steeper than the down slope, especially with contrast administration protocols for CTA characterized by a high injection rate. PME, peak of maximum enhancement; tPME, delayed time to peak. *Adapted from*: Cademartiri F, Nieman K. Contrast material injection techniques for CT angiography of the coronary arteries. In: Schoepf UJ, ed. CT of the Heart. Principles and Applications. New Jersey: Humana Press, 2005, with permission.

the injection, with the peak arterial enhancement occurring nearly at completion of the injection. An ideal bolus shape during uniphasic injection would correspond to a rapid rise in attenuation with maintenance of this level allowing timing of the acquisition beginning at peak and continuing during this 'plateau' phase. The peak of contrast enhancement is typically reached at the end of the injection of the contrast agent followed by a decline in attenuation values. With the biphasic injection protocol, the initial higher speed injection is followed by a slower injection rate. The advantage of such an injection protocol is that the duration of contrast enhancement is enhanced. The third method of changing bolus shape is the exponentially decelerated injection. This involves an exponential decline in the injection rate all the time. This has been previously tested in mathematical models as well as in animals. However, this is not currently used in clinical protocols. Uniform contrast enhancement is more or less desirable in CTA applications in the periphery. One of the advantages of using such a protocol is that it becomes less critical to time the acquisition correctly for the peak arterial contrast enhancement.

A number of factors influence the bolus geometry, as shown in Figure 5.6. The three main factors include:

Injection speed: by increasing the rate of delivery of contrast agent, the peak enhancement is shifted upwards and towards the left (earlier peak) (Figure 5.6b). Rapid rates are preferred in CTA to allow an ascending limb and higher attenuation values. Thus rates of ≥4 ml/s are common. Higher rates (>6 ml/s) may cause complications such as contrast extravasation.

Injection volume: increasing the injection volume delays peak contrast enhancement, prolongs the duration of the bolus, and shifts the peak contrast enhancement upwards and to the right (Figure 5.6c). Therefore increasing the duration of the bolus has the effect of prolonging the bolus curve (increasing the area under the curve while also increasing the peak enhancement). With single-slice and 4-slice scanners, it is acceptable to match the injection duration to the scan duration. However, with the introduction of faster scanners, this approach may not be acceptable. An injection duration equal to the scan duration results in very poor arterial enhancement owing to the fact that imaging may occur during the descending limb of the contrast enhancement curve. One option is to reduce the duration of attainment of peak arterial enhancement by using higher injection rates; however, there are practical limitations to this, and, for most practical purposes, injection rates >5 ml/s may have safety implications. Another option is to ensure that the duration of contrast enhancement persists for the most part stably during the acquisition by extending the bolus duration.

Iodine concentration: use of contrast material with higher concentrations of iodine has the effect of accomplishing higher degrees of peak contrast enhancement. Figure 5.6c illustrates enhancement curves attained in a large conduit vessel by using three different concentrations of iodinated contrast agents (300, 350, and 400 mg iodine/ml), while keeping the total iodine load constant. When one uses the same injection rate of 5 ml/s, the contrast material with the highest concentration of iodine delivers more iodine mass per second, resulting in greater peak arterial enhancement. Thus, besides increasing the injection speed, another way of obtaining higher levels of arterial enhancement is by changing the iodine concentration of the contrast material. Thus, in patients who have poor intravenous access, that precludes placement of a large-bore intravenous cannula (less than or equal to 20 gauge), an alternate method to increase peak arterial contrast is by using contrast agents with higher iodine loads. It should be noted that as iodine concentration increases, viscosity increases and osmolality increases. As a general principle, the minimal amount of contrast material needed to perform a diagnostic study should be used to ensure patient safety and benefits.

Saline flush: usage of the saline flush immediately following contrast injection has several potential advantages. It flushes out contrast material that would otherwise be left behind in the injection tubing. It also eliminates the extra step of flushing the vascular access site of residual contrast agents after injection. By pushing the contrast bolus forward, it may create a more desirable bolus shape (Figure 5.6d). It also increases the amount of contrast available to use in image acquisition and may reduce artifact. Typically, a dual power injector is required for a saline flush.

Minor factors include the cardiac output and body surface area. A lower cardiac output (low ejection fraction) results in higher peak arterial enhancement and a longer time to peak arterial enhancement. Large body surface area may result in dilution of the contrast and reduction in peak arterial enhancement. Thus the 'large' patient may require larger doses of contrast to accomplish the same peak attenuation. Factors such as age, gender, and hemodynamic parameters (blood pressure and heart rate) typically do not affect geometry.

CONTRAST ARRIVAL TIMING

In CTA determination of the appropriate scan timing is important in obtaining satisfactory images. Determination of the appropriate time for image acquisition can be obtained by a test bolus sequence or by using bolus-tracking methods. The purpose of determining the appropriate scan delay is that patient-related factors, for example low cardiac output and other physiologic variables such as concomitant disease states, will alter the time of the arrival of contrast agent in the vascular territory of interest. Different timing and synchronization techniques are shown in Figure 5.7.

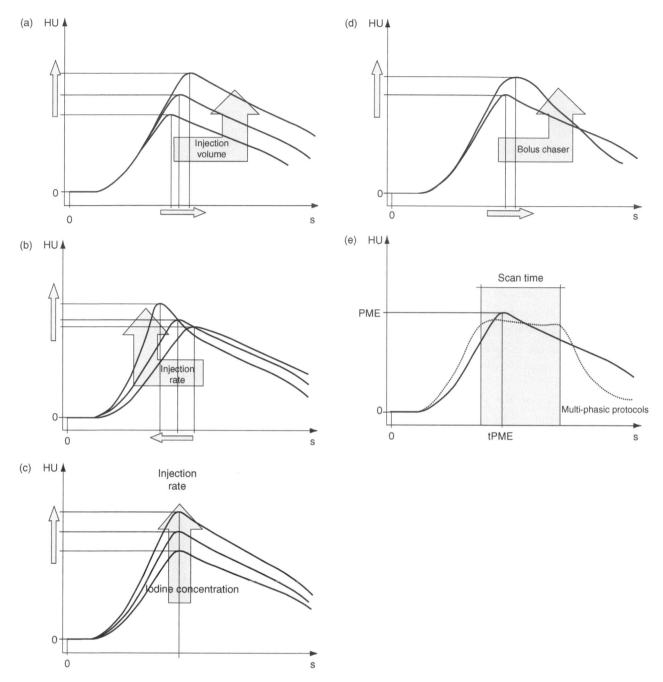

Figure 5.6   Parameters affecting bolus geometry. (a) The influence of contrast material (CM) volume. Increasing the volume of injected CM produces an increase in the peak of maximum enhancement (PME), and a delayed time to peak (tPME). (b) The influence of CM injection rate. Increasing the rate of injected CM produces an increase in PME, and an earlier tPME. (c) The influence of CM iodine concentration. Increasing the iodine concentration of the injected CM produces an increase in PME, without any influence on tPME. (d) The influence of the saline chaser. The saline chaser pushes the injected contrast medium through the veins of the forearm, providing a result similar to the injection of a larger contrast volume. The example shows the effect of a 50 ml saline chaser (thicker curve), using a bolus with the same volume, rate, and iodine concentration. Moreover the saline chaser prevents the decrease of the CM in the arm veins, which may normally cause an increase in the CM concentration after the end of contrast injection. (e) The influence of scan time are consistent, but with a shorter scan time, as with 16-row multi-slice CT, the importance of a lone plateau enhancement is reduced if compared to the impact of a very high PME. *Adapted from*: Cademartiri F, Nieman K. Contrast material injection techniques for CT angiography of the coronary arteries. In: Schoepf UJ, ed. CT of the Heart. Principles and Applications. New Jersey: Humana Press, 2005, with permission.

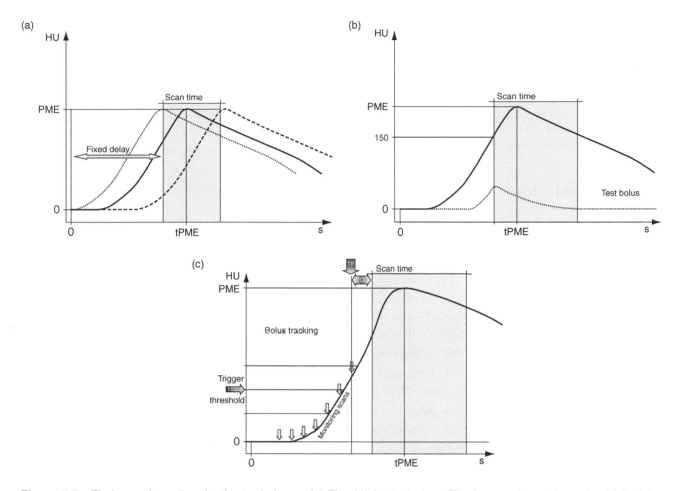

Figure 5.7 Timing and synchronization techniques. (a) Fixed delay technique. The image shows the main pitfall of the fixed delay technique. The continuous curve shows the ideal situation where the fixed delay and bolus geometry correspond to perfectly making for optimal imaging. In some cases the bolus geometry of the patient can be different from the expected one. If the actual bolus geometry is faster than fixed delay (dotted curve), the enhancement of vascular structures will still be present but reduced, and prominent venous enhancement may be evident. If the actual bolus geometry is slower than fixed delay (dashed curve), the risk is to scan the passage of contrast material (CM) only in the distal portion of the scan range with poor contrast enhancement of the arteries. (b) Test bolus technique. The correlation between test bolus time to peak maximum enhancement (tPME) and main bolus tPME is displayed. In this case, the test bolus correlates with the time to reach 150 HU (Hounsfield units) in the main bolus. A main scan based on this information will be successful, even though not optimal for CTA. In fact the vascular attenuation of 150 HU at the beginning of the scan is too low for optimal CTA. Worse results are obtained when the correlation is with the time to reach 50 HU or 100 HU. The test bolus actually has a different geometry from the main bolus. The lack of injection power after injection of the test bolus determines a pooling of the test bolus system without any *vis a tergo*. In other words, the test bolus is left alone in the venous system of the arm, without the help of saline solution (bolus chaser) or adjunctive contrast medium (main bolus) that pushes it forward. (c) Bolus tracking technique. The sequence of real time bolus tracking is displayed. After the topogram is acquired, the monitoring scan is set at the level of the aortic root and the region of interest (ROI) inside the lumen of the ascending aorta. The trigger threshold is set at 100 HU. Then, CM administration and the monitoring sequence are started at the same time, and when the attenuation in the ROI reaches a value greater than 100 HU at the triggering point (TP) a transition delay (TD – generally 4 s are enough for this procedure) starts while the table reaches its starting position and the patient receives breath holding instructions. *Adapted from*: Cademartiri F, Nieman K. Contrast material injection techniques for CT angiography of the coronary arteries. In: Schoepf UJ, ed. CT of the Heart. Principles and Applications. New Jersey: Humana Press, 2005, with permission.

Fixed delay

This involves usage of an empirically derived delay to predict bolus arrival. As such this should be rarely used as it may result in inappropriate timing of contrast arrival and because there are better ways to predict bolus arrival. Practically however, usage of empiric delays has been used routinely in CTA with very good results in the majority of patients.

Test bolus technique

In this method, a small test bolus (5 ml of iodinated contrast) is injected, followed by a saline bolus of the same volume and speed used in the actual CTA protocol (usually 50 ml of normal saline). The time to peak enhancement is calculated and is used to predict the true contrast arrival by using an empiric correction factor (usually 6–8 s). This is because the bolus geometry of the test bolus (being smaller) is different from the actual contrast injection (larger volume). The latter is going to be shifted to the right and thus one needs to add an arbitrary duration that corresponds to this delay. There is very poor correlation between the time to peak enhancement of the test bolus and the time to peak enhancement of the actual contrast injection. In contrast, there is good correlation between peak enhancement of the test bolus and attainment of a predetermined threshold such as 100 or 150 HU on the main injection protocol. Thus beginning the acquisition on the ascending limb of the contrast curve may be advantageous if the arterial bed is located in the mid portion of the scan range, which will actually correspond to peak arterial opacification. In contrast, if the vessels are located at the beginning of the scan range, this may result in starting the scan too early.

Bolus tracking

A better approach to timing the scan is the use of bolus tracking techniques. This involves a real-time tracking technique based on a user-defined area of interest within the lumen of the artery to be imaged. A threshold attenuation is chosen at which to trigger the actual CTA acquisition. This arbitrary threshold can vary depending upon the application and the goals of the study. Thus, the scan is initiated on attainment of this empiric threshold. Furthermore, there is a small time delay dependent on the scanner, between detection of the threshold enhancement and actual initiation of scanning (2 to 9 s, depending upon the table position and CT scanner). During this delay, it may be actually beneficial to ensure that adequate arterial enhancement is accomplished at the time of initiation of the scan and continues throughout the duration of the CT angiographic image acquisition. Thus, in bolus tracking algorithms, the injection duration should at least equal the scan duration added to the time delay between detection of the threshold and the actual initiation of scanning (2 to 9 s, as indicated previously). Amongst the advantages of using a bolus tracking technique as opposed to the test bolus technique is that a separate injection is not required. Additional advantages include the fact that this protocol is very easy to standardize.

LIMITATIONS

Adverse reactions

Adverse reactions to contrast agents range from mild reactions such as itching associated with hives, to life-threatening emergencies such as laryngeal edema and even death. Renal toxicity is a well known adverse reaction associated with the use of any intravenous contrast material. Other forms of adverse reactions include delayed allergic reactions, anaphylactoid reactions, and local tissue damage. Prior history of allergic reactions to contrast material, asthma, and known multiple allergies are factors associated with an increased risk of developing an adverse reaction.

PROPHYLACTIC MEDICATIONS

If the patient had a previous severe reaction with a cardiorespiratory component, an alternate imaging study should be considered. However if it is still necessary to proceed with CTA, the following prophylactic regimen may be considered. Either methylprednisolone, one 32 mg tablet, may be orally administered 12 and 2 hours before the study, or prednisone, one 50 mg tablet, may be orally administered 13 hours, 7 hours, and 1 hour before the study. In addition, antihistamines or an H1 blocker such as diphenhydramine, one 50 mg tablet, should be orally administered 1 hour before the study and an H2-histamine receptor blocker, such as cimetidine, 300 mg, or ranitidine, 50 mg, may be orally administered 1 hour before study.

CONTRAST NEPHROPATHY

Patients should be well hydrated prior to a contrast enhanced study, and hydration should be continued for several hours after a contrast-enhanced procedure is performed. Other potentially nephrotoxic drugs should be discontinued whenever possible prior to contrast administration. The minimal amount of contrast material, preferably a non-ionic, low-, or iso-osmolar agent, needed to perform a diagnostic study should be used. If multiple studies are required, several days should be allotted between studies to allow the kidneys to recover fully from the first injection. *N*-Acetylcysteine with hydration may reduce the risk of contrast nephropathy in patients with chronic renal insufficiency and should be considered in appropriate patients.

PRACTICAL PEARLS

- The two major clinically important attributes of a contrast agent are its iodine dose and osmolality.

- CTA requires tailoring the delivery of iodinated contrast by adjusting volume, concentration and rate, to optimize timing of the scan.

- There is poor correlation between the time to peak enhancement of test bolus and time to peak enhancement of the contrast injection while there is good correlation between peak enhancement of test bolus and attainment of a threshold such as 100 or 150 HU.

- The rate of injection and volume of injected contrast depend on the vascular bed being studied, the scanner, number of detectors and pitch.

- While bolus tracking the injection duration should at least equal the scan duration plus an additional time delay between detection of the threshold and initiation of scanning (2 to 9 seconds).

- Low-osmolar agents are the most commonly used contrast agents for CTA.

- Injection speed, volume, and iodine concentration are the main factors that influence bolus geometry.

- Factors such as age, gender and hemodynamics do not affect geometry.

- The best approach to scan timing is usage of bolus tracking techniques which involves a real-time tracking technique based on a user-defined area of interest within the lumen of the artery to be imaged.

FURTHER READING

Birck R, Krzossok S, Markowetz F et al. Acetylcysteine for prevention of contrast nephropathy: meta-analysis. Lancet 2003; 362(9384): 598–603.

Cademartiri F, Nieman K. Contrast material injection techniques for CT angiography of the coronary arteries. In: Schoepf UJ, ed. CT of the Heart. Principles and Applications. New Jersey: Humana Press; 2005.

Masui T, Katayama M, Kobayashi S, et al. Intravenous injection of high and medium concentrations of computed tomography contrast media and related heat sensation, local pain, and adverse reactions. J Comput Assist Tomogr 2005; 29(5): 704–8.

Matthai WH Jr, Kussmaul WG 3rd, Krol J et al. A comparison of low- with high-osmolality contrast agents in cardiac angiography. Identification of criteria for selective use. Circulation 1994; 89(1): 291–301.

Mukherjee D. Diagnostic catheter-based vascular angiography. In: Rajagopalan S, Mukherjee D, Mohler E, eds. Manual of Vascular Medicine. Philadelphia, PA: Lippincott Raven, 2004, 28–47.

Rosioreanu A, Alberico RA, Litwin A et al. Gadolinium-enhanced computed tomographic angiography: current status. Curr Probl Diagn Radiol 2005; 34(6): 207–19.

Weinmann HJ, Platzek J, Schirmer H et al. Contrast media: future aspects. Eur Radiol 2005; 15(Suppl 4): D70–3.

6

CT angiography of the extracranial and intracranial circulation with imaging protocols

Marja Berg, Marko Kangasniemi, Hannu Manninen, and Ritva Vanninen

INTRODUCTION

Catheter-based angiography has been the reference standard for imaging the cerebral and cervical vasculature for decades. The technique is invasive and is associated with a small but definite risk for neurologic and other complications such as puncture site hematomas and pseudo-aneurysms. There is thus a need for less invasive imaging modalities for the evaluation of this vascular territory. Multi-detector row computed tomography (MDCT) angiography technology fulfills many of the requirements for an optimal imaging modality for this territory, being robust, non-invasive, and providing versatility in a range of attributes over traditional catheter-based angiography. These include superior lesion characterization (presence of calcification, ulcerations, lipid, and fibrotic components), and perfusion-based measures that may be useful in providing 'at-risk areas' in the stroke patient and in intervention planning. The focus of this chapter is to help the reader build an understanding of this imaging modality, delineate clinical protocols, and provide practical pointers when using computed tomography (CT) angiography (CTA) for the assessment of the extracranial and intracranial circulations.

INDICATIONS

See Table 6.1.

FUNDAMENTALS AND GENERAL APPROACH

Compared to sequential imaging or single-detector CT imaging, fast spiral scanning using MDCT with thin detector collimation markedly improves volume coverage with superb spatial resolution and substantially fewer artifacts. The orientation of extracranial carotid arteries is favorable for CTA, since CTA can delineate arteries running perpendicular to the scanning plane better than arteries running parallel to the scanning plane (for example renal arteries). However, with near-isotropic or isotropic imaging available with current CT scanners the orientation of the vessels is no longer such a limitation.

Table 6.1 Indications for CTA of the extracranial and intracranial circulations

Extracranial circulation

Atherosclerosis

Fibromuscular dysplasia

Aneurysms, pseudoaneurysms, or dissection in the carotid, subclavian, vertebrobasilar system, and aorta

Cervical tumors (carotid body)

Follow-up after carotid stenting and endarterectomy

Intracranial circulation

Intracranial aneurysms

Arteriovenous malformations

Extracranial–intracranial bypasses

Contrast considerations

The inherent nephrotoxicity of contrast media must be considered, especially in individuals with pre-existing renal function impairment (e.g. diabetes mellitus, chronic kidney disease). For these individuals, except in emergency situations, creatinine clearance should be tested before scheduling the patient. Other contraindications for contrast studies including allergies to iodinated contrast should be evaluated, and patients given appropriate pre-medication, if necessary. Fasting is not mandatory, with the exception of patients with previous contrast-induced gastro-intestinal reactions.

MDCT angiography sequence planning and considerations

When scanning cervicocranial arteries, the patient is in the supine position with the upper arms along the body. The right antecubital vein is the preferred site for the venous access and contrast infusion to avoid 'streak artifacts' related to a high concentration of contrast medium in the left subclavian vein. The imaging volume is planned based on the topogram, with the duration of scan determining the contrast medium bolus duration (Chapter 5). The guiding principle when performing CTA in general is to maintain high concentrations of contrast agent in the target vessels during the arterial phase of the bolus. This can be achieved with the usage of automated dual injectors that provide high flow rates, followed by a saline bolus to compact the contrast bolus and to flush it from the peripheral to the central circulation. An automated bolus tracking algorithm or the use of a test bolus is equally accepted for synchronizing contrast media arrival and scanning. Although scans with a fixed delay time (15–18 s) can be used, this is not recommended, especially in individuals with low cardiac output or in the elderly. The use of thin collimation (0.5–1.25 mm) is preferable when imaging the cervicocranial arteries to assure high spatial resolution. Tube rotation time and the length of the table feed per second in relationship to the width of the collimation define the pitch p (see Chapters 1 and 2). The pitch value indicates the degree of gaps in the acquisition ($p > 1$) or the extent of data overlap ($p < 1$). For imaging the cervicocranial vessels, pitch values close to unity are important when using fast scanners (≥ 16 detector scanners, Table 6.2). When reconstructing axial images from a CTA exam, a smooth convolution kernel is preferable (B25f or B30f). The reconstruction increment defines the overlap of the axial images during reconstruction. An overlap of 20–50% (reconstruction increment of 0.5–0.8) has been recommended for peripheral angiographic applications.

DETAILED CLINICAL PROTOCOL

Extracranial circulation

Table 6.2 provides the acquisition parameters for 16, 32×2, and 64 slice detector scanners. We recommend reading up

Table 6.2 Scanning protocols for extracranial arteries (carotid and vertebrals)

	Siemens		General Electric		Philips		Toshiba	
Detectors	16	32×2	16	64	16	64	16	64
mAs	160	200	380 mA	Smart mA	250	250	300 mA	SUREExposure™ mA
kV	120	120	140	120	120	120	120	120
Rotation time (s)	0.5	0.33	0.5	0.4	0.75	0.75	0.5	0.5
Detector collimation (mm)	0.75	0.6	0.625	0.625	0.75	0.625	0.5	0.5
Slice thickness (mm)	0.75	0.75	0.625	0.625	1.0	0.9	1	0.5
Translation speed (mm/s)								
Table speed (Philips)	24	51.8	13.75	51.6	15	64	15	21
Pitch[a]	1	0.9	0.5625	0.516	0.938	1.2	0.938	0.656
Kernel/filter	B30f	B20f	Standard	Standard	Standard/B	Standard/B	Standard	FC04

[a]Pitch=table feed per rotation/total width of the collimated beam.
Philips parameters provided by Don Boshela BS, RT(R) (CT), Senior CT Product Development Specialist, Philips Medical Systems.
Toshiba parameters provided by Toshiba America Medical Systems.

the manuals of the CT device used for CTA, as well as additional sources. Although empiric timing for the extracranial circulation can be used, it is recommended that the precise time interval to optimize arterial enhancement be determined either through a test bolus approach or through a bolus triggering protocol.

Test bolus

A test bolus of 10 ml of contrast is administered at the same flow rate as is being planned for the CTA. A premonitoring slice with 5 mm collimation may be obtained at the level of the ascending aorta, arch, or common carotid arteries. Repeated scans are obtained with the lowest possible kV after a scan delay of 6–10 s (total duration being 30 s). The time to peak enhancement is evaluated from the scans. The scan delay for the CTA is calculated using the time to peak enhancement to which another 2–5 s are added; the longer the time to peak enhancement, the longer the time delay for contrast infusion.

Bolus triggering protocol

A region of interest is placed in the aortic arch image with a predefined threshold of 50–70 Hounsfield units (HU) to initiate the CTA acquisition. The contrast medium infusion and the scanner are activated at the same time, with monitoring scans starting after a scan delay of 6–10 s in order to allow contrast to travel from the peripheral circulation to the central venous system. The CTA acquisition mode is automatically activated from the bolus tracking algorithm after a short pause (5–6 s, depending of the CT device). The breathing instructions are given to the patient during this pause. With 64-slice scanners it is possible to trigger from the left ventricle, with coverage of the entire thoracic aorta and cervico-cranial circulation.

Scan volume

The prescribed scan volume depends on the clinical question. A scan volume in a caudo-cranial direction, covering the aortic arch to a level above the circle of Willis, allows comprehensive evaluation of the intracranial circulation.

Acquisition slice thickness (detector or slice collimation)

For cranio-cervical applications submillimeter detector collimation (0.6–0.75 mm) is preferable in view of the size of

the anatomic structures that may need to be characterized (e.g. small aneurysms, etc.).

Contrast agent bolus considerations

Low osmolality, non-ionic contrast agents are generally preferable (350–400 mg of iodine/ml). A volume of 60–100 ml (depending on the flow rate and the scan duration) at a flow rate of 3–5 ml/s is typically used. The use of bolus triggering or a test bolus approach is preferable. The use of high iodine concentrations (350 mg I/ml or greater) of contrast material for carotid CTA is supported by practical considerations and published data. Higher concentrations enable rapid infusion of the contrast bolus for an early arterial phase acquisition, and the results from multiple studies reveal improved arterial enhancement or visualization using concentrations of 350–400 mg I/ml when compared with both disparate and equal iodine loads using 300 mg I/ml, infused at the same rate.

Other instructions

Breath holding of the patient should be used as the scan typically covers the aortic arch, which moves with respiration. For dyspneic patients, and when imaging of the carotids and/or carotid bifurcation only is required, then shallow breathing may be allowed. The patient is also instructed not to swallow during the acquisition. To avoid the artifacts related to dental amalgam or metal over the carotid bifurcation region, the patients may need to be instructed to lift the chin and to keep the jaw closed. Lead shielding can be used over female breasts outside the scanning area.

Reconstruction width and increment

Smooth or medium smooth reconstruction kernels are recommended for the reconstruction of the axial slices in order to ensure high quality reformatted slices. A reconstructed slice thickness of 1 mm with a 50–80% reconstruction increment is often acceptable for initial assessment of the carotid circulation. Thicker sections may be generated for the purposes of archiving, but in the current environment of cheap archiving options, the axial images themselves may be archived.

Analysis

Interactive analysis in our practice involves the evaluation of raw data (axial images) and multidirectional multi-planar reformations (MPRs) using a workstation. The interpreting physician reconstructs coronal and oblique sagittal thin slab maximum intensity projections (MIPs) of both carotid bifurcations at 1.5 mm thickness, leading to approximately 40–50 images, which may be archived in picture archiving and communication system (PACS) together with axial MPR images, specially reconstructed for archiving purposes at 1.5 mm section width. Volume-rendered (VR) images may be used to provide gross anatomic detail to the referring physician, but are seldom necessary for diagnostic purposes (Figure 6.1). Additional findings such as anatomic variants or concomitant findings in the arch and vertebrobasilar circulation should also be reported.

Evaluation of the intracranial circulation

Dedicated CTA of the intracranial arterial circulation is performed mostly for the evaluation and treatment of intracranial aneurysms. The acquisition in these cases is performed during free breathing from the level of the first cervical vertebra to beyond the roof of the lateral ventricles. Timing for the CTA is usually derived using a test bolus or bolus triggering system. We use a standard dose of 120 ml of the contrast medium (300 mg I/ml) injected into the antecubital vein using an automated injector with an injection speed of 4 ml/s. This protocol has proven to be reliable in providing optimal contrast medium concentration for high quality CTA images of cerebral artery aneurysms. In a small percentage of cases, the delay time may need to be extended (in cases with slow flow into the intracranial vessels after a major intracranial hemorrhage) by 2–4 s, or the CTA may need to be repeated with additional contrast medium

injection (usually 30–60 ml). In the latter case, the residual contrast medium in the circulation from the 120 ml injection in conjunction with the additional 60 ml secondary bolus results in a high quality CTA. With the advent of 64-slice scanners with appropriate improvements in volume coverage, the acquisition time and the amount of contrast used have been dramatically reduced. The adoption of bolus tracking algorithms with these scanners provides optimal visualization of the intracranial circulation. Table 6.3 provides the acquisition parameters for 16, 32×2, and 64 slice detector scanners.

Analysis

As previously described, analysis involves the evaluation of raw data as axial, sagittal, and coronal MPRs using a workstation. The interpreting physician then constructs MIP reconstructions of the entire volume or subvolume along with three-dimensional (3D) volume rendered or surface shaded images using dedicated workstations (Figure 6.2). The anatomic focuses of these reformatted images are the standard locations for cerebral artery aneurysms. These include the origins of the posterior inferior cerebellar artery (PICA), the basilar artery, the posterior cerebral artery, and the internal carotid artery (ICA), emphasizing the origins of the ophthalmic arteries, the posterior communicating

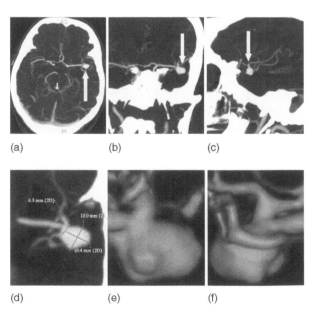

Figure 6.2 Reformatted 22 mm thick slab reformat images in axial (a), coronal (b) and sagittal (c) planes, together with two-dimensional (2D) multi-projection MIP volume reconstruction with measurements for aneurysm length and width, and the width of neck (d). Additional 3D volume rendered surface shaded images demonstrate the aneurysm (e and f).

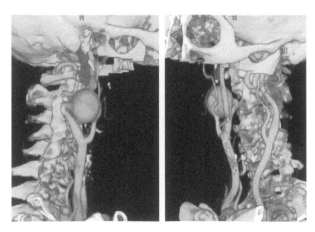

Figure 6.1 CT angiography with volume rendered images illustrates a fusiform aneurysm of the right internal carotid artery in the cervical portion.

Table 6.3 Scanning protocols for intracranial arteries

	Siemens		General Electric		Philips	
Detectors	16	32×2	16	64	16	64
mAs	100		420 mA	335 mA	400	300
kV	120		120	120	120	120
Rotation time (s)	0.5	0.33	0.5	0.4	0.75	0.75
Detector collimation (mm)	0.75	0.6	0.625	0.625	0.75	0.625
Slice thickness (mm)	0.75	0.75	0.625	0.625	1.0	0.625
Translation speed (mm/s)						
Table speed (Philips)	*	*	5.625	26.55	11	49.38
Pitch[a]	*	*	0.5625	0.531	0.688	0.926
Kernel/filter	B60s	B20f	Standard	Standard	Standard/B	Standard/B

[a]Pitch=table feed per rotation/total width of the collimated beam.
Philips parameters provided by Don Boshela BS, RT(R) (CT), Senior CT Product Development Specialist, Philips Medical Systems.
*Manufacturers do not have a recommended value in these cases.

arteries, and the anterior choroidal arteries. Additional locations include the tip of the ICA, the middle cerebral artery (MCA, particularly the first branch of the M1 segment and the MCA bifurcation), the anterior communicating artery, and the origin of the callosomarginal artery from the pericallosal artery. The diagnosis and interpretation of the anatomy, such as the relation of the aneurysm to associated arterial branches, are made from the raw data or from the two-dimensional (2D) reformatted images. Also the measurements (aneurysm length, width, and the width of the aneurysm neck) are always made from the 2D reformatted images. The 3D images are used for appreciating gross anatomic and spatial relationships and only in very rare cases provide additional information that is helpful from a diagnostic standpoint.

CLINICAL APPLICATION AND DIAGNOSTIC PERFORMANCE OF CTA

Extracranial circulation

The most frequent indication for CTA of the extracranial circulation is evaluation of a suspected stenosis caused by carotid artery atherosclerosis, in symptomatic patients with transient ischemic attacks or stroke (Figure 6.3), or in asymptomatic individuals. Nonetheless, in the latter situation duplex ultrasonography should probably represent the first line approach, with CTA or magnetic resonance angiography (MRA) being considered in those individuals where duplex

provides conflicting or inadequate data (high bifurcation lesions, arch disease, vertebral artery disease, or significant intracranial disease, etc.). For the comprehensive evaluation of the patients with acute stroke, CTA with non-enhanced brain CT, CT perfusion imaging, and CTA have proven to be valuable tools (see below). A less common cause for carotid stenosis is fibromuscular dysplasia (Figure 6.4). Another indication for cervico-cranial CTA is the evaluation of aneurysms, pseudoaneurysms, or dissection in the carotid, subclavian, vertebrobasilar system, and aorta (Figures 6.1 and 6.5). Individuals with suspected spontaneous or trauma-related carotid artery dissection might benefit from CTA evaluation

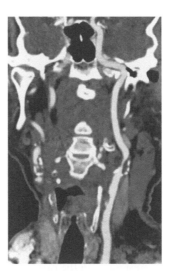

Figure 6.3 Curved planar reformation from the left carotid artery shows significant stenosis and non-calcified plaque with minor calcifications at the bifurcation, and hemodynamically insignificant but ulcerated plaque at the common carotid artery.

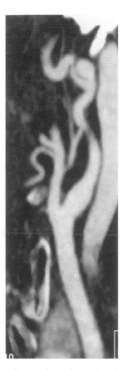

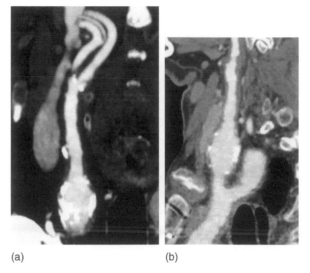

(a)   (b)

Figure 6.5 CT angiography with multiplanar reformat (a) and curved planar reformat (b) of the right carotid artery. The multiplanar reformat shows significant stenosis and mural calcification at the symptomatic bifurcation, while curved planar reformation gives less severe estimation of the stenosis degree. Both images demonstrate a fusiform aneurysm of the common carotid artery.

Figure 6.4 CT angiography with thin slab MIP reconstruction demonstrates a pseudoaneurysm and two stenosed segments in the internal carotid artery distal to the bulb, suggestive of fibromuscular dysplasia.

in view of its superior spatial resolution compared to MRA. MDCT angiography may also be used for the evaluation of cervical tumors, especially carotid body tumors owing to the complex vascular supply of these lesions and involvement of contiguous structures. CTA may also be used for the follow-up after carotid endovascular stenting over MRA, owing to its ability to assess complications such as in-stent restenosis (Figure 6.6).

The diagnostic performance of CTA is discussed as it pertains mainly to extracranial carotid disease.

Single-slice CT angiography

In a meta-analysis by Koelemay et al, the pooled sensitivity and specificity for the detection of severe carotid stenosis (70–99%) of CTA with single-slice CT was 85% and 93%, respectively. For the detection of an occlusion, the accuracy of CTA was even higher, reaching 100% sensitivity and specificity in most studies. Moll and Dinkel have shown that CTA has higher sensitivity than duplex ultrasonography for the detection of severe (70–99%) stenosis in the carotid artery. In this study, the results of the imaging modalities were compared with the findings on operative evaluation. CTA was as sensitive and specific as digital subtraction angiography (DSA) for the detection of severe stenosis.

MDCT angiography

With the advent of MDCT scanners, these have effectively replaced single-slice scanners in light of significant improvements in volume coverage and spatial resolution. Chen et al compared 4-slice CTA with DSA and reported 100% accuracy in diagnosing total versus near occlusions. Further, CTA showed 100% correlation with catheter angiography for the location of tight stenoses. Interobserver agreement (κ value) in evaluating total versus near occlusion, stump length, retrograde ICA flow, and the location of the stenotic site was 1.0, 0.94, 0.86, and 0.89, respectively. In addition, CTA was helpful in distinguishing the underlying pathology such as dissection or thrombosis.

Our group has evaluated the diagnostic performance of CTA using a 4-slice scanner at the Kuopio University Hospital during 2001–2002. The main focus of the study was to evaluate the diagnostic performance of CTA compared with conventional X-ray DSA and rotational DSA as reference standards. A total of 36 consecutive, symptomatic patients with cerebrovascular disorders such as minor stroke, transient ischemic attack, amaurosis fugax, and dizziness underwent CTA. The degree of stenosis was calculated by the North American Symptomatic Carotid Endarterectomy Trial criteria. In this study, the degree of stenosis was slightly underestimated with CTA, with mean differences ($\pm$standard deviation) per observer of 6.9$\pm$17.6% and 10.7$\pm$16.1% for cross-sectional and 2.8$\pm$19.2% and

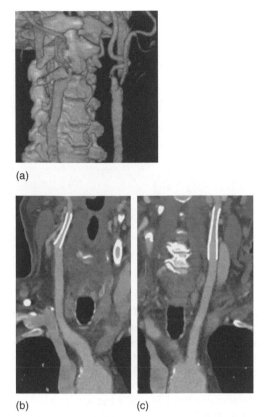

Figure 6.6 CT angiography volume rendered image (a) demonstrates an occlusion of the right internal carotid artery (ICA) and severe stenosis of the left ICA with bilateral stenosis of external carotid arteries. The left ICA and the right external carotid artery giving ophthalmic and leptomeningeal collateral branches (not shown) were treated with stents. Post-procedural control CT angiography with curved planar reformations shows the patent lumen of the stent in the right external carotid artery (b) and in the left internal carotid artery (c).

9.1±16.8% for oblique sagittal MPRs compared with rotational angiography. CTA was somewhat inaccurate for measuring the absolute minimal diameter of high-grade stenoses. For symptomatic lesions, interactive CTA interpretation combined with MPR measurements for lesions with a visual estimate of ≥50% diameter narrowing achieved a sensitivity of 95% and specificity of 93% in the detection of carotid stenosis compared with DSA. Based on these results we concluded that the diagnostic performance of CTA with interactive interpretation is sensitive for detection of significant carotid artery stenosis and underscores the clinical utility of this test for the evaluation of symptomatic and asymptomatic disease.

Zhang et al from our group have shown that the semiautomatic 3D CTA analysis method is highly reproducible for the assessment of degree of carotid stenosis, but it proved to have low sensitivity and therefore may not lend itself for use in routine clinical practice. However, in the future the use of

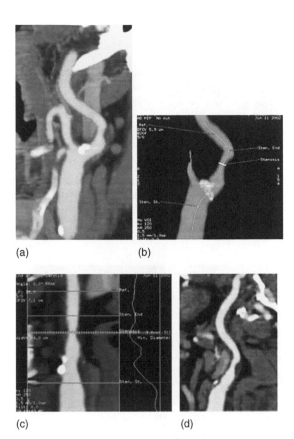

Figure 6.7 CT angiography with thin slab MIP (a) shows moderate stenosis in the left internal carotid artery above the bulb. Assessment of carotid stenosis degree can be made using semiautomated software (b–d), which in this case calculated 41% diameter stenosis and 31% area stenosis.

area stenosis might be an alternative for diameter stenosis in the assessment of stenosis degree in the carotid artery (Figure 6.7).

Intracranial circulation

MDCT angiography has become the primary diagnostic method to detect intracranial aneurysms or arteriovenous malformations (AVMs) in many hospitals (Figure 6.8). MDCT angiography can be performed immediately after subarachnoid or intracerebral hemorrhage is diagnosed on non-contrast CT (Figure 6.9). It may also be used if a non-ruptured cerebral artery aneurysm has been found on MRA, to provide better spatial resolution (submillimeter) images for treatment planning, and to evaluate whether the patient has additional cerebral artery aneurysms that were not detected by MRA. Another application for MDCT angiography is the follow-up of extracranial–intracranial bypasses (Figure 6.10).

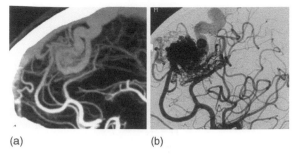

(a)   (b)

Figure 6.8 CT angiography (a) and digital subtraction angiography (b) of arteriovenous malformation, lateral view.

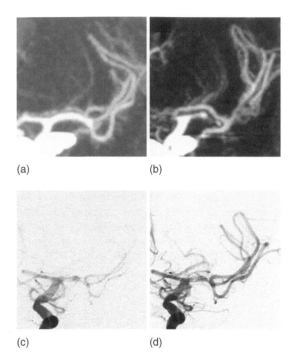

(a)   (b)

(c)   (d)

Figure 6.9 CT angiography from a patient with subarachnoid hemorrhage showing a normal middle cerebral artery (MCA; a) and follow-up CT angiography showing vasospasm on the M1 segment and distal MCA branches (b); digital subtraction angiography of the same patient verifying the vasospasm (c) and showing release of the vasospasm after local injection of papaverin into the M1 segment (d).

MDCT in the evaluation of acute stroke

CTA using MDCT is also useful for the assessment of patients with acute stroke (Figure 6.11). Compared with magnetic resonance imaging, CT is more accessible, fast, and relatively inexpensive. In early trials of thrombolysis, unenhanced CT alone was used to exclude patients with brain hemorrhage or large infarctions. However, it is now apparent that this approach alone is insensitive to early signs of cerebral ischemia or infarction and does not

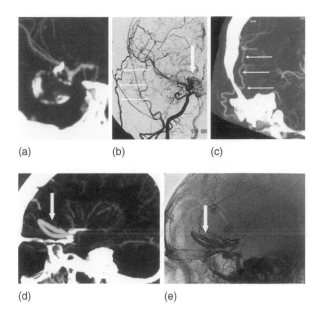

(a)   (b)   (c)

(d)   (e)

Figure 6.10 CT angiography of a large, partially calcified, and totally thrombosed aneurysm of the right middle cerebral artery (MCA) bifurcation (a); digital subtraction angiography of a patient suffering from right internal carotid artery (ICA) moya-moya (large arrow) imaged after superficial temporal artery (STA)–MCA bypass (small arrows; b); CT angiography showing the STA–MCA bypass from the same patient shown on (b); CT angiography (c) and digital subtraction angiography (d) of a patient with ICA–MCA bypass with a venous graft (arrow).

provide any insights into stroke pathophysiology. A contemporary approach utilizing the superior spatial and temporal resolution (rotation times ≤ 500 ms) with current generation MDCT scanners will afford the possibility of incorporating perfusion CT together with non-contrast CT evaluation and CTA for hyperacute stroke imaging. CTA can define the occlusion site, depict arterial dissection, grade collateral blood flow, and characterize atherosclerotic disease, whereas perfusion CT may allow the accurate depiction of infarct core and the ischemic penumbra. Using such an approach, early stroke within the window of thrombolytic therapy may potentially be identified. Parameters derived from perfusion CT maps such as cerebral blood flow, volume, mean transit time, and time-to-peak contrast may be helpful in assessing the infarcted area and the ischemic penumbra.

LIMITATIONS OF CTA

Although the performance and advantages of MDCT angiography provide a powerful argument for its widespread utilization for the evaluation of the cervico-cranial circulation, there are multiple limitations that may on

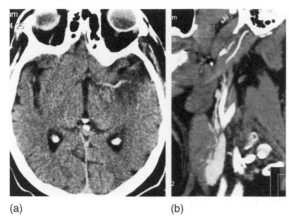

(a) (b)

Figure 6.11 CT of the brain (a) shows a dense cerebri media sign and an infarction in the left middle cerebral artery territory. CT angiography of the patient (b) confirms dissection of the left internal carotid artery as the etiology of the acute brain infarction.

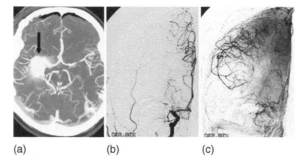

(a) (b) (c)

Figure 6.12 Axial thick slab reformatted CT angiography image after surgical clipping of a right middle cerebral artery (MCA) aneurysm. Large artifacts arise from multiple steel clips (arrow), distal MCA branches appear similarly filled with contrast medium on both the right and left sides (a); the digital subtraction angiography picture shows that clips completely occlude the MCA (b) and the right distal branches of the MCA are filled via collaterals from the interior cerebral artery (c).

occasion limit its usefulness. Calcification in segments can obscure the lumen due to blooming artifact and on occasion can lead to overestimation of stenosis severity. Mural calcification in the ICA, especially the petrous segments, where these calcifications are common, can be problematic. Sometimes a thin web-like stenosis may be difficult to diagnose in axial slices and may be obscured in reconstructed MIP images. In such cases, thin MPR reconstructions may be useful. As always, experience in interpreting these frequently complex lesions is mandatory. In addition, the radiation dosage associated with MDCT protocols is also a consideration, especially in individuals who may require multiple studies on different occasions. The radiation dose with aorto-cervical CTA varies between 1.7 and 3.0 mSv, depending on the imaged volume and the type of scanner.

CTA images are obtained when arteries and/or veins are filled with contrast medium and CTA does not show flow dynamics. Thus, there may be overlapping veins that prevent the detection of small cerebral artery aneurysms by CTA, or after surgical clipping of a cerebral artery aneurysm, arterial branches distal to the clip may be filled retrogradely via collateral arteries but appear normally filled with contrast medium on CTA (Figure 6.12). There are usually large blooming artifacts from steel clips (Figure 6.12), but aneurysm wall calcification can often be well identified (Figure 6.10).

evaluation of the vessels simultaneously with delineation of soft tissues, including atherosclerotic plaque, and associated abnormalities such as aneurysms and AVMs. In conjunction with CT-based perfusion maps with current generation MDCT scanners, CT has the capability of providing detailed evaluation of the stroke patient and clinically valuable information regarding stroke mechanisms and prognosis, including patient selection for thrombolytic therapy.

PRACTICAL PEARLS

- Use thinnest detector collimation to provide high spatial resolution in the z-direction and approach isotropic spatial resolution wherever possible.

- Use automated bolus tracking or test bolus techniques to avoid timing-related issues.

- For the interpretation of CTA always rely on source images (axial and MPRs) and review these in various planes. Use MIP projections in conjunction with source images.

- For the analysis of complex anatomy, and for the demonstration of the findings, 3D reconstructions are useful for demonstrating general anatomic and spatial relationships, as long as these are not often used for diagnostic purposes.

CONCLUSIONS

CTA is a powerful tool for the assessment of the entire cervico-cranial circulation. The advantages include comprehensive

FURTHER READING

Bendzus M, Koltzenburg M, Burger R et al. Silent embolism in diagnostic cerebral angiography and neurointerventional procedures: a prospective study. Lancet 1999; 354(9190): 1594–7.

Berg M, Zhang, Z, Ikonen A et al. Multi-detector row CT angiography in the assessment of carotid artery disease in symptomatic patients: comparison with rotational angiography and digital subtraction angiography. AJNR 2005; 26(5): 1022–34.

Chen CJ, Lee TH, Hsu HL et al. Multi-slice CT angiography in diagnosing total versus near occlusions of the internal carotid artery: comparison with catheter angiography. Stroke 2004; 35(1): 83–5.

Esteban JM, Cervera V. Perfusion CT and angio CT in the assessment of acute stroke. Neuroradiology 2004; 46(9): 705–15.

Flohr TG, Schaller S, Stierstorfer K, Bruder H, Ohnesorge BM, Schoepf UJ. Multi-detector row CT systems and image-reconstruction techniques. Radiology 2005; 235(3): 756–73.

Hoh BL, Cheung AC, Rabinov JD, Pryor JC, Carter BS, Ogilvy CS. Results of a prospective protocol of computed tomographic angiography in place of catheter angiography as the only diagnostic and pretreatment planning study for cerebral aneurysms by a combined neurovascular team. Neurosurgery 2004; 54: 1329–40.

Josephson SA, Bryant SO, Mak HK, Johnston SC, Dillon WP, Smith WS. Evaluation of carotid stenosis using CT angiography in the initial evaluation of stroke and TIA. Neurology 2004; 63(3): 457–60.

Kangasniemi M, Mäkelä T, Koskinen S, Porras M, Poussa K, Hernesniemi J. Detection of intracranial aneurysms with two-dimensional and three-dimensional multislice helical computed tomographic angiography. Neurosurgery 2004; 54(2): 336–41.

Koelemay MJ, Nederkoorn PJ, Reitsma JB, Majoie CB. Systematic review of computed tomographic angiography for assessment of carotid artery disease. Stroke 2004; 35(10): 2306–12.

Matsumoto M, Kodama N, Sakuma J et al. 3D-CT arteriography and 3D-CT venography: the separate demonstration of arterial-phase and venous-phase on 3D-CT angiography in a single procedure. AJNR 2005; 26: 635–41.

Moll R, Dinkel HP. Value of the CT angiography in the diagnosis of common carotid artery bifurcation disease: CT angiography versus digital subtraction angiography and color flow Doppler. Eur J Radiol 2001; 39(3): 155–62.

Prokop M, Galanski M, eds. Spiral and Multislice Computed Tomography of the Body. Stuttgart, New York: Thieme, 2003.

Rubin GD. Techniques for performing multidetector-row computed tomographic angiography. Tech Vasc Interven Radiol 2001; 4(1): 2–14.

Wintermark M, Flanders AE, Velthuis B. Perfusion-CT assessment of infarct core and penumbra. Receiver operating characteristic curve analysis in 130 patients suspected of acute hemispheric stroke. Stroke 2006. 37(4): 979–85.

Zhang Z, Berg M, Ikonen A, Vanninen R, Manninen H. Carotid artery stenosis: reproducibility of automated 3D CT angiography analysis method. Eur Radiol 2003; 14(4): 665–72.

Zhang, Z, Berg M, Ikonen A et al. Carotid stenosis degree in CT angiography: assessment based on luminal area versus luminal diameter measurements. Eur Radiol 2005; 15(11): 2359–65.

7

CT angiography and venography of the pulmonary circulation with imaging protocols

Prachi Agarwal and Ella A Kazerooni

INTRODUCTION

CT vascular imaging techniques are commonly used to evaluate both the pulmonary arterial and venous circulation. CT pulmonary angiography (CTPA) is a well established and often first-line diagnostic test performed in the evaluation of pulmonary vascular disease and may be combined with indirect CT venography (CTV) of the lower extremities as part of comprehensive evaluation for venous thromboembolic disease. Table 7.1 lists the common indications for CTPA and CTV.

ACUTE PULMONARY EMBOLISM

Untreated acute pulmonary embolism (PE) is associated with significant mortality and is the third most common cause of cardiovascular death after myocardial infarction and stroke. This necessitates prompt diagnosis, so that appropriate treatment can be started in a timely fashion. A high specificity of diagnosis is desirable to avoid unnecessary anticoagulation, due to the 7% risk of major hemorrhage with the later. PE most commonly results from thrombi dislodged from veins in the pelvis and lower extremities, with deep venous thrombosis (DVT) and PE representing manifestations of the same disease process (venous thromboembolism).

The clinical manifestations of PE are non-specific, making the diagnosis challenging. Thus there are various diagnostic tests that have been traditionally used in the diagnosis of PE.

d-Dimer: this is a breakdown product of cross-linked fibrin and is an inexpensive, non-invasive test with a high negative predictive value (99%) for PE. A negative d-dimer can play an important role in reducing the need for further tests in patients with a low clinical suspicion of PE. However, when d-dimer is high it is not specific for PE, and may be elevated in conditions such as myocardial infarction, pneumonia, heart failure, cancer, and recent surgery.

Chest radiography: although chest radiographs are often the first imaging test performed, they have a limited role in diagnosing PE. The classic radiographic findings such as the Westermark sign (pulmonary oligemia – distal to obstructing embolus, Fleischner sign – large pulmonary artery due to central thrombus with abrupt tapering, Hampton hump – wedge-shaped pleural-based opacity, often along the diaphragmatic pleura with the apex pointing towards the hilum (Figure 7.1a and b) are rarely seen with PE. More commonly, the radiographic findings are non-specific and include atelectasis and pleural effusion.

Ventilation perfusion (V/Q) scintigraphy: scintigraphy has long been the mainstay in the diagnostic algorithm for suspected PE.

Perfusion scintigraphy is performed after the intravenous injection of Tc-99m-labeled albumin macroaggregates, while the ventilation scintigraphy may be obtained with the inhalation of Xe-133, Tc-99m diethylenetriaminepentaacetic acid or Tc-99m pyrophosphate. The PIOPED (Prospective Investigation of Pulmonary Embolism Diagnosis) study, conducted in 1985–6, evaluated the sensitivity and specificity of V/Q scintigraphy using pulmonary angiography as the reference standard. In PIOPED, 14% of the V/Q scans were normal or near-normal, 34% were low probability for PE, 39% were intermediate probability, and 13% were high probability. Though normal and high probability V/Q scans are quite useful in excluding or confirming pulmonary emboli, a large proportion of the scans were low or intermediate probability, which usually requires additional diagnostic tests to definitively confirm or exclude the diagnosis of PE. Additionally, there is high interobserver variability in the interpretation of V/Q scans, particularly low and intermediate probability scans. V/Q scans are more likely to be diagnostic when the chest radiograph is normal and there is no pre-existing cardiopulmonary disease.

Catheter pulmonary angiography: this has long been considered the reference test for the diagnosis of PE. This invasive technique is underutilized, and associated with a small but definite risk of morbidity and mortality. With the rapid developments in multi-detector CT over the last decade, the imperfect nature of this reference standard test has become more readily apparent, particularly for PE at the subsegmental level. Considerable interobserver variability is also seen in the interpretation of pulmonary angiograms at the subsegmental level.

Duplex studies: since DVT and PE are manifestations of the same disease process and require similar treatment, ultrasound studies of the lower extremity are an important part of the diagnostic algorithm for PE. However, patients with negative leg veins for DVT who are being evaluated for PE require additional tests to diagnose PE, as DVT is found in less than half of patients with angiographically proven PE. Also, Doppler can be technically challenging in obese patients, particularly for evaluating pelvic veins.

CT pulmonary angiography (CTPA)

Recent advancement in CT technology with shorter gantry rotation (0.33–0.4 s) and faster acquisition speeds has resulted in improved visualization of the small pulmonary arteries, particularly the subsegmental pulmonary arteries. PIOPED II, a prospective multi-center study, was designed to determine whether multi-detector CTPA can reliably detect and rule out acute PE and whether the addition of CTV improves this ability. The role of a validated clinical assessment (the Wells score) in improving the ability to rule out PE by CTA or CTA–CTV was also tested. A composite

---

Table 7.1 Indications for CTPA and CTV

- Acute and chronic thromboembolic pulmonary vascular disease
- Pulmonary arteriovenous malformations, pulmonary artery aneurysms, and pseudoaneurysms
- Preprocedure planning and follow-up of patients undergoing atrial fibrillation ablation

---

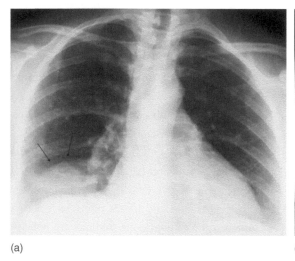

(a)

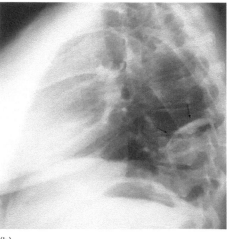

(b)

Figure 7.1 35-year-old woman with acute pulmonary embolism. Chest radiographs in the (a) postero-anterior and (b) lateral projections demonstrate a focal pleural based opacity in the right lower lobe (arrows) representing a Hampton's hump of a pulmonary infarct.

reference standard was used to diagnose or rule out PE and required one of the following conditions: V/Q scan showing high probability in a patient with no history of pulmonary embolism, abnormal pulmonary DSA, new abnormal lower extremity ultrasound studies, and non-diagnostic V/Q. The study was performed with predominantly 4 detector scanners (very few performed with 16-detector scanners). Diagnostic criteria for acute PE by CTPA were similar to those listed in Table 7.4 while the criterion for CTV was a complete or partial central filling defect in a proximal deep vein (IVC, pelvic, or thigh vein). Among 824 patients with a reference diagnosis and a completed study, CTA was inconclusive in 51 because of poor image quality. Excluding such inconclusive studies, the sensitivity of CTA was 83% and the specificity was 96%. Positive predictive values were 96% with a concordantly high or low probability on clinical assessment, and 92% with an intermediate probability on clinical assessment (Table 7.3). The sensitivity of CTA–CTV for PE was 90%, and specificity was 95%. Thus in patients with suspected PE, multidetector CTA–CTV has a higher diagnostic sensitivity than does CTA alone, with similar specificity. Positive results on CTA in combination with a high probability or intermediate probability of PE on the basis of clinical assessment or normal findings on CTA with a low clinical probability had a predictive value (positive or negative) of 92 to 96% in PIOPED II.

CTV only requires a few additional minutes to perform and utilizes the same contrast administered for CTPA. Radiation dose can be reduced by using a sequential technique for CTV as outlined in Table 7.2. An advantage of CTV over compression venous ultrasound is the better visualization of the pelvic veins and inferior vena cava, especially in large individuals.

Table 7.2 Acquisition protocol for CT pulmonary angiography and indirect CT venography

CTPA	16-slice	64-slice
Scan type	Helical	Helical
Rotation time (s)	0.6	0.6
Detector configuration	16×0.625	64×0.625
Beam collimation (mm)	10	40
Slice thickness (mm)	1.25	1.25
Pitch	1.375:1	0.984:1
Table speed (mm/s)	13.75	39.37
Interval (mm)	0.625	0.625
kVp	120	120
mA	400	500
Contrast	125 ml contrast 20 ml saline chaser	125 ml contrast 20 ml saline chaser
Rate	4 ml/s	4 ml/s
Venous scan: iliac crest to tibial plateau		
Scan type	Helical	Helical
Rotation time (s)	1	1
Detector configuration	16×0.625	64×0.625
Beam collimation (mm)	20	40
Slice thickness (mm)	7.5	5
Pitch	1.375:1	1.375:1
Table speed (mm/s)	27.5	55
Interval (mm)	7.5	7.5
kVp	120	120
mA	190	190
Delay (s)	180	180

Technique (CTPA and CTV)

CT acquisition parameters for CTPA are dependent on the type of scanner used. Example scan protocols for CTPA and CT venography (CTV) using 16- and 64-row multidetector CT scanners are described in Table 7.2. Use of multi-detector CT allows for faster scan acquisition, improved z-axis coverage, and less partial volume averaging. Optimal contrast enhancement of the pulmonary arteries is critical for diagnosing emboli because of poor inherent contrast between unopacified blood and intraluminal clot. There are several methods that can be used to optimize peak pulmonary arterial enhancement, with the most commonly used being a fixed scan delay, a timing bolus to determine individual patient peak enhancement, and automatic scan triggering with bolus tracking. Initially, and perhaps most commonly, a fixed preset scan delay time was and is used. Since this was not optimal in a number of patients, this evolved to patient individualized scan delays (time delay between the start of contrast injection and the start of scan acquisition) calculated using a timing bolus of 15–20 ml. A region of interest is placed in the pulmonary trunk and repeated scans are acquired at the same level every 2 to 4 seconds. A time density curve is then obtained, allowing for calculation of the scan delay. Hartmann et al compared the image quality of CTPA obtained using an individualized scan delay versus a fixed scan delay of 20 s and found no significant difference between them. Another approach is to use a bolus tracking method, which automatically initiates the scan once a preset attenuation threshold is achieved in the target vessel, which in this case is the main pulmonary artery.

Table 7.3   PIOPED II results: CTA vs CTPA using additional clinical assessment

Positive and negative predictive values of CTA, as compared with previous clinical assessment[*]

Variable	High clinical probability		Intermediate clinical probability		Low clinical probability	
	No/Total No	Value (95% CI)	No/Total No	Value (95% CI)	No/Total No	Value (95% CI)
Positive predictive value of CTA	22/23	96 (78–99)	93/101	92 (84–96)	22/38	53 (40–73)
Positive predictive value of CTA or CTV	27/28	95 (81–99)	100/111	90 (82–94)	24/42	57 (40–72)
Negative predictive value of CTA	9/15	60 (32–83)	121/136	89 (82–93)	158/164[†]	96 (92–98)
Negative predictive value of both CTA and CTV	9/11	82 (48–97)	114/124	92 (85–96)	146/151[†]	97 (92–98)

[*]The clinical probability of pulmonary embolism was based on the Wells score: less than 2.0, low probability; 2.0 to 6.0, moderate probability; and more than 6.0, high probability, CI denotes confidence interval.
[†]To avoid bias for the calculation of the negative predictive value in patients deemed to have a low probability of pulmonary embolism on previous clinical assessment, only patients with a reference test diagnosis by ventilation–perfusion scanning or conventional pulmonary DSA were included.
From Stein P et al. N Engl J Med 2006; 354: 2317–27, with permission from the New England Journal of Medicine.

Type of contrast medium

The pulmonary arteries are evaluated with the first pass of the intravenously administered contrast agent, while the veins of the pelvis and lower extremities are examined in the equilibrium phase with a scan delay of 2.5–3.5 minutes. Theoretically, use of an iso-osmolar contrast agent should reduce osmotic diuresis and hemodilution, thereby leading to improved retention of contrast beyond the first pass, contributing to better first pass enhancement. However, this has not been substantiated by clinical studies.

CT findings of acute PE

The CTPA findings of acute PE can be divided into arterial findings and ancillary findings, as summarized in Table 7.4 and illustrated in Figures 7.2–7.6. Filling defects in the arteries may partially or completely occlude a pulmonary artery, sometimes enlarging the artery. When an acute embolus is adjacent to an artery wall it forms acute angles with the wall, in contrast to chronic pulmonary emboli which are adherent to the wall, and form obtuse angles. Acute pulmonary emboli frequently straddle the bifurcation of the pulmonary arteries. The larger emboli straddling the bifurcation of the main pulmonary artery are referred to as 'saddle emboli' (Figure 7.5). Lung findings in acute PE include lung infarcts (Figure 7.6b), atelectasis, and oligemia of affected territory. Rarely, PE may be visualized on a non-contrast CT as focal hyper- or hypoattenuation in the pulmonary arteries. CTPA examinations should be interpreted on a workstation using scrolling mode. Optimized window settings, which are wider than conventional mediastinal settings, should be used while scrolling, to ensure that partially occlusive thrombi are not obscured by high attenuation contrast material. Active scrolling in and out each main, lobar, segmental, and subsegmental artery avoids confusion with veins or mucus-filled bronchi. Multi-planar reformats of the pulmonary arteries can be generated, either automatically at the CT scanner itself, or when viewing on a workstation in multiple planes. Use of these images may improve reader confidence for subtle or questionable findings, but added diagnostic accuracy using these techniques has not been validated. An important fact to keep in mind while interpreting a CTPA study is that most pulmonary emboli are larger than 1–2 mm. Therefore, filling defects seen on only one 1.25 mm image are more likely to be artifactual than true emboli. Pulmonary emboli most commonly result from dislodgement of thrombi from their sites of formation in deep veins of the pelvis and lower extremities. Sometimes the source of emboli can be found in the thorax by inspection of the superior vena cava, brachiocephalic and subclavian veins, right atrium (Figure 7.7), and neck veins. This is particularly true for patients with indwelling venous catheters.

CT venography findings of acute deep venous thrombosis

The findings of acute DVT include partial and/or complete filling defects, which often enlarge the occluded vein. There

Table 7.4 CTPA findings of acute pulmonary embolism

Arterial findings	Ancillary findings
• Complete filling defect (Figure 7.2b) • Partial filling defect • Rim sign: in cross-section (Figure 7.3) • Railway track sign: in long axis (Figure 7.4) • Enlargement of the occluded artery	*Lung parenchymal:* • Infarcts (Figures 7.2b, 7.6b) • Pulmonary hemorrhage • Mosaic perfusion (oligemia/hyperemia) • Atelectasis *Other:* • Pleural effusion • Large right ventricle and straightening of the interventricular septum (acute right heart strain)

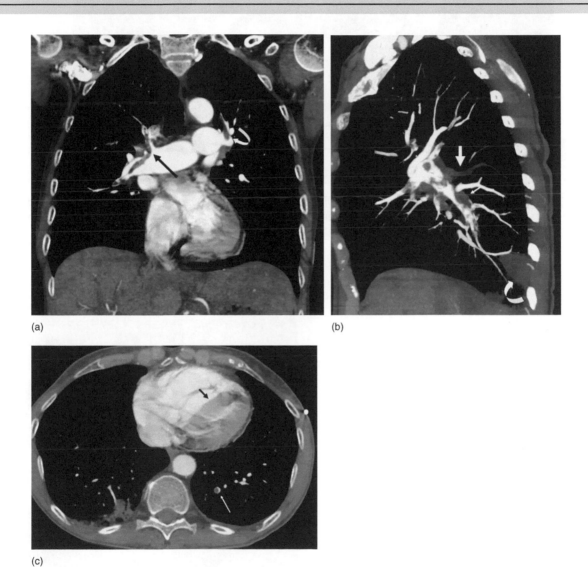

(a)

(b)

(c)

Figure 7.2 50-year-old man with pleuritic chest pain and prolonged immobilization due to recent knee replacement surgery, diagnosed with acute pulmonary embolism. (a) Coronal reformatted CT image demonstrates bilateral central intravascular filling defects consistent with acute pulmonary emboli (arrows). The right-sided embolus straddles the bifurcation of the pulmonary artery (straight arrow). (b) Sagittal reformatted CT image demonstrates right pulmonary emboli with a corresponding wedge-shaped subpleural parenchymal lesion (curved arrow) representing a pulmonary infarct. Some of the pulmonary emboli are partial filling defects (thin arrow), while others cause complete occlusion (thick arrow). (c) Axial CT image demonstrates marked dilatation of the right ventricle (RV) with leftward deviation of the interventricular septum (black arrow) due to elevated RV pressures. A pulmonary embolus is also seen in the left lower lobe (white arrow).

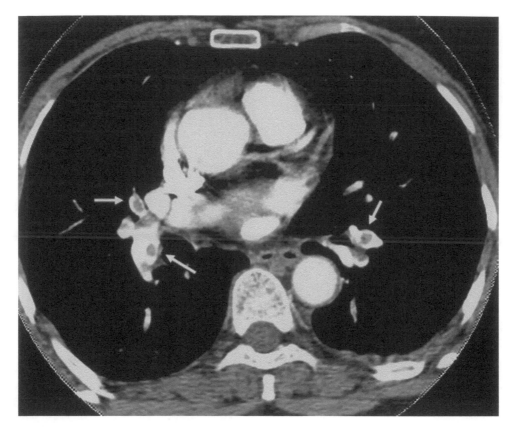

Figure 7.3 35-year-old woman on oral contraceptives with acute onset of shortness of breath. Axial CT image demonstrates multiple bilateral segmental pulmonary emboli demonstrating the 'rim' sign in cross-section through the arteries (arrows).

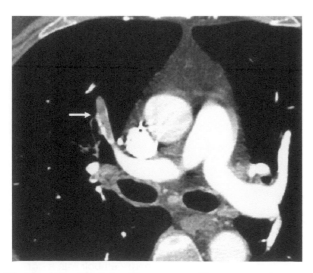

Figure 7.4 45-year-old woman with acute pulmonary embolism in a segmental branch of the right upper lobe pulmonary artery with tram track sign (arrow) in the long axis of the artery.

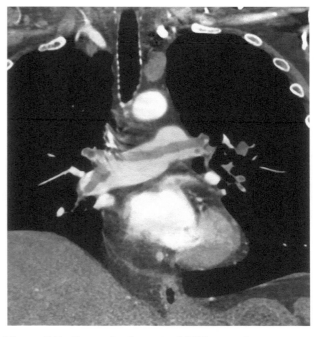

Figure 7.5 Coronal reformatted CT image demonstrates a 'saddle' pulmonary embolus straddling the bifurcation of the main pulmonary artery.

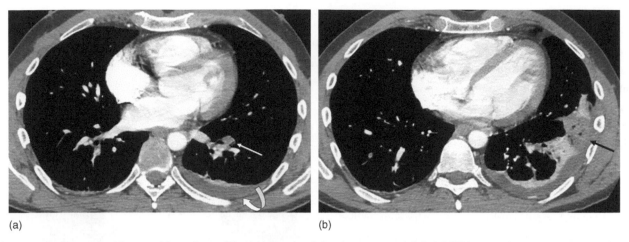

(a)   (b)

Figure 7.6 45-year-old man with prolonged immobilization following trauma. (a) Axial CT image demonstrates segmental left lower lobe pulmonary emboli (straight arrow) and small left pleural effusion (curved arrow). (b) Wedge-shaped subpleural low attenuation abnormality in left lower lobe is a pulmonary infarct, with less enhancement (arrow) than the adjacent atelectatic lung.

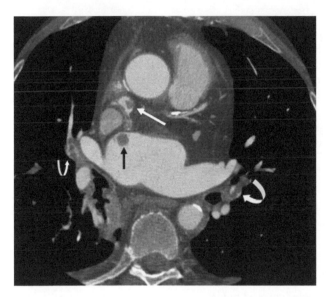

Figure 7.7 Axial CT image demonstrates filling defects within the right atrium consistent with thrombi (straight white arrow) and bilateral pulmonary emboli (curved arrows). An incidental left atrial myxoma is noted (straight black arrow).

may also be perivenous edema and generalized leg edema (Figure 7.8a and b).

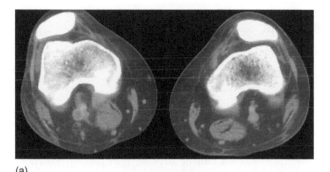

(a)

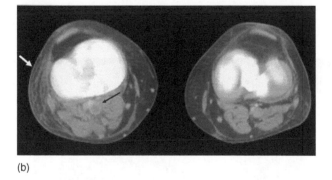

(b)

Figure 7.8 40-year-old woman with acute deep venous thrombosis. There is (a) enlargement of the right popliteal vein that contains a central filling defect, and (b) right popliteal vein thrombus (black arrow) with perivenous stranding and subcutaneous edema (white arrow) in the right leg.

CTPA predictors of patient outcome

Massive acute PE can cause right ventricular strain, which manifests as right ventricular dilatation, deviation of the interventricular septum towards the left ventricle, and reflux of contrast material into the inferior vena cava. A short axis diameter ratio of right ventricle to left ventricle of 1.5 : 1 or greater indicates severe right ventricular strain. Adverse events, such as need for resuscitation, mechanical ventilation, pressors, surgical and percutenous intervention and mortality are more common when the ratio of right ventricle to left ventricle diameter on reconstructed 4-chamber views is 0.9 or greater. Qanadli et al described a CT index that can be used to quantify the severity of obstruction caused by emboli. It is calculated as $\Sigma(n \cdot d)/40 \times 100$, where n is the value of the proximal clot site, equal to the number of segmental branches arising distally, and d is the degree of obstruction (no thrombus=0, partial thrombus=1, complete thrombus=2). 'n' is calculated by assuming that the pulmonary arteries of each lung have 10 segmental arteries (three for the upper lobes, two for the middle lobe and lingula, five for the lower lobes). Embolus in a segmental artery is given 1 point and emboli in the most proximal arterial level are given a value equal to the number of segmental arteries arising distally. The maximum possible value of $\Sigma(n \cdot d)$ is therefore 40. To obtain a percentage, $\Sigma(n \cdot d)$ is divided by 40 and multiplied by 100. In this study, the authors found that a CT index greater than 40% correlated well with echocardiographic findings of right ventricular dilatation. Wu et al showed the CT index to be an important predictor of patient outcome. Using a cut-off of 60%, the index identified 52 of 53 (98%) patients who survived (CT index <50%), and 5 of 6 (83%) patients who died (CT index >60%).

Pitfalls in diagnosing pulmonary emboli on CT

The pitfalls of CTPA can be divided into patient-related factors (Figure 7.9), technical factors (Figure 7.10), and interpretative pitfalls (Table 7.5).

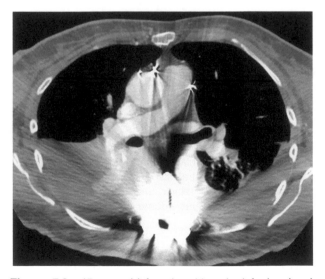

Figure 7.9 45-year-old female with spinal fusion hardware. Significant streak artifacts are noted emanating from the orthopedic spinal hardware and mediastinal surgical clips, making the examination suboptimal for assessment of PE.

Patient-related factors

Pseudo filling defects can arise from motion artifacts due to volume averaging with surrounding lung or bronchus. This can be recognized by observing the chest wall for respiratory

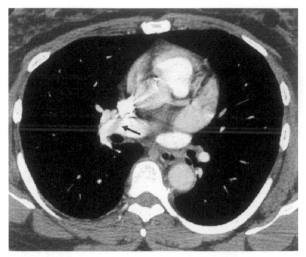

Figure 7.10 Beam hardening artifacts due to the very high attenuation of contrast material in the superior vena cava, creating streak artifacts traversing the right pulmonary artery that could be confused for a pulmonary embolism (arrow).

Table 7.5 Pitfalls in the diagnosis of pulmonary emboli on CTPA

Patient-related factors
1. Respiratory motion artifact
2. Large body habitus with poor signal-to-noise ratio
3. Streak artifact from lines, tubes, or other metallic orthopedic hardware
4. Patent foramen ovale or atrial septal defect

Technical factors
1. Poor contrast bolus
2. Beam hardening artifact from dense contrast in superior vena cava
3. Inappropriate window/level settings
4. High spatial frequency algorithm
5. Stair-step artifact
6. Partial volume averaging

Interpretive pitfalls
1. Perihilar or bronchopulmonary lymph nodes
2. Vascular bifurcation
3. Mistaking pulmonary veins for arteries
4. Mucoid plugging

Pathophysiologic factors
1. Transient interruption of contrast enhancement
2. Unilateral increase in pulmonary vascular resistance

motion. In large patients, images are frequently grainy, which may contribute to a suboptimal study. In such cases, using a thicker slice collimation (2.5 mm rather than 1.25 mm), or reconstructing the 1.25 mm acquired data as 2.5 mm thickness, can improve the visualization of the pulmonary vessels. Streak artifacts from metal in lines, tubes, or other orthopedic hardware can obscure or even mimic pulmonary emboli (Figure 7.9). Whenever possible, withdrawing a catheter or indwelling line prior to the examination is recommended, so that its tip is farther away from the pulmonary artery. This is particularly important for Swan–Ganz catheters.

Additionally, decreased attenuation of pulmonary arteries in combination with early abnormal enhancement of the aorta in CTPA studies performed at deep inspiration may be caused by a patent foramen ovale (PFO). The physiologic basis is the increase in right atrial pressure with deep inspiration. This, coupled with contrast injection using a power injector, causes a sudden rise in right atrial pressure, which exceeds the left atrial pressure and results in a right-to-left shunt. Some contrast material is thus shunted to the left atrium, bypassing the pulmonary artery and leading to decreased attenuation. Henk et al studied 244 CTPA studies done at deep inspiration and found 45 patients with equal or greater enhancement of the aorta than the main pulmonary artery. The mean attenuation in the aorta and pulmonary artery was 248±69 Hounsfield units (HU) and 221±72 HU, respectively, 39 of the 45 patients underwent echocardiography, which confirmed a PFO in 36 patients and an atrial septal defect in 3 patients. In the remaining 199 of 244 patients, attenuation values were higher in the main pulmonary artery (mean 273±66 HU) than in the ascending or descending aorta (mean 206±67 HU).

Technical factors

Suboptimal contrast opacification of the pulmonary arteries limits the evaluation for pulmonary emboli. Hence, good timing of the bolus is of paramount importance. Dense contrast in the superior vena cava may result in a beam hardening artifact (Figure 7.10) that obscures arteries in the adjacent right upper lobe. Using a saline push of 20–25 ml immediately after the contrast injection and scanning in the caudo-cranial direction can reduce this artifact. Appropriate window settings while scrolling are important to avoid missing emboli that may be obscured by contrast. A window width equal to the mean attenuation of the pulmonary artery plus 2 standard deviations, and a window level of half

this value is usually satisfactory. Similarly, a standard algorithm should be used while evaluating emboli rather than a high spatial frequency algorithm, which can create artifacts that masquerade as emboli. Stair-step artifacts manifest as lines traversing a vessel, and are easy to identify. These can be reduced by using overlapping reconstructions. However, this may not help if the artifact is secondary to cardiac or respiratory motion. Partial volume averaging is the result of imaging an axially oriented vessel. However, this is usually not seen on contiguous sections, and has ill-defined margins. Use of a narrow detector width can decrease partial volume averaging.

Interpretative pitfalls

Normal anatomic structures and other disease processes can sometimes be mistaken for pulmonary emboli. These include lymph nodes, pulmonary veins (mistaken for arteries), mucoid impaction in bronchi, and vascular bifurcations. Knowledge of anatomy is essential in the interpretation of CTPA studies. Use of lung windows can help in differentiating pulmonary veins from arteries (which are accompanied by bronchioles) at the segmental and subsegmental level. Remember, the arteries and bronchi run together, and the veins run separately. Also, scrolling can help determine whether the vessel drains into the left atrium (vein) or converges towards the hilum (artery). Transient interruption of contrast ('TIC') in the pulmonary arteries may occur due to an inspiration that occurs immediately prior to imaging, resulting in a mixture of contrast opacified blood from the superior vena cava with a bolus of unopacified blood entering the right atrium from the inferior vena cava. TIC manifests as a short segment loss of pulmonary arterial opacification, usually in the lower lobes, and is also referred to as 'stripe sign'.

Lung consolidation may lead to reactive vasoconstriction and shunting of blood elsewhere in the pulmonary arterial circulation, thereby resulting in *asymmetric vascular resistance*. The poorly enhanced vessels can mimic pulmonary emboli. Recognition of this phenomenon is important and a second acquisition using a longer scan delay can be performed for further assessment.

Indeterminate CTPA examinations

Even though CTPA has a high sensitivity for acute PE, some examinations are 'indeterminate' or non-diagnostic. Motion and poor contrast enhancement are the most important factors. Other factors, such as beam hardening artifact due to body habitus, parenchymal disease such as collapse, consolidation, tumor, and streak artifacts, are somewhat less common. In PIOPED II, of 824 patients with a reference diagnosis and a completed CT study, the quality of the CTA was insufficient for conclusive interpretation in 51 (6% of studies).

Pitfalls in indirect CT venography

Flow artifacts can be seen due to suboptimal timing of contrast. Arterial inflow problems, usually due to peripheral vascular occlusive disease, can also cause poor opacification of deep veins. While CTPA can be tailored to use as little as 70–80 ml for patients with impaired renal function, this low-contrast volume is insufficient for CTV. In addition, streak artifacts from orthopedic hardware, arterial calcification, or dense contrast in the bladder may obscure veins. Interpretive pitfalls include mistaking native arteries, bypass grafts, lymph nodes, tendons, and the sciatic nerves as veins. Such errors can be avoided by a thorough knowledge of the anatomy in this region and active scrolling during interpretation.

Chronic pulmonary embolism

Most acute pulmonary emboli resolve without sequelae. However, less than 5% of patients may develop chronic PE, which can result in pulmonary hypertension and eventually cor pulmonale. The acute emboli undergo recanalization and retraction, contributing to pulmonary vascular stenosis and arterial remodeling seen in chronic PE.

Imaging findings

Chest radiograph. It is an insensitive technique, but can show enlarged central pulmonary arteries with rapid tapering, peripheral oligemia, and right ventricular enlargement.

V/Q scan. Multiple patchy segmental or lobar mismatched defects are seen in chronic thromboembolic pulmonary hypertension (CTEPH). This is in contrast to primary pulmonary hypertension, where the V/Q scan is either normal or shows patchy non-segmental perfusion defects. The V/Q scan may be a sensitive test for CTEPH based on some studies, but provides no indication on hemodynamics.

2D echo. This is extremely useful in the initial assessment of CTEPH and in assessing RV function. Hemodynamic assessment and estimation of peak PA systolic and diastolic

pressures are its strengths. The portability and non-invasiveness also make it ideally suited for follow-up of patients, at least from the hemodynamic perspective.

MRI/MRA. The role of MRI/MRA is discussed in detail in Chapter 16. MRI provides superb detail on RV geometry in chronic pulmonary hypertension and may be helpful in prognostication of these patients. The PA and branches can also be assessed at the same time. Large prospective studies are, however, lacking.

CTPA. CT is the imaging modality of choice in suspected CTEPH. The imaging features on CT parallel those seen on angiography. However, CT has the advantage of depicting peripheral smoothly marginated thrombi, which may not cause significant luminal irregularity and can be difficult to visualize on angiography. The CT findings of CTEPH consist of mural adherent thrombi contiguous with the vessel wall (Figures 7.11 and 7.12). Recanalized thrombi appear as intra-arterial webs (Figure 7.13), or become retracted, manifesting as narrowing and irregularity. Parenchymal signs include mosaic perfusion (Figure 7.14) and non-specific scars, likely from previous pulmonary infarction. Mosaic perfusion refers to geographic areas of low and high attenuation, with the low attenuation areas representing hypoperfusion, and high attenuation areas representing redistributed blood flow. Bronchiectasis has also been reported with chronic PE, often associated with pulmonary arterial stenosis. Another feature of CTEPH is bronchial hypervascularity, which consists of increased proximal bronchial artery diameter to greater than 1.5 mm and arterial tortuosity. The CT features of chronic PE are summarized in Table 7.6.

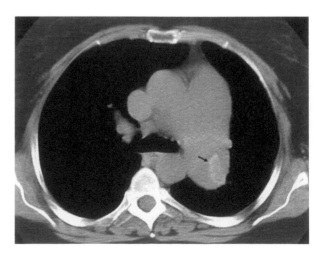

Figure 7.11 Non-contrast CT image demonstrates dilated central pulmonary arteries with a rim of calcification within chronic mural thrombi.

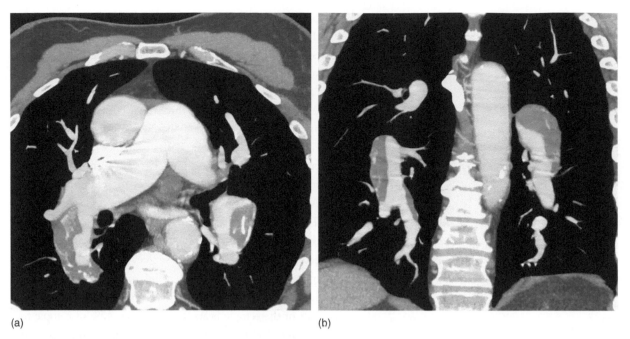

(a)   (b)

Figure 7.12 55-year-old woman with chronic pulmonary embolism and dilated pulmonary arteries due to secondary pulmonary hypertension. (a) Oblique axial CT image demonstrates partially calcified mural filling defects. (b) Coronal reformatted image demonstrates peripheral partially calcified filling defects adherent to the arterial walls that form obtuse angles with the arterial wall, in contrast to the central filling defects and peripheral defects with acute angles found with acute emboli.

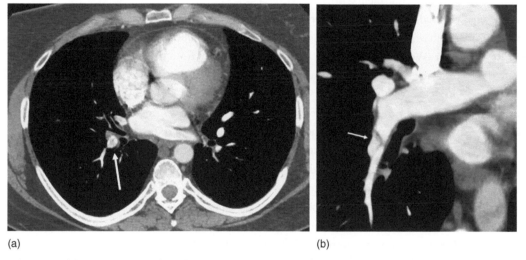

(a)   (b)

Figure 7.13 45-year-old man with chronic pulmonary embolism manifesting as intra-arterial webs. (a) Axial CT image and (b) oblique reformatted image show intra-arterial webs (arrows) in the right lower lobe artery.

Presurgical assessment

Currently, chronic thrombi which extend proximally into the main, lobar, and segmental pulmonary arteries are amenable to surgical thromboendarterectomy, while those that begin more distally are not. Extensive central disease and limited small vessel involvement have been postulated to be predictors for good response to pulmonary thromboendarterectomy. Schwickert et al reported a CT sensitivity of 77% and accuracy of 80% in depicting central thromboembolism and concluded that pre-operative conventional angiography may not be needed in all patients.

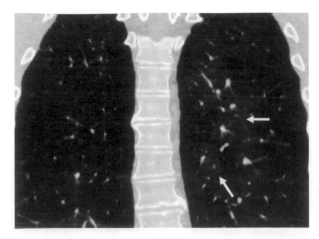

Figure 7.14 50-year-old man with chronic PE. Coronal images of the lungs show mosaic attenuation. The hyperattenuating areas with dilated pulmonary arteries are due to redistributed blood flow (arrows) from the lower attenuation areas with small arteries where there is chronic pulmonary embolism.

Other indications

CTPA provides an excellent demonstration of the pulmonary circulation and can be used to non-invasively diagnose pulmonary arteriovenous malformations (AVMs), pulmonary artery aneurysms, and pseudoaneurysms.

Pulmonary AVMs can be single, multiple, or can occur as part of systemic disorders such as hereditary hemorrhagic telangiectasia and Rendu–Osler–Weber disease. CTPA can clearly demonstrate the feeding artery and draining vein in pulmonary AVM (Figure 7.15).

Pulmonary artery aneurysms are rare and can be congenital (post-valvular or arterial stenosis with post-stenotic dilatation); degenerative (Marfan's syndrome, hereditary hemorrhagic telangiectasia); infectious (mycotic) secondary to syphilis, tuberculosis (Rasmussen aneurysm), pyogenic organisms, and rarely fungi; vasculitic (Behçet's disease); pulmonary hypertension (left-to-right shunt); and idiopathic (Hughes–Stovin syndrome). Aneurysms secondary to trauma are better described as pseudoaneurysms as the wall of these lesions is composed of blood clot. Pseudoaneurysms develop as a result of trauma to the chest or directly to the vessel (e.g. iatrogenic – from a pulmonary artery catheter).

CT imaging of the pulmonary veins and left atrium

CT imaging of the pulmonary veins and left atrium is commonly performed in patients before and/or after ablation procedures performed for atrial arrhythmias, to both map the venous anatomy as well as to look for post-procedure complications. Atrial fibrillation (AF) is the most common sustained cardiac arrhythmia and is associated with significant morbidity, and mortality. The major complication of AF is the formation of thrombi in the atrium or atrial appendage, which can embolize systemically, increasing the risk for embolic stroke. Radiofrequency ablation (RFA), cryoablation, and surgical ablation are techniques used to manage AF, especially in recurrent or refractory AF, and AF resistant to pharmacologic therapy or cardioversion. The left atrial myocardium extends a variable distance into the distal pulmonary veins, and is a frequent source of ectopic foci causing AF. These sleeves are generally longer in the superior pulmonary veins, and longest in the left superior pulmonary vein, which alone accounts for almost half of the ectopic beats. In one series, 47% of ectopic foci originated in the left superior pulmonary vein, 37% in the right superior pulmonary vein, 8% in the right inferior pulmonary vein, and 5% in the left inferior pulmonary vein. In addition, ectopic foci can originate in the right atrium, around the crista terminalis and the orifice of the coronary sinus.

CT in pre-RFA planning

RFA of the pulmonary veins is performed to electrically disconnect them from the left atrium, thereby interrupting the source of ectopic foci. A percutaneous femoral venous approach is used and a catheter is advanced under fluoroscopic guidance through the inferior vena cava, right atrium, and then into the left atrium, either through a transseptal puncture or a patent foramen ovale, if present. Pulmonary veins are selectively cannulated, electrically mapped, and selected for ablation based on clinical and electrophysiologic assessment. Generally, all of the pulmonary veins are empirically ablated, to reduce the need for a repeat procedure. Ablation is targeted at approximately 5 mm outside the ostium of the pulmonary veins to reduce the incidence of pulmonary vein stenosis. Successful RFA necessitates preprocedural knowledge of the number of pulmonary veins, their ostial orientation, and the distance from the veno-atrial junction to the first bifurcation of the vein, to minimize complications. The exact prevalence of pulmonary vein variations is not well known. However, based on observations of the human heart at autopsy, common ostia were identified in 25% of hearts, and the veins were separated by muscle tissue less than 3 mm wide in an additional 40%.

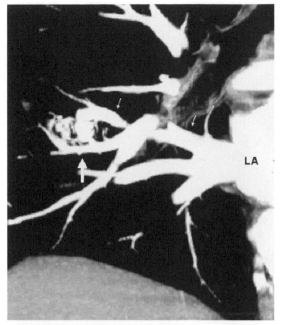

(a)

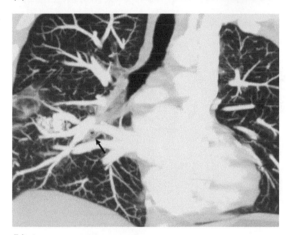

(b)

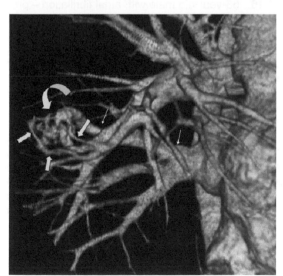

(c)

Table 7.6 CT findings of chronic pulmonary embolism and chronic thromboembolic pulmonary hypertension

Arterial

Eccentric filling defect forming obtuse angles with the vessel wall

Irregular contour of the intimal surface

Abrupt cut-off and narrowing of vessel diameter

Marked variation in size of segmental vessels

Webs, bands, and stenosis with post-stenotic dilatation

Calcification in chronic thrombi

Lung parenchymal

Mosaic perfusion

Parenchymal scarring

Bronchiectasis

Systemic collateral supply

Abnormal dilatation of bronchial arteries

Cardiac abnormalities

Pulmonary hypertension and right ventricular hypertrophy

Thrombi (occasionally calcified) in right heart cavities

Information provided on CT

CT is used to delineate the pulmonary vein anatomy, demonstrating the number of pulmonary veins and the distance from the veno-atrial junction to the first bifurcation for each vein (V1, distance from the veno-atrial junction to the first bifurcation). Shaded surface displays from the posterior projection together with endoscopic images of the posterior wall of the left atrium demonstrate the course of each pulmonary vein. Measurement of the venous ostial diameter is useful to establish a baseline for early recognition of venous stenosis

Figure 7.15 40-year-old female with dyspnea and a pulmonary arteriovenous malformation. (a) Coronal maximum intensity projection (MIP) image demonstrates the right lower lobe pulmonary arteriovenous malformation with the feeding pulmonary artery (thick arrow) and draining pulmonary vein (thin arrows) emptying into the left atrium (LA). (b) Coronal reformat with lung windows shows the arteriovenous malformation. Note the bronchus (arrow) accompanying the pulmonary artery. Recognition of an accompanying bronchus allows for easy differentiation between pulmonary veins and arteries. (c) Three-dimensional volume-rendered CT image clearly depicts the arteriovenous malformation with a nidus (curved arrow), feeding artery (thick arrows), and draining vein (thin arrows).

post-procedure. The left atrial appendage should be scrutinized for the presence of thrombus, which is an absolute contraindication to RF ablation. Lastly, left atrial volume and contractility can be calculated using EKG-gated techniques.

Pulmonary vein anatomy

CT provides an excellent assessment of the pulmonary venous anatomy. Conventionally, there are four pulmonary veins, two on each side, which drain through four separate ostia into the left atrium. The right superior pulmonary vein drains the right upper and middle lobe, the left superior pulmonary vein drains the left upper lobe (including the lingula) and the inferior pulmonary veins drain their respective lower lobes. Accessory pulmonary veins are more common on the right, the commonest being a separate drainage of the right middle lobe vein (Figure 7.16). Accessory veins are usually smaller than the remaining veins and may be difficult to identify on angiography. Conjoined veins (with a single trunk draining into the left atrium) are more common on the left side (Figure 7.17). Pulmonary veins draining into the right side of the heart constitute an anomalous pulmonary venous return and can be partial or total. The commonest partial anomalous pulmonary venous return (PAPVR) is the right superior pulmonary vein draining into the superior vena cava (Figure 7.18).

Some of the commonly used terms and their definitions are as follows:

1. *V1 segment*: pulmonary vein segment from the ostium to the first branch point.

2. *Ostial branch*: venous branch within 5 mm of the atrio-pulmonary venous junction or, in other words, V1<5 mm.

3. *Intervenous saddle*: portion of left atrial wall between ipsilateral pulmonary veins (Figure 7.17b).

4. *Intravenous saddle*: portion of vein wall interposed between branches of a single pulmonary vein.

5. *Pulmonary vein inflow vestibule*: includes the intervenous saddle and the ipsilateral pulmonary vein ostia.

CT technique

CT pulmonary venous mapping is performed on multi-detector helical CT scanners. The acquisition covers the entire thorax, to ensure coverage and recognition of anomalous pulmonary venous return. EKG gating is recommended as it

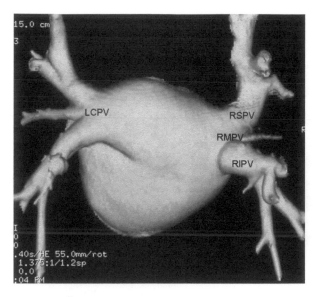

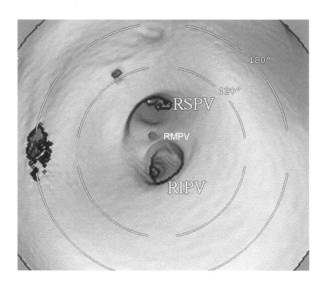

Figure 7.16 53-year-old male with atrial fibrillation – pre-ablation procedure. (a) Three-dimensional shaded surface display model of the left atrium from a posterior view of the heart demonstrates three right pulmonary veins: a right superior pulmonary vein (RSPV), a separate drainage of the right middle pulmonary vein (RMPV), and a right inferior pulmonary vein (RIPV). On the left, the left superior and inferior pulmonary veins form a common trunk (LCPV, left common pulmonary vein) before draining into the left atrium. Conjoined veins are much more common on the left side, while accessory veins are more common on the right. (b) Endocardial navigator view from within the left atrium directed at the right pulmonary veins shows the three pulmonary vein ostia. Note that the opening of the RMPV is much smaller than the RSPV or RIPV, which makes the detection of accessory veins difficult on fluoroscopy.

provides better quality 3D reformations and at the same time also allows for calculation of left atrial function. Scanning in the cranio-caudal direction minimizes respiratory motion artifacts, especially for patients unable to hold their breath for

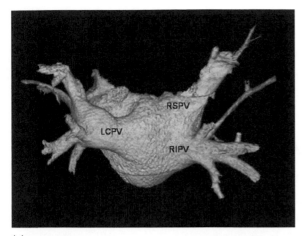

(a)

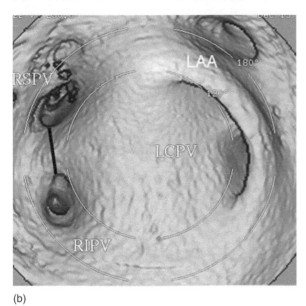

(b)

Figure 7.17 45-year-old male with atrial fibrillation – pre-ablation procedure. (a) Three-dimensional volume-rendered model of the left atrium from a posterior view demonstrates common ostia of the left pulmonary veins. The right superior (RSPV) and inferior pulmonary (RIPV) veins drain normally. (b) Endocardial navigator view from within the left atrium directed at the posterior wall of the left atrium shows a common opening of the left pulmonary veins (LCPV) and normal separate openings of the right superior (RSPV) and right inferior pulmonary (RIPV) veins. The solid black line between the RSPV and RIPV represents the intervenous saddle.

prolonged periods, and reduces streak artifacts from contrast in SVC. A fixed time interval or a test bolus can be used to calculate the appropriate scan delay prior to administration of non-ionic intravenous contrast using a power injector and a rate of 4 ml/s. Bolus tracking for optimal timing is preferable in situations where there is significant variation in the heart rate and cardiac output. Examples of scan parameters used are depicted in Table 7.7.

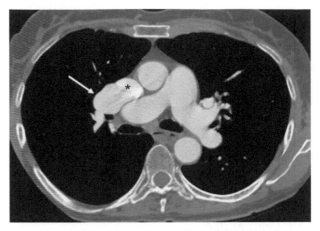

Figure 7.18 40-year-old male with atrial fibrillation and anomalous drainage of the right superior pulmonary vein (arrow) into the superior vena cava (asterisk), as demonstrated on an axial CT image.

Table 7.7 CT scan protocol for pulmonary vein mapping

	16-Slice scanner	64-Slice scanner
Rotation time (s)	0.5	0.35
Detector configuration	16×0.625	64×0.625
Beam collimation (mm)	10	40
Slice thickness (mm)	1.25	1.25
Interval (mm)	1.25	1.25
kVp/Ma	120/440	120/800
Contrast	100 ml	100 ml
	50 ml saline chase	50 ml saline chase
Rate of injection (ml/s)	4	4
Scan delay	Peak+3 s	Peak+6 s

Post-processing

Post-processing is done to obtain volume-rendered (VR) epicardial and endocardial views of the left atrium and pulmonary veins and surface-rendered views of the left atrium. In addition, multi-planar reformations (oriented perpendicular to the pulmonary veins) are done for accurate measurement of the ostial diameters.

Epicardial volume-rendered views. These provide an excellent depiction of the left atrium and pulmonary veins and provide 'angiographic images' (Figures 7.16a and 7.17a). Sufficient views are obtained to clearly demonstrate the number of pulmonary veins, their angulation, and any ostial branches.

Endocardial volume-rendered views. A 'navigator tool' is used to generate the endocardial view of the left atrium. These views (Figures 7.16b and 7.17b) show the anatomy from an intra-atrial perspective with depiction of the pulmonary vein ostia, intervenous saddle, and any prominent endocardial ridges. Two standard views are obtained for the right and left pulmonary vein inflow vestibules.

Complications of RFA

Complications can occur during or after RFA and these include pulmonary vein stenosis, pulmonary vein thrombosis, hemothorax/hemopericardium and stroke are some of the known serious complications post RFA necessitating follow-up imaging with multi-detector CT for early detection (Table 7.8).

CONCLUSIONS

RFA is a commonly used procedure for the treatment of refractory AF. Multi-detector CT is an excellent tool for pre-RFA planning, and provides a road map for successful ablation, thereby reducing the fluoroscopy time and minimizing the risk of complications. Additionally, it provides a baseline for early detection of pulmonary vein stenosis, a known complication of the procedure.

PRACTICAL PEARLS

- CT vascular imaging techniques is commonly used to evaluate both the pulmonary arterial and venous circulations.

- CT pulmonary angiography in conjunction with indirect CT venography (CTV) provides a comprehensive test for evaluation of suspected venous thromboembolic disease based on PIOPED II results.

- Most pulmonary emboli are >1–2 mm. Therefore, filling defects seen on only one 1.25 mm image are more likely to be artifactual.

- Normal anatomic structures, such as viens, and other disease processes may sometimes be mistaken for pulmonary emboli. An easy way to distinguish veins is that arteries and bronchi run together while the veins run separately.

- Early enhancement of the aorta in CTPA studies with deep inspiration may be caused by a PFO.

- Transient interruption of contrast with CTPA may occur due to inspiration that results in a mixture of contrast from SVC with a bolus of unopacified blood from the IVC. This manifests as a loss of pulmonary arterial opacification in the lower lobes ('stripe sign').

- Accessory pulmonary veins are more common on the right, the commonest being a separate drainage of the middle lobe vein while conjoined veins are more common on the left side.

Table 7.8 Complications of radiofrequency ablation (RFA)

During RFA
1. Endocardial charring
2. Pulmonary vein dissection
3. Atrial/pulmonary vein perforation
4. Bradyarrhythmias due to stimulation of vagal fibers in walls of pulmonary veins
5. Other complications associated with cardiac catheterization

Post RFA:

(a) Mild
1. Hemodynamically insignificant pulmonary vein stenosis
2. Pleural or pericardial effusions
3. Transient small atrial septal defects

(b) Severe
1. Hemodynamically significant pulmonary vein stenosis, leading to venous infarction and development of pulmonary hypertension over a period of time
2. Pulmonary vein thrombosis
3. Hemothorax/hemopericardium
4. Stroke
5. Esophageal perforation

FURTHER READING

Bedard JP, Blais C, Patenaude YG, Monga E. Pulmonary embolism: prospective comparison of iso-osmolar and low-osmolarity nonionic contrast agents for contrast enhancement at CT angiography. Radiology 2005 Mar; 234(3): 929–33.

Brink JA, Woodard PK, Horesh L et al. Depiction of pulmonary emboli with spiral CT: optimization of display window settings in a porcine model. Radiology 1997; 204: 703–8.

Chiles C, Carr J. Vascular disease of the thorax: Evaluation with multidetector CT. RCNA 2005; 43: 543–69.

Cobelli R, Zompatori M. Visualization of hypoattenuation clots on unenhanced CT of the thorax [letter]. AJR 2004; 182: 530–1.

Cronin P, Sneider MB, Kazerooni EA. MDCT of the left atrium and pulmonary veins in planning radiofrequency ablation for atrial fibrillation. AJR 2004; 183: 767–78.

Ghaye B, Szapiro D, Dacher et al. Percutaneous ablation for atrial fibrillation: the role of cross-sectional imaging. Radiographics 2003; 23 Spec No: S19–33.

Gosselin MV, Rassner UA, Thieszen SL, Phillips J, Oki A. Contrast dynamics during CT pulmonary angiogram: analysis of an inspiration associated artifact. J Thorac Imaging 2004; 19(1): 1–7.

Hartmann IJ, Lo RT, Bakker J, de Monye W, van Waes PF, Pattynama PM. Optimal scan delay in spiral CT for the diagnosis of acute pulmonary embolism. J Comput Assist Tomogr 2002; 26(1): 21–5.

Henk CB, Grampp S, Linnau KF et al. Suspected pulmonary embolism: enhancement of pulmonary arteries at deep-inspiration CT angiography-influence of patent foramen ovale and atrial-septal defect. Radiology 2003; 226(3): 749–55.

Ho SY, Cabrera JA, Tran VH, Farre J, Anderson RH, Sanchez-Quintana D. Architecture of the pulmonary veins: relevance to radiofrequency ablation. Heart 2001; 86(3): 265–70.

Jones SE, Wittram C. The indeterminate CT pulmonary angiogram: imaging characteristics and patient clinical outcome. Radiology 2005; 237(1): 329–37.

Kazerooni EA, Gross BH. Pulmonary vascular disease. In: Cardiopulmonary Imaging. Philadelphia, PA: Lippincott Williams and Wilkins, 2004; 583.

Kim KI, Muller NL, Mayo JR. Clinically suspected pulmonary embolism: utility of spiral CT. Radiology 1999; 210: 693–7.

Lacomis JM, Wigginton W, Fuhrman C et al. Multi-detector row CT of the left atrium and pulmonary veins before radiofrequency catheter ablation for atrial fibrillation. Radiographics 2003; 23: S35–S50.

Patel S, Kazerooni EA. Helical CT for the evaluation of acute pulmonary embolism. AJR 2005; 185: 135–49.

Qanadli SD, El Hajjam ME, Vieillard-Baron A et al. New CT index to quantify arterial obstruction in pulmonary embolism: comparison with angiographic index and echocardiography. AJR 2001; 176: 1415–20.

Remy-Jardin M, Remy J, Mayo JR, Muller NL. Pulmonary hypertension. In: Remy-Jardin M, Remy J, Mayo JR, Muller NL, eds. CT Angiography of the Chest. Philadelphia, PA: Lippincott Williams and Wilkins, 2001; 67–81.

Stein PD, Fowler SE, Goodman LR et al. PIOPED II Investigators. Multidetector computed tomography for acute pulmonary embolism. N Engl J Med 2006; 354: 2317–27.

The PIOPED Investigators. Value of the ventilation/perfusion scan in acute pulmonary embolism. Results of the prospective investigation of pulmonary embolism diagnosis (PIOPED). JAMA 1990; 263(20): 2753–9.

Wittram C, Maher M, Yoo A et al. CT Angiography of pulmonary embolism: Diagnostic criteria and causes of misdiagnosis. Radiographics 2004; 24: 1219–38.

8

CT angiography of the thoracic aorta with protocols

Sanjay Rajagopalan, Javier Sanz, Vasco Gama Ribeiro, and Santo Dellegrottaglie

INTRODUCTION

Multi-slice CT angiography (CTA) with current generation scanners allows large volume coverage in single breath holds at isotropic voxel resolution (Chapter 1). In this chapter, CTA of the thoracic aorta refers to performance of this procedure using multi-slice systems (16-detector scanners and beyond).

The speed, ready availability, and superb spatial resolution ($\approx 0.6 \times 0.6 \times 0.6$ mm) of CTA makes it the examination of choice for evaluation of the thoracic aorta in the acute setting (dissection, rupture, and intramural hematoma) and in the evaluation of chronic aortic disease, both pre- and post-intervention (surgical and percutaneous). The other advantages of CTA are those inherent to the technique as discussed in Chapter 1, such as acquisition of volumetric data that can be manipulated in infinite planes, allowing a comprehensive evaluation of thoracic structures (vascular and non-vascular). A particular advantage of CTA over MR angiography is that it allows simultaneous evaluation of the lung parenchyma, and, if indicated, an evaluation of the coronary arteries. Coronary MR angiography, although feasible, is time consuming and does not lend itself to a comprehensive evaluation of the circulation (proximal and distal coronaries including grafts). These considerations are important in a patient presenting with chest pain syndrome, where comprehensive evaluation of the coronaries, the aorta, and pulmonary arteries can be performed in one session. Table 8.1 outlines the current indications of CTA when evaluating the thoracic aorta. This chapter will not

include coronary artery or graft imaging and the reader is referred to other texts.

ANATOMIC CONSIDERATIONS

Normal anatomy

Thoracic aorta

The size and shape of the aorta differ significantly among individuals and even within the same individual at different ages. The thoracic aorta may be divided into different segments (Figure 8.1): (1) ascending aorta including the root, (2) proximal and distal aortic arch, and (3) descending thoracic aorta. The ascending aorta extends from the root to the origin of the right brachiocephalic artery. The aortic root is a portion of the ascending aorta containing the valve, the annulus, and the sinuses. The aortic arch begins at the origin of the right brachiocephalic artery and ends at the attachment of the ligamentum arteriosum and may be divided into a proximal and a distal segment (extending from the origin of the left subclavian artery to the attachment of the ligamentum arteriosum). The distal arch is occasionally narrower than the proximal descending thoracic aorta, and is referred to as the 'isthmus'. The descending thoracic aorta begins after the ligamentum arteriosum and extends to the aortic hiatus in the diaphragm. The portion of the descending thoracic aorta immediately after the

Table 8.1 Indications for CT angiography for thoracic aortic diseases

Aortic dissection
- Acute
- Chronic
- Pre- and post-surgical
- Pre- and post-percutaneous stenting (endoleak assessment)

Evaluation of thoracic aortic aneurysm
- Follow-up
- Pre- and post-surgical
- Pre- and post-percutaneous stenting (endoleak assessment)
- Assessment of inflammatory aortic disease (immune, infectious)
- Evaluation of congenital anomalies of the thoracic aorta
- Evaluation of thoracic atherosclerosis
- Assessment of complications (embolization)
- Penetrating aortic ulceration

Connective tissue diseases
- Marfan's syndrome, Ehlers–Danlos syndrome, annulo-aortic ectasia, etc.

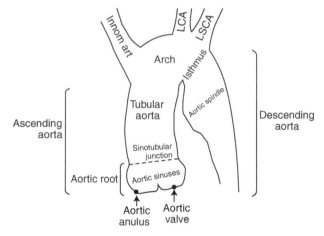

Figure 8.1 Anatomic segments of the thoracic aorta and relationships.

Table 8.2 Aortic diameters (cm) at various thoracic levels as measured by CT angiography

Location	Female (cm)	Male (cm)	Average (cm)
Aortic sinuses	2.9±0.4	3.0±0.5	3.0±0.5
Ascending aorta (max)	2.9±0.3	3.2±0.4	3.1±0.4
Proximal to innominate	2.8±0.4	3.0±0.4	2.9±0.4
Proximal transverse arch	2.7±0.3	2.8±0.4	2.8±0.4
Distal transverse arch	2.4±0.3	2.7±0.4	2.6±0.4
Aortic isthmus	2.3±0.4	2.6±0.4	2.5±0.4
Diaphragm	2.8±0.3	2.4±0.3	2.4±0.4

Adapted with permission from Hager et al. J Thorac Cardiovasc Surg 2002; 123: 1060–6.

insertion of the ligamentum arteriosum may appear slightly dilated and is referred to as the 'aortic spindle'. The aortic wall is normally 1–2 mm in thickness on CT and is usually smooth in appearance. Table 8.2 lists normal reference diameters (wall-to-wall) for the various segments of the thoracic aorta by CTA.

Superior vena cava (SVC) and inferior vena cava (IVC)

The SVC is an important structure to recognize. It is formed at the confluence of the brachiocephalic (innominate) veins and travels posterior to the right lateral margin of the sternum. A persistent left SVC arises due to incomplete resorption of embryonic vasculature and occurs as an inci-

dental abnormality in 2–5% of individuals, and sometimes with congenital heart disease. It arises from the left subclavian vein and travels inferiorly to enter the left atrium through the oblique vein of Marshall. The IVC begins at the confluence of the iliac veins. After receiving the hepatic veins it traverses the diaphragm through a foramen in the central tendon at the level of T8. Vena caval interruption can sometimes occur.

Azygos, hemiazygos, and accessory hemiazygos veins

These vessels are opacified in routine imaging and it is important to recognize them. The azygos, hemiazygos, and accessory hemiazygos systems together provide a large-caliber pathway for venous drainage to the right heart. The azygos forms after the right subcostal vein joins the ascending lumbar vein and enters the thoracic cavity through the aortic hiatus and finally ends at the SVC after crossing the right mainstem bronchus. The hemiazygos vein ascends on the spine, crossing from the left side to join the azygos. The accessory hemiazygos vein is confined to the thorax and receives many intercostal veins, and communicates with both the azygos and hemiazygos systems. These vessels usually become conspicuous in the setting of high-grade SVC obstruction but the azygos vein may also enlarge with congenital vena cava interruption.

Variant (normal) anatomy

Aortic spindle. The aortic spindle appears as a smooth, circumferential bulge below the region of the isthmus (Figure 8.2). This should not be mistaken for an aortic aneurysm at this level.

Ductus diverticulum. The ductus diverticulum is the term applied to a focal convex bulge along the anterior aspect of the isthmus. This needs to be distinguished from a pseudo-aneurysm (post-traumatic). The two differentiating aspects include the fact that the ductus diverticulum usually creates an obtuse angle with the aortic wall, while a pseudo-aneurysm has acute angles. Contrast may further 'hang' in a pseudoaneurysm.

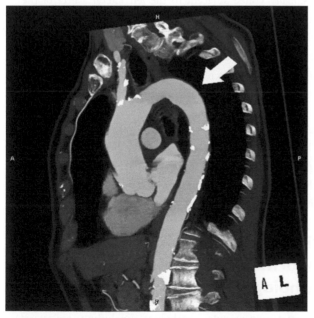

Figure 8.2 CTA of the thoracic aorta. The aortic spindle is visible as a circumferential bulge of the first portion of the descending aorta (arrow).

Variant anatomy of the aortic arch

The typical order of vessels shown in Figure 8.1 is seen in two-thirds of individuals. In the remaining, the arch vessels may show a great deal of variation, as illustrated in Figure 8.3. A bovine configuration and origin of the left common carotid artery (CCA) from the distal brachiocephalic trunk consti-tutes a common anomaly. The left vertebral artery may origi-nate directly from the arch in 0.5% of individuals, usually between the left common carotid and the left subclavian, and is often hypoplastic. Another not uncommon (0.5%) anomaly is a left-sided arch with an aberrantly originating right subcla-vian artery. In this anomaly, the first branch is the right CCA, followed by the left CCA and the left subclavian artery. The right subclavian is the last vessel and crosses from left to right behind the esophagus, and may sometimes be associated with an aneurysm at its origin (Kommerell's diverticulum). Finally, a right aortic arch may be associated with an aberrant left sub-clavian artery which also courses posterior to the esophagus and may be compressed by the latter.

Anatomic structures that can cause diagnostic dilemmas

Normal vascular and extravascular structures in close prox-imity to the aorta may often be mistaken for pathologies such as dissection or signs associated with traumatic aortic injury. Most commonly, pericardial recesses, the left brachiocephalic vein, the left inferior pulmonary vein, the left superior inter-costal vein, the right atrial appendage, and normal thymus constitute the most frequently encountered normal anatomic structures that may simulate aortic pathology.

Pericardial recesses. The pre-aortic and retro-aortic portions of the superior pericardial recesses are intimately related to the ascending aorta and may occasionally simulate dissection or hematoma. The pre-aortic recess is located in the anterior aspect of the ascending aorta (see Chapter 17, Figure 17.12) while the retro-aortic portion of the superior pericardial recess is located posterior to the ascending aorta at the level of the left pulmonary artery (Figure 8.4). The homogeneous water attenuation and characteristic locations are clues to the proper diagnosis.

Left inferior pulmonary vein. The left inferior pulmonary vein is in close proximity to the descending thoracic aorta near its entry into the left atrium. This can sometimes mimic a subtle abnormality in the aortic wall such as an intramural hematoma involving the descending thoracic aorta (Figure 8.5).

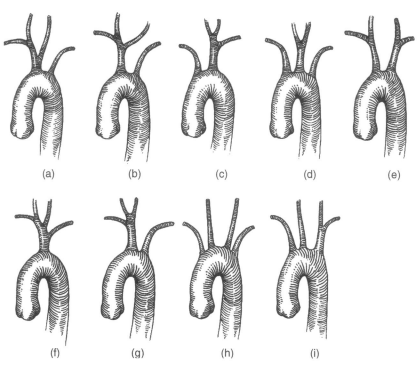

(a)   (b)   (c)   (d)   (e)

(f)   (g)   (h)   (i)

Figure 8.3 Variations in the origins of the aortic arch vessels. (a) and (b) account for 73 per cent of all arch vessel anomalies. (a) Common origin of left common carotid and brachiocephalic arteries (approximately 15% of individuals). (b) Left common carotid originating from mid to upper brachiocephalic artery (approximately 7% of individuals). (c) Common carotid trunk giving off the left subclavian artery. (d) Common carotid trunk. (e) Left and right brachiocephalic arteries. (f) Single arch vessel (the brachiocephalic artery) gives off the left common carotid and left subclavian arteries. (g) Common carotid trunk gives off the right subclavian artery, or origin of left common carotid artery from the right common carotid artery. (h) Independent origin of all vessels; i.e., no brachiocephalic artery is present. (i) Left brachiocephalic artery. Adapted from Kadir S. Regional anatomy of the thoracic aorta from Atlas of Normal and Variant Angiographic Anatomy. Philadelphia, PA: WB Saunders,1991.

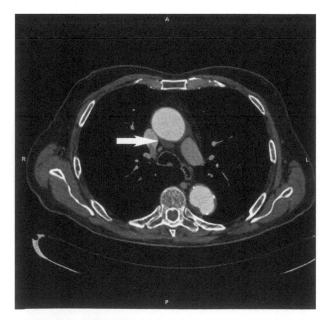

Figure 8.4 Axial CTA image showing the relationship between the retro-aortic portion of the superior pericardial recess (arrow) and the ascending aorta.

Left superior intercostal vein. The left superior intercostal vein is occasionally visible adjacent to the left lateral aspect of the aortic arch as it courses anteriorly to the left brachiocephalic vein (Figure 8.6). If the left upper extremity is used for contrast delivery, the opacification of this vessel may cause an abnormality of the aortic arch that may mimic a focal abnormality involving the wall of the aortic wall termed the aortic nipple.

Right atrial appendage. The right atrial appendage is normally visible on CTA studies anteriorly to the proximal ascending aorta just above the aortic root, where it may simulate aortic pathology. Following this structure into the right atrium on contiguous images demonstrates its true nature (Figure 8.7).

Miscellaneous non-vascular abnormalities mimicking aortic pathology

Periaortic non-vascular pathology, including atelectasis involving the medial basal left lower lobe segment, left-sided

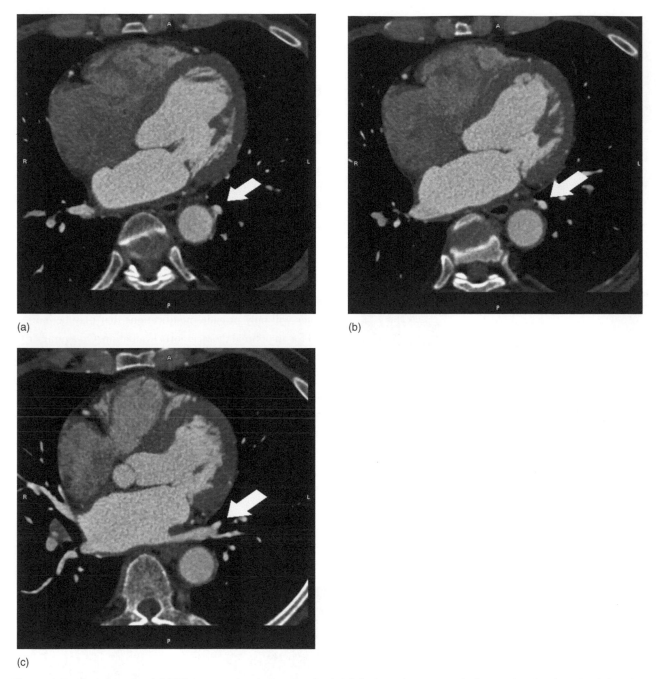

(a)

(b)

(c)

Figure 8.5 A series of axial CTA images (a–c) showing the left inferior pulmonary vein (arrows) going into the left atrium and its relationship with the descending thoracic aorta.

pleural effusion, mediastinal masses, pericardial effusion, and thymus may all simulate aortic abnormalities. Specific features including clinical history may help in differentiating these from aortic pathology. For instance, the presence of air bronchograms visible on lung windows may suggest the proper diagnosis of lung tissue in a para-aortic abnormality. A small left-sided pleural or pericardial effusion adjoining the descending thoracic aorta may resemble peri-aortic hematoma in the acutely injured patient, but attenuation meas-

urements may be useful for distinguishing these conditions. Mediastinal masses and adenopathy may mimic hematoma in the trauma patient. The focal, lobulated appearance and location may suggest the correct diagnosis. Often a fat plane between the mass and the aorta may be present, but almost never with a hematoma. The thymus is usually seen in young adults and is located anterior to the aortic arch and ascending aorta and may mimic a mediastinal hematoma. The age of the patient (young), characteristic location,

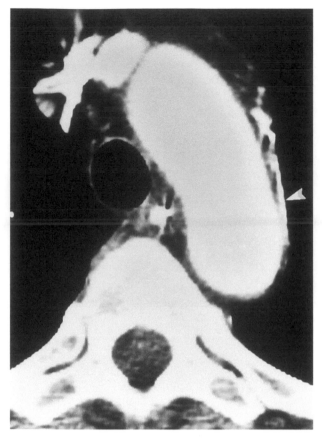

Figure 8.6 Axial CTA image showing the left superior intercostal vein (arrow) and its relationship with the aortic arch.

triangular shape, and lack of mass effects are clues to its differentiation.

PROTOCOL AND TECHNICAL CONSIDERATIONS IN THORACIC CTA

A number of general technical considerations involving performance of CTA have been outlined in Chapter 1. These include field-of-view (FOV), detector collimation, tube voltage (kV), tube current pitch, kernel, and reconstruction increment. These variables must be optimized to provide the highest possible scan quality for a thoracic aortic examination. The basics of contrast agent selection and contrast kinetics have been outlined in Chapter 6 and this chapter will only provide modifications that may be indicated for an optimal thoracic aorta evaluation. On a number of occasions, these parameters may need to be adjusted to find a balance between the volume of coverage and the clinical question being addressed. Table 8.3 provides commonly used parameters for thoracic aortic evaluation. An unenhanced scan may be performed prior to a contrast-enhanced scan, especially if acute aortic injury is present, to evaluate for intramural hematoma. This can be done using relatively thick (5 mm) collimation.

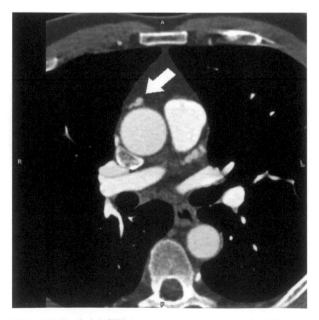
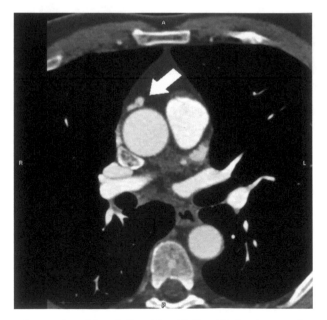

Figure 8.7 Axial CTA images showing the right atrial appendage (arrows) and its relationship with the proximal ascending aorta.

Table 8.3   Protocol for CT angiography of the thoracic aorta (non-gated acquisition[a])

	Siemens		General Electric		Philips		Toshiba	
Scan direction	Cr-Ca	Cr-Ca	Cr-Ca	Cr-Ca	Cr-Ca	Cr-Ca	Cr-Ca	Cr-Ca
Detectors	16	32 x 2	16	64	16	64	16	64
mAs	225	250	370 mA	Auto mA	250	250	250	250
kV	120	120	120	120	120	120	120	120
Rotation time (s)	0.5	0.33	0.5	0.4	0.5	0.75	0.5	0.75
Detector collimation (mm)	0.75	0.6	0.625	0.625	0.75	0.625	0.75	0.625
Slice thickness (mm)	1	0.75	0.625	0.625	1.0	0.9	1	2
Table speed (mm/s)	30	42.4	27.5	137.5	22.51	57.38	22.51	100.18
Pitch[b]	1.25	0.7	1.375	1.375	0.938	1.076	0.938	1.174
Kernel/filter	B30f or B20f	B20f or B30f	Standard	Standard	Standard/ B	Standard/ C	Standard/ B	Standard/ B

[a]For gated acquisition use the appropriate pitch suggested by the individual manufacturer.
[b]Pitch=table feed per rotation/total width of the collimated beam.
Philips parameters provided by Don Boshela BS, RT(R) (CT), Senior CT Product Development, Specialist Philips Medical Systems.
Cr-Ca, Cranio-caudal.

Scanner settings

Field of view and volume of coverage

A wide field of view (50 cm) to allow imaging of the entire thoracic cavity is used. A useful landmark to set the FOV is outer rib to outer rib at the widest portion of the thorax. The superior extent of coverage is variable but should always include the thoracic inlet and extend to the aortic bifurcation, especially if one is evaluating for aneurysmal disease or aortic dissection. In cases where the primary consideration is evaluation of coronary disease, one may stop below the level of the diaphragm, but, in the event an aneurysm or dissection is seen, due consideration to performing an additional run must be given.

Kilovoltage and milliampere values

The kV value need not be adjusted in most patients and a value of 120 provides the best attenuation. There are recent data suggesting that 100 kV may also suffice, and this may be used if radiation dose reduction is important (Chapter 1). Tube current may need to be increased in the obese patient, from the standard setting in most scanners, due to significant attenuation with a corresponding increase in noise. The metric to express tube current is different in some vendors (Table 8.3 and Chapter 1). Increases in mA may often prompt additional adjustment of FOV and coverage in order to reduce the effective dose (Chapter 3).

EKG gating

EKG gating is required for most thoracic aorta evaluations that include simultaneous assessment of the coronary arteries and to rule out subtle abnormalities (focal dissection flaps and intramural hematoma (IMH)) involving the proximal ascending aorta. The latter area, in contrast to the distal ascending aorta and arch, is prone to excessive pulsatility artifact (Figure 8.8). The entire thoracic aorta including the abdominal aorta can be covered in <10s without EKG gating. If EKG gating is a requisite for the reasons mentioned, a dedicated second station involving the abdominal aorta may need to be performed as it may not be possible to perform both of these satisfactorily in one breath hold.

Collimation

The minimum detector collimation feasible is used (usually 0.6 mm) to allow high-resolution isotropic imaging of the thoracic aorta. Narrow collimation provides for excellent quality image post-processing.

Pitch

Non-gated aortic evaluations typically involve a higher pitch. A gated evaluation that involves concomitant assessment of the coronaries has a low pitch to allow overlapping coverage, and this proportionately increases acquisition time (Chapter 1).

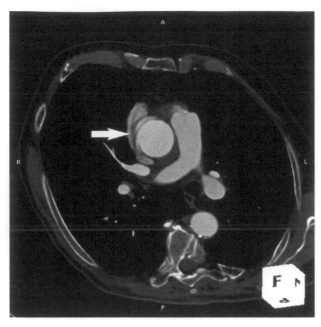

Figure 8.8 Axial CTA image showing pulsatility artifacts involving the ascending aorta (arrow).

Reconstruction increment

A 50% overlap is usually recommended (Chapter 1). This corresponds to a reconstruction increment of half of the detector collimation, or 0.3 mm (assuming a detector collimation of 0.6 mm). Increasing the degree of overlap beyond this does little to increase the longitudinal resolution (Chapter 1).

Contrast considerations in thoracic aortic imaging

Rate

A rate of 4 ml/s of a 350 mg/ml solution of iodinated contrast agent is usually sufficient, although some investigators use rates as high as 5 ml/s These rates can be accomplished by placement of a large bore catheter (≥20 gauge). The right forearm is preferred over the left to avoid streaking artifacts from the left brachiocephalic vein that may obscure neighboring arteries.

Timing and location of contrast arrival

Timing considerations are described in Chapter 5. Empiric timing approaches, although they may work in the vast majority of patients (usually a delay of 25 s), are not recommended. If one were using a timing bolus or a bolus tracking

approach, the region of interest, where the arrival of contrast will be determined, needs to be decided beforehand. This may vary depending on the clinical question. For most thoracic aorta evaluations, timing contrast arrival at the level of the distal ascending aorta or arch should be adequate to provide complete delineation of the aorta, proximal arch vessels. In the event that a concomitant coronary evaluation is being performed, timing in the proximal ascending aorta is critical. For comprehensive evaluation of the thoracic and abdominal aorta (non-EKG-gated) timing may be performed in the proximal descending aorta as well. Bolus timing software programs are preferred over timing approaches for CTA examination of the thoracic aorta, because they are standardizable and one can almost always ensure excellent opacification of the thoracic aorta. The threshold and the locus used to trigger can vary depending on which part of the thoracic aorta one is trying to 'optimally' opacify and the volume coverage.

Volume of contrast

The volume of contrast injected is predominantly dictated by the acquisition time, which in turn is dependent on anatomic coverage and pitch (Chapter 1). The length of the bolus at the very least should correspond to the acquisition time (Chapter 5). In the event a 'care bolus' approach is being used, an additional delay before the machine switches to the high-resolution mode (4–5 s) may be required. If a timing bolus run is used, an empiric period of 6–7 s is added to the time to peak bolus, as the contrast arrival time.

Post-processing

The entire data set should be carefully examined, making sure to examine MPR images (raw data) in multiple orientations including the axial plane. The aortic wall should be carefully examined, especially in segments that are classic sites for dissection.

CLINICAL APPLICATIONS

Chronic atherosclerotic vascular disease

Aortic atherosclerotic vascular disease is a common incidental finding in thoracic aortic examinations but is being recognized as an important etiology for stroke, coronary, and peripheral vascular manifestations. Features of aortic atherosclerotic vascular disease include intimal plaques that may be smooth or complex with varying degrees of calcification. Advanced plaques may demonstrate evidence of ulceration, thrombus formation and may at times protrude into the lumen (Figures 8.9 and 8.10). Plaques ≥4 mm have been associated with an increased risk of stroke. Protruding atheromas are prone to embolize (Figure 8.11). Various plaque components may be distinguished according to their distinct X-ray attenuation properties. Areas rich in lipid components within the plaque, often associated with increased plaque vulnerability, have lower attenuation coefficients than fibrotic tissue (Table 8.4).

Acute aortic syndromes

Classic aortic dissection, aortic IMH, and penetrating aortic ulcer have similar clinical manifestations, and the term 'acute aortic syndrome' was recently proposed to describe this condition. CT and MRI are the preferred modalities for comprehensive evaluation of the aorta.

Penetrating aortic ulceration

Penetrating atherosclerotic ulcers occur when atherosclerotic plaque penetrates through the intima and internal elas-

tic membrane of the aorta, allowing blood to gain access to the aortic media. This may result in IMH and can progress to dissection, aneurysm, or frank aortic rupture. The CTA findings of an aortic ulceration that has penetrated the aortic wall include focal contrast 'out pouching' or projection of contrast beyond the confines of the lumen. Aortic wall enhancement and, rarely, contrast extravasation may also be encountered. Aortic ulceration can be multiple, and evidence of complications, such as dissection and pseudo-aneurysm, may coexist. Aortic ulceration secondary to atherosclerosis is less likely to progress to dissection, due to reparative fibrosis in the aortic wall that tends to limit the progression. Some studies have suggested a malignant course for atherosclerotic aortic ulceration, whereas others have indicated that these ulcers may have an indolent course. Patients who are symptomatic (chest pain, embolization), or remain symptomatic after the initiation of therapy, and ulcers that are wider than 2 cm, or greater than 1 cm in depth, represent a high-risk group and should be managed aggressively by surgical therapy. Medical therapy is generally recommended for ulcerations involving the descending thoracic aorta that is stable or asymptomatic.

Aortic dissection

Aortic dissection is a split or separation of the intimal and medial layer of the aortic wall from the adventitia, resulting

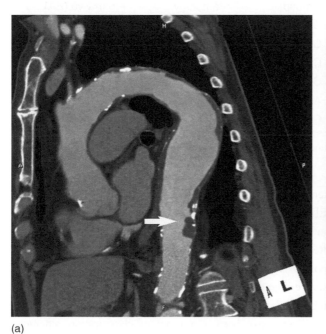

(a)

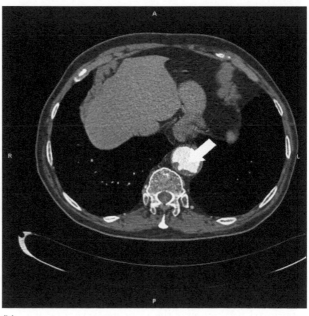

(b)

Figure 8.9 Sagittal and axial MIP images from a CTA of the thoracic aorta showing diffuse atherosclerotic plaques (arrows). The plaques are particularly prominent in the descending thoracic aorta. Note that the plaques have calcifications but are predominantly non-calcified.

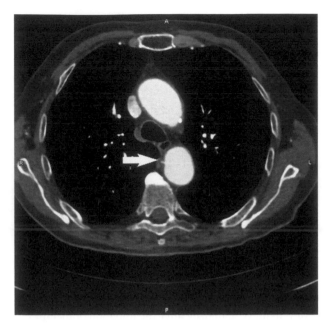

Figure 8.10 Axial CTA image showing an ulcerated atherosclerotic plaque (arrow) at the level of the proximal descending aorta.

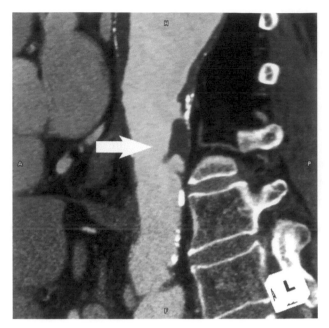

Figure 8.11 Coronal MIP image from a thoracic CTA showing a protruding atheroma at high risk for embolization (arrow). This is immediately below an aneurysmal segment. Note diffuse plaque throughout the aorta.

Table 8.4 Differences in attenuation coefficients between predominantly lipid-rich versus fibrous atherosclerotic plaques

| Reference source | Attenuation (HU) | | Methods | | |
	Lipid-rich	Fibrous	Territory	Reference test	Other
Estes et al.	39 ± 12	90 ± 24	Carotid	Pathology	In vivo (EA)
Schroeder et al.	14 ± 26	91 ± 21	Coronary	IVUS	In vivo
Becker et al.	49 ± 22	91 ± 22	Coronary	Pathology	Ex vivo
Nikolaou et al.	47 ± 13	87 ± 29	Coronary	Pathology	Ex vivo
Schroeder et al.	42 ± 22	70 ± 21	Coronary	Pathology	Ex vivo
Viles-Gonzalez et al.	51 ± 25	116 ± 27	Aortic	Pathology, MRI	In vivo (rabbit)
Leber et al.	49 ± 22	91 ± 22	Coronary	IVUS	In vivo

HU: Hounsfield units; EA: endarterectomy; IVUS: intravascular ultrasound; MRI: magnetic resonance imaging.

in a propagated flap or septum that divides and often impedes blood flow. The region of the right anterolateral wall is frequently the proximal entry site (Figure 8.12). The false lumen created from the tear may or may not re-enter the true aortic lumen (re-entry tear) at a point removed from the primary intimal tear. The intimal tear itself may be a primary inciting factor in aortic dissection or it may be the result of primary weakening of the aortic media because of a spontaneous IMH or other causes of aortic medial weakening. Predisposing factors for aortic dissection include hyper-

tension, connective tissue disorders (e.g., Marfan syndrome, Ehlers–Danlos syndrome), aneurysm, trauma, surgery, infections (syphilis), and arteritis. Based on the International Registry of Acute Aortic Dissection (IRAD), a large contemporary registry of dissection patients, the abrupt onset of severe chest or back pain is the single most common presenting complaint.

There have been a number of classification schemes proposed (Figure 8.13). Fundamentally, the most important clinical distinction is whether the ascending aorta or arch is involved (Stanford type A dissection), or just the segment beyond the left subclavian artery (Stanford type B dissection) as most proximal (type A) dissections are treated surgically, whereas type B dissections are usually managed medically (provided evidence of end-organ ischemia is not present). Type A dissection comprises about 60–70% of all dissections and is the most common aortic emergency. More proximal

tears such as those involving the aortic root are associated with ~37% early mortality compared to those starting from the arch (~23%), and less than 15% beyond the left subclavian artery (type B). A newer classification scheme incorporates subtle forms of dissection that have been recognized with the availability of sensitive imaging modalities (Figure 8.14).

The objectives during the CTA imaging evaluation of a dissection are (1) identification of the dissection flap/confirmation of diagnosis, (2) assessing the extent and size of the aorta, (3) assessing the patency of the false lumen and degree of true lumen compression, and (4) evaluating for evidence of end-organ ischemia, branch vessel involvement (great vessels, mesenteric and renal arteries) and complications such as pericardial effusion or pleural effusion that may indicate rupture or imminent rupture. The most reliable criterion for the diagnosis of aortic dissection on CTA studies is the demonstration of an intimal flap separating the true and false lumen. In cases when an intimal flap is not seen, the diagnosis of aortic dissection must be made on the basis of ancillary criteria, such as distortion of the aortic contour, intramural high attenuation, periaortic hematoma, or displaced intimal calcifications.

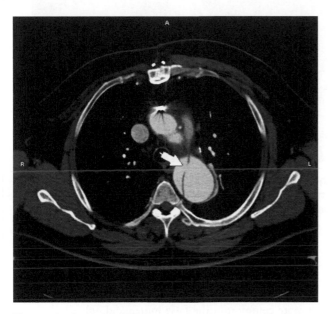

Figure 8.12 Axial CTA image showing an aortic dissection involving the arch. The region of the right anterolateral wall is frequently the proximal entry site (arrow).

True vs. false lumen on CTA: The false lumen is often larger than the true lumen, and the intimal flap may be flat or curved towards the true lumen, although not always.

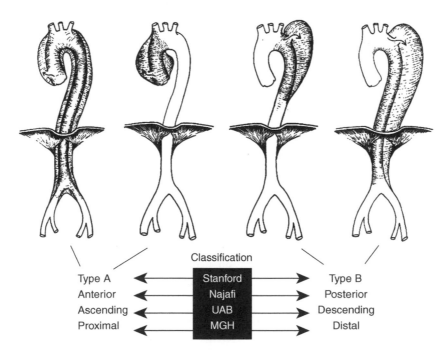

Figure 8.13 Classification schemes for aortic dissection. From Morissey et al.

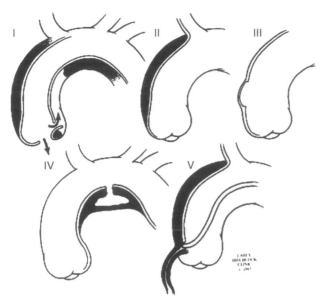

Figure 8.14 A variants of aortic dissection: I, Classic dissection with flap/septum between true and false aneurysm; II, intramural hematoma; III, limited intimal tear with eccentric bulge at tear site; IV, Penetrating atherosclerotic ulcer with surrounding hematoma, usually subadventitial; V, Iatrogenic or traumatic dissection illustrated by coronary catheter causing dissection. From Svensson.

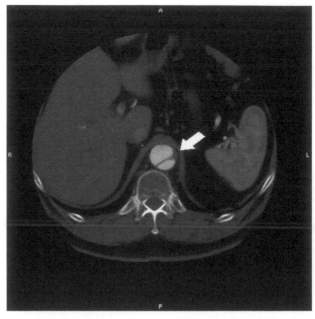

Figure 8.15 Axial CTA image showing the area of junction of the intimal flap to the outer wall of the false lumen ('beak sign', arrow).

On cross-sectional imaging, the junction of the intimal flap and the outer wall of the false lumen forms an acute angle, created as the sharp wedge of the hematoma cleaves the aortic media, and has been referred to as the 'beak sign' (Figure 8.15). The space formed by the acute angle may be filled with either high-attenuation contrast-enhanced blood, or low-attenuation hematoma. Another indicator of the false lumen is the presence of aortic 'cobwebs', which are irregular strands that represent fragments of sheared media and can be seen attached to the wall and projecting to the lumen. The true lumen is frequently located along the left posterolateral aspect of the descending thoracic aorta and abdominal aorta (Figure 8.16), explaining the tendency of thoraco-abdominal dissection to involve the left renal and common iliac arteries preferentially. A false lumen with a convex orientation towards the true lumen is indicative of high pressure within the false lumen, which may in turn be associated with increased incidence of complications. LePage et al. found that the most reliable signs of the false lumen were the 'beak' sign and a larger area. Aortic cobwebs, although specific, are not sensitive (9% of acute and 17% of chronic dissections). Outer wall calcification is seen only in the true lumen and never in the false lumen in acute dissection, however in chronic dissection, outer wall calcification may be seen in false lumens. Intraluminal thrombus is much more common in the false lumen and only rarely in the true, in both acute and chronic dissection.

Intramural hematoma

Intramural hematoma represents localized hemorrhage within the aortic media and is a type of early dissection. IMH may result from trauma, as a consequence of an ulceration extending into the media (penetrating aortic ulcer) or from rupture of the vasa vasorum. The formation of an IMH may presage eventual rupture, dissection, or aneurysm formation. IMH is an important pathway involved in the genesis of aneurysms. IMH appears as a focal thickening of the aortic wall that has high attenuation, and may be better appreciated in non-contrast images, if these have been obtained. If there is adjoining calcium, this may often be displaced. Differentiation of IMH from intraluminal thrombus on a contrast-enhanced CT may be difficult. Intraluminal thrombus is often localized, and within a dilated aorta, whereas IMH may extend over a longer distance, within a non-dilated aorta. In some studies, IMH has involved a 8.5 ± 5 cm length of the aorta. The location of IMH may also determine prognosis, with IMH in the ascending aorta having a poorer prognosis than other locations. Direct flow

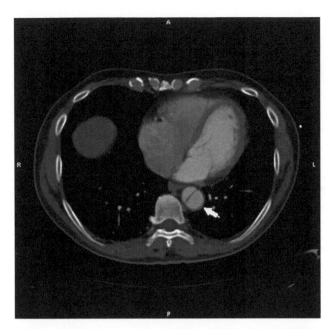

Figure 8.16 Axial CTA image showing a dissection involving the descending thoracic aorta. The true lumen in this case is located along the right anterolateral aspect of the descending aorta. The arrow depicts the false lumen.

communication between the aortic wall and the lumen and older age are risk markers for adverse events with IMH.

Outcome of IMH: The most common outcome with IMH may be progression to aortic aneurysm or pseudoaneurysm. The former may occur in >50% of patients, at least in some series. IMH in the ascending aorta should be managed surgically, while IMH involving the descending thoracic aorta is managed in a fashion similar to type B dissections. Imaging every 3 months in the first year after diagnosis and continued long-term follow-up to detect the development of fusiform aneurysms may be indicated.

Focal dissection/tears without IMH: These have been discovered at surgery in up to 5% of individuals at autopsy and are often detected as incidental abnormalities in patients undergoing thoracic CTA for unrelated reasons.

Thoracic aortic aneurysms

Aneurysm of the aorta is defined as dilation of the aorta involving all three wall layers. Aortic aneurysms may have multiple etiologies including degenerative, inherited disorders of collagen, traumatic and infectious (mycotic). Certain etiologies tend to have a predilection for certain locations.

For example, Marfan's syndrome and its variants (annulo-aortic ectasia) typically affect the ascending aorta, whereas atherosclerotic aneurysms most often affect the descending thoracic aorta. The risk of rupture rises with increasing aneurysm size, with rupture risk increasing dramatically for thoracic aneurysms beyond 5 cm. Since the risk of rupture increases with increasing size, and elective aneurysm repair is associated with a lower mortality than emergent repair, criteria for operative intervention have been suggested. Size thresholds for operative intervention are 5.5 and 7.0 cm for ascending and descending thoracic aortic aneurysms, respectively. The presence of an inherited collagen vascular defect or the presence of concomitant risk factors such as aortic regurgitation and left ventricular dilation may argue for earlier intervention (5.0 cm in ascending and 6.0–6.5 in descending aneurysms). Thoracic aortic aneurysms have been associated with growth rates of 0.10–0.12 cm/year, in contrast to the 0.2 cm/year growth rate suggested for abdominal aortic aneurysms. Thoracic aneurysms may frequently extend into the abdomen. Thoraco-abdominal aneurysms have the same etiology as those of thoracic aneurysms and are classified according to the Crawford classification (Figure 8.17).

CT evaluation of thoracic aortic aneurysms

CTA can clearly delineate the size, spatial extent, tortuosity, and morphologic features of the aneurysm, including the presence of calcification and thrombus in the aneurysm. The involvement of branch vessels and the effect on surrounding structures are clearly seen owing to the excellent spatial resolution. CTA findings of thoracic aortic aneurysm rupture, or impending rupture, include high-attenuation fluid in the pleural or pericardial spaces. When evaluating an aneurysm, it is important to assess its size along the long axis of the vessel. The maximal diameter, superior–inferior extent, and involvement of the branch vessels should be commented on.

Infectious aneurysms

Infectious (mycotic) aneurysms are the result of hematogenous seeding of the aortic wall, with development of focal aortitis and formation of a false aneurysm. These are usually saccular in configuration, may involve any location, and are prone to rupture. Predisposing factors include indwelling catheters, infective endocarditis, infected prosthetic valves and intravenous drug use. An infectious etiology of a

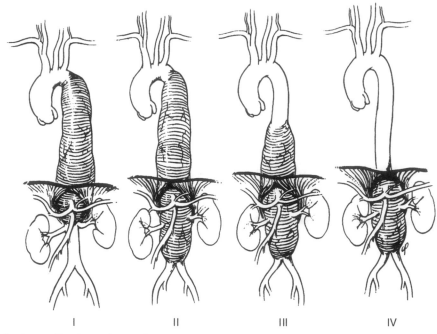

I   II   III   IV

Figure 8.17 Crawford classification scheme for aortic aneurysms. Type I aortic aneurysms involve most of the descending thoracic aorta from the left subclavian artery down to vessels in the abdomen (arresting before the origin of the renal arteries). Type II aneurysms begin at the left subclavian artery and reach the infrarenal abdominal aorta. Type III aneurysms involve the distal half or less of the descending thoracic aorta and substantial segments of the abdominal aorta (the arch is preserved). Finally, type IV aneurysms are those that involve the abdominal aorta and all or none of the infrarenal aorta. From Faber et al.

saccular aneurysm is suggested when an aneurysm is found in an atypical location.

Aortic root abscess: These are almost always seen in conjunction with infective endocarditis and are a consequence of extension of the infection to the aortic root. This is associated with a high mortality and is an indication for immediate surgery. CTA in a patient with a root abscess is an increasingly common indication for CTA as the presence of a root abscess makes a diagnostic catheter coronary angiography more risky. The exam in these cases should be performed with EKG gating and concomitant imaging of the coronaries is mandatory to provide the surgeon with additional information regarding concomitant bypass grafting.

Acute traumatic aortic injury

Aortic injury is typically with deceleration injuries due to high-speed motor vehicle accidents or falls from significant heights. The most common site of injury is the aortic isthmus (90%), followed by the ascending aorta (5–10%), and the descending thoracic aorta, near the diaphragmatic hiatus (1–3%). Great vessel injuries may coexist, including

transection, dissection, and thrombosis. CTA findings of aortic injury are classified as direct or indirect. One of the most commonly encountered direct signs is a pseudo-aneurysm. Other direct findings include abnormal aortic contours, abrupt caliber changes, pseudocoarctation, occlusion of a segment of aorta, and an intimal flap. Rarely, intravenous contrast extravasation may be encountered. Indirect findings include mediastinal hematomas. Although indirect findings suggest the possibility of aortic injury these are not specific and may be the result of venous bleeding. When a mediastinal hematoma is encountered, its relationship to the aorta is of paramount importance. Hematomas that obliterate the fat plane surrounding the aorta or great vessels remain suspicious for occult aortic trauma. Those mediastinal hematomas that do not directly contact the aorta or great vessels may represent mediastinal venous bleeding, and aortography is not required. The performance of CTA using older scanners (single detector) approached 100% sensitivity and 82% specificity. There are recent data supporting 100% sensitivity and 100% negative predictive value in aortic trauma for multi-slice CTA. Isolated abnormalities such as aortic bands or vessel contour abnormalities (in the absence of indirect signs such as mediastinal hematoma) raise the possibility of artifacts or non-traumatic etiologies. In cases of isolated mediastinal hematoma other possible sources of bleeding should be considered before directing patients to thoracic aortography.

Post-operative aorta

The post-operative aorta often poses a diagnostic dilemma as it can assume a number of appearances that appear identical to pathology (Figure 8.18). Prior to evaluation of a surgically manipulated aorta, it is helpful to familiarize oneself with the history and the operative details of the patient as these can be invaluable in avoiding an erroneous diagnosis. The two most common techniques involve placement of an interposition graft or an inclusion graft. In the former technique, the aortic root, ascending aorta, and aortic arch are replaced, with excision of the diseased segment. The inclusion graft technique involves closure of the remaining diseased aorta around the graft, creating a potential space between the graft and the aortic wall. This perigraft space may contain thrombus, flowing blood, or both. When an interposition graft is used, necessary vasculature, such as the coronary arteries, is re-implanted into the graft. Occasionally, high-attenuation felt rings are used to reinforce the anastomosis of interposition grafts; these rings indicate the site of anastomosis. If such rings are not used, the site of the anastomosis may be surmised by noting an abrupt change in caliber of the aorta or an abrupt change in

an atherosclerotic native aorta versus a disease-free graft. Felt pledgets also are sometimes used with interposition grafts to reinforce the sites of cannula placement. These felt pledgets should be differentiated from a pseudoaneurym as they have high attenuation.

The coronary arteries are reimplanted into the aortic graft in the modified Bentall procedure. The tip of the coronary where it is anastomosed to the graft often has a hood of native aortic root. These hoods can once again appear prominent and resemble an anastomotic pseudoaneurysm. The use of inclusion graft technique, entails insertion of graft material within the native, diseased aorta. This form of reconstruction creates a potential space between the graft material and aorta. This gap between the graft and native aorta may thrombose, but may often contain flowing blood. Blood flow within the peri graft space does not mandate surgery unless the situation is associated with hemodynamic instability. Complications that should be monitored in the post-operative patient include dehiscence of the surgical suture line and pseudoaneurysm formation. Pseudoaneurysm at the site of coronary artery re-implantation may result in myocardial ischemia and infarction. Aneurysm formation and dissection may also occur, particularly in patients with cystic medial necrosis. CT or MR imaging surveillance of aortic grafts is routinely recommended. The Stage I elephant trunk technique is employed in patients with a diffuse aneurysmal process, which may warrant

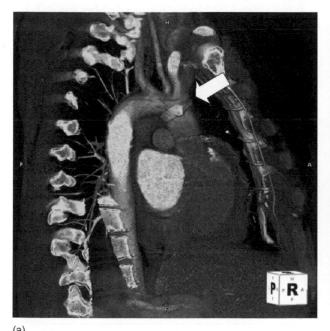

(a)

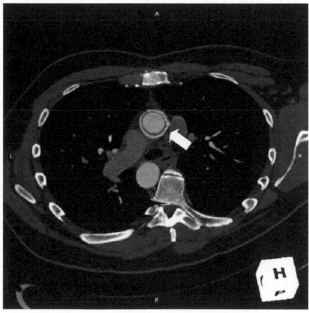

(b)

Figure 8.18   Volume rendered 3D image and axial images showing the typical appearance of the thoracic aorta in a patient treated with a Bentall procedure (arrows).

replacement of the entire aorta at some stage. This procedure involves graft replacement of the ascending aorta and aortic arch with or without a separate valve replacement. A free segment of graft material is left projecting into the proximal end of an invariably diseased descending aorta. This allows repair of the descending aorta at a later date.

CT in endovascular thoricaortic repair (EVAR)

EVAR of the thoracic aorta may be currently indicated as an alternative to surgical intervention of the thoracic aorta in poor surgical candidates or in the event of an emergency. In such cases, EVAR may be an excellent alternative to surgical treatment, especially since the latter may be associated with complications such as paraplegia in 5–10% of individuals. EVAR requires (1) adequate vascular access (sufficient diameter of the iliac artery and abdominal aorta without severe tortuosity) and (2) an aortic lesion without excessive tortuosity and whose neck extends more than 15 mm above the celiac artery and is more than 5 mm distal to the left subclavian artery, without excessive mural thrombus. CTA allows reliable assessment of diameter and the status of the aortic branches as well as evaluation of the iliac and femoral arteries (diameter, tortuosity) for vascular access prior to EVAR of the thoracic aorta. Stent graft diameter is currently determined on the basis of CT findings rather than MR findings. Generally, 10–15% oversizing of stent grafts is required to prevent migration and provide good apposition to the aortic wall. Ideally, stent grafts should cover the lesion and at least 1.5 cm of the normal aorta (landing zone) at each extremity. Whenever possible, greater proximal and distal coverage should be used to prevent late stent graft migration and endoleak due to aortic disease progression. Post-procedure, CTA is performed at the time of discharge, 3, 6, and 12 months after stent graft insertion, and annually thereafter. Chest radiographs are obtained at the same time intervals to assess for metallic failure of the stent graft.

The most common complication following endovascular repair of an abdominal aortic aneurysm is an endoleak. An endoleak is defined as contrast deposit or enhancement in the aneurysm sac outside the graft. CT studies show that up to 20% of patients have an endoleak. Leaks are classified according to Table 8.5. In contrast to the infrarenal aorta, type II endoleaks are uncommon in EVAR of the thoracic aorta. Because of the modular nature of device components, type I and III endoleaks are much more prevalent.

CTA in endoleak detection

The protocol for endoleak detection typically involves acquiring a CTA during the arterial phase and repeating a delayed phase after a few minutes. Endoleak is defined as the extravasation of contrast material outside of the graft during the delayed phase. Type 1 endoleaks result from incomplete sealing of the stentgraft at the proximal or distal attachment site and these, along with type 3, are far more common than type 2 endoleaks (more common in the infrarenal aorta). Many type 1 and type 3 endoleaks may be treated with insertion of a longer stent graft. There is some emerging data from van der Laan et al to suggest MR techniques may be more sensitive that CT in detecting endoleaks, but less specific in precisely locating the site of the leak.

Congenital disorders of the aorta

The diagnosis and treatment of aortic coarctation are based on clinical and imaging findings. There is little need for

Table 8.5   Revised classification of endoleaks
Type of endoleak
I. Leak at attachment site
A Proximal end of graft
B Distal end of graft
C Iliac occluder
II. Branch leaks
A Simple or to-and-fro (from only one patent branch)
B Complex or flow-through (with two or more patent branches)
III. Graft defect
A Junctional leak or modular disconnect

B Fabric disruption (midgraft hole)
    Minor (<2 mm; e.g. suture hole)
    Major (>or =2 mm)

IV. Graft wall (fabric) porosity
(<30 days after graft placement)
Adapted from Pearce et al.

aortography except at the time of a potential percutaneous intervention for the purposes of treatment planning. MRA provides both physiologic and angiographic information, including collateral flow, and may be considered the preferred modality in coarctation (Chapter 17). CTA directly depicts both the stenosis and the collateral circulatory pathways, but does not provide physiologic indices of severity like MR (Chapter 17). It is well known that the degree of anatomic narrowing in coarctation does not provide an adequate index of severity. Other concomitant disorders such as cardiac malformations or aortic stenosis cannot be adequately imaged with CTA. CTA may be useful for planning stent graft implantation and for post-operative follow-up examination, although even in these cases MR may be the preferred modality.

Pseudocoarctation

Pseudocoarctation of the aortic arch is a rare congenital anomaly characterized by one or more stenoses of the descending thoracic aorta immediately distal to the origin of the left subclavian artery. This condition is differentiated from true coarctation of the aorta by the absence of hemodynamic obstruction. Pseudocoarctation is usually benign, but aneurysmal dilatation may develop in the affected areas and must be monitored and treated.

PERFORMANCE OF CTA

CTA for acute aortic syndromes

In the IRAD study, CT was the most commonly utilized imaging modality (93%) followed by TEE and MRI. In this study, which utilized predominantly single detector technology, overall sensitivity of CT for dissection was 93% compared with 100% for MR (very few patients were included). A comparison of spiral CT, transesophageal echocardiography, and MR imaging in 49 patients who had clinically suspected aortic dissection showed 100% sensitivity for aortic dissection for all three techniques, a specificity of 100% for CT, and 94% for both transesophageal echocardiography and MR imaging. In the diagnosis of aortic arch vessel involvement, CT was clearly superior, with a sensitivity and specificity of 93% and 97% compared with transesophageal echocardiography (60% and 85%) and MR imaging (67% and 88%). Large studies detailing the accuracy of multi-slice CTA (≥16 detectors) for aortic dissection are not yet available, but the improved speed and spatial res-

olution suggest that it should be equal or superior to results obtained with single-detector scanners. Disadvantages include the inability to evaluate the aortic valve and assess stenotic or regurgitant involvement.

CTA in the diagnosis of inflammatory aortic disease

CTA can be used to obtain a generalized survey of the aorta and its proximal branches for areas of stenosis and may be diagnostic for inflammatory involvement of the thoracic aorta and its branches. Detection of luminal stenosis and aneurysm formation is exceptional. In addition, CTA can characterize the aortic wall and provide an estimate of wall thickness that can then be used for follow-up studies. Arterial phase wall enhancement has been suggested as a marker of disease activity in conditions such as Takayasu's arteritis, but this may be neither specific nor sensitive for activity. CTA is more effective in depicting mural calcification and intraluminal thrombus, and it can be used to evaluate the supra-aortic vessels, the thoraco-abdominal aorta and its visceral branches, and the pulmonary artery in a single imaging session. Some work suggests that CTA can be helpful in following disease response to therapy. Wall thickness and degree of arterial phase enhancement may both be used as surrogates. The main limitation with CTA pertains to the toxicity associated with contrast agents and the risk for cumulative radiation in these conditions, many of which require repeated scanning.

ARTIFACTS

Streak artifact

Streak artifact results from dense, highly concentrated contrast causing beam hardening and obscuring photon transmission. Streak artifact commonly affects the left brachiocephalic vein and superior vena cava, potentially obscuring the aortic arch and ascending aorta, respectively (Figure 8.19). Streak artifacts may also result from pacemakers, surgical staples, external monitoring devices, or positioning the patient's arms at their sides during the scan (Figure 8.20). These artifacts are readily recognized by identifying their source. Streak artifacts may be reduced by injecting the right upper extremity, using a compact bolus followed by a saline chaser, and sometimes by using dilute contrast mixtures.

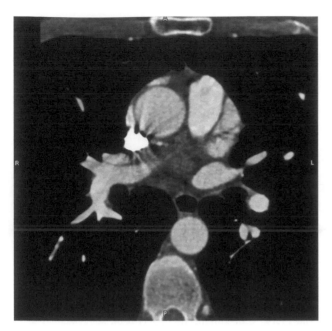

Figure 8.19 Axial CTA image showing streak artifacts produced by high contrast concentration in the superior vena cava, limiting the visualization of the ascending aorta.

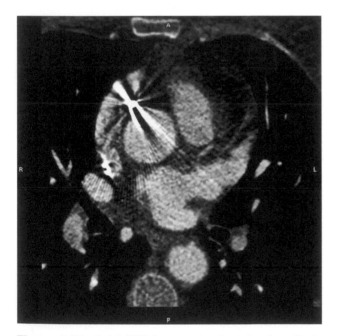

Figure 8.20 Axial CTA image showing streak artifacts produced by a pacemaker lead and severely affecting the adequate visualization of the ascending aorta.

Motion artifact

Motion artifacts can occasionally be problematic, particularly at the base of the heart surrounding the ascending aorta. Motion artifacts may simulate the appearance of aortic dissection (Figure 8.21). EKG gating is a good way to prevent artifacts and should be incorporated if one is interested in

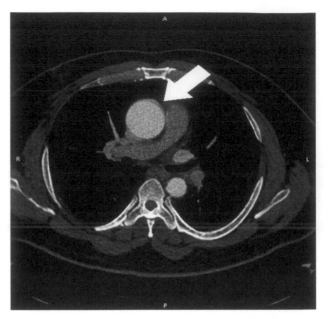

Figure 8.21 Axial CTA image showing motion artifact simulating a dissection involving the ascending aorta (arrow).

high resolution, cardiac motion minimized imaging of the heart and great vessels. If one is using EKG gating, multiple reconstructions may be needed (especially in diastole, at 60–70% of the R-R interval) to rule out motion-related artifact. Noting motion elsewhere on the scan, and the fact that the artifact is usually absent or markedly different at immediately adjacent levels, may allow recognition.

CONCLUSIONS

CTA represents a major advance in the non-invasive evaluation of thoracic aortic disease and is often the first-line investigation for rapid and complete (arch vessels to iliac bifurcation) imaging of the aorta. The widespread availability and ease of use have allowed CTA to become the modality of choice in the initial investigation of acute aortic syndromes. Although the protocols for CTA are very standardized, requiring little physician interaction at the scanner console, paying special attention to various technical parameters may help acquire high-quality images. Further, familiarity with common artifacts and diagnostic is necessary for accurate diagnosis.

PRACTICAL PEARLS

- Consider gated thoracic evaluations when wishing to evaluate the ascending aorta and coronaries.

- Pericardial recesses, the left brachiocephalic vein, and the left superior intercostal vein may frequently mimic aortic wall abnormalities.

- The entire data set should be carefully examined, making sure to examine MPR images (raw data) in multiple orientations including the axial plane.

- Intramural hematoma (IMH) may be differentiated from a thrombus of the aorta by its attenuation and extension over a longer distance, within a non-dilated aorta.

- Direct findings of aortic trauma include IMH, abnormal aortic contours, abrupt caliber changes, pseudo-coarctation, occlusion of a segment of aorta, and an intimal flap.

- Aortic ulcerations and IMH have a worse prognosis when they involve the ascending aorta and often demand surgical treatment.

- The reliable signs to identify false lumen are the 'beak' sign and a larger area vs the true lumen. Aortic cobweb, although specific, is not sensitive. Outer wall calcification is seen only in the true lumen and never in the false lumen in acute dissection.

- Thoracic aortic aneurysms have normal growth rates of 0.12 cm/year, in contrast to the 0.2 cm/year growth rate for abdominal aortic aneurysms.

FURTHER READING

Batra P, Bigoni B, Manning J et al. Pitfalls in the diagnosis of thoracic aortic dissection at CT angiography. Radiographics 2000; 20: 309.

Becker C, Soppa C, Haubner M et al. Spiral CT angiography and 3D reconstruction in patients with aortic coarctation. Eur Radiol 1997; 7: 1473–7.

Becker CR, Nikolaou K, Muders M et al. Ex vivo coronary atherosclerotic plaque characterization with multi-detector-row CT. Eur J Radiol 2003; 13: 2094–8.

Estes JM, Quist WC, Lo Gerfo FW et al. Noninvasive characterization of plaque morphology using helical computed tomography. J Cardiovasc Surg 1998; 39: 527–34.

Evangelista A, Mukherjee D, Mehta RH et al. International Registry of Aortic Dissection (IRAD) Investigators. Acute intramural hematoma of the aorta: a mystery in evolution. Circulation 2005; 111(8): 1063–70.

Faber MA, Mauro MA, Tan WA. Thoracic aortic aneurysm and dissection. In: Rajagopalan S, Mukhergee D, Mohler ER III, eds. Manual of Vascular Diseases. Philidelphia, PA: Lippincott, Williams and Wilkins 2005; 186.

Fisher RG, Sanchez-Torres M, Thomas JW et al. Subtle or atypical injuries of the thoracic aorta and brachiocephalic vessels in blunt thoracic trauma. Radiographics 1997; 17: 835.

Hagan PG, Nienaber CA, Isselbacher EM et al. The International Registry of Acute Aortic Dissection (IRAD): new insights into an old disease. JAMA 2000; 283(7): 897–903.

Hager A, Kaemmerer H, Rapp-Bernhardt U et al. Diameters of the thoracic aorta throughout life as measured with helical computed tomography J Thorac Cardiovasc Surg 2002; 123: 1060–6.

Kadir S. Regional anatomy of the thoracic aorta. In: Kadir S, eds. Atlas of Normal and Variant Angiographic Anatomy. Philadelpia, PA: WB Saunders 1991.

Leber AW, Knez A, Becker A et al. Accuracy of multidetector spiral computed tomography in identifying and differentiating the composition of coronary atherosclerotic plaques: a comparative study with intracoronary ultrasound. J Am Coll Cardiol 2004; 43: 1241–7.

LePage MA, Quint LE, Sonnad SS et al. Aortic dissection: CT features that distinguish true lumen from false lumen. AJR 2001; 177: 207.

Matsunaga N, Kuniaki H, Sakamoto I, Ogawa Y, Matsumoto T. Takayasu arteritis: protean radiologic manifestations and diagnosis. RadioGraphics 1997; 17: 579–94.

Moore AG, Eagle KA et al. Choice of computed tomography, transesophageal echocardiography, magnetic resonance imaging, and aortography in acute aortic dissection: International Registry of Acute Aortic Dissection (IRAD). Am J Cardiol 2002; 89(10): 1235–8.

Morissey NJ, Hamilton IN, Hollier LH. Thoracoabdominal aortic aneurysms. In: Moore WS, eds. Vascular Surgery. Philadeplphia, PA: WB Saunders 2002.

Nikolaou K, Becker CR, Muders M et al. Multidetector-row computed tomography and magnetic resonance imaging of atherosclerotic lesions in human ex vivo coronary arteries. Atherosclerosis 2004; 174: 243–52.

Pearce WH. What's new in vascular surgery? J Am Coll Surg 2003; 196(2): 253–66.

Rajagopalan S. Approach to the management of non-dissecting thoracic and thoraco-abdominal aneurysms. In: Rajagopalan S, Mukherjee DM, Mohler ER III, eds. Manual of Vascular Diseases. Philadelphia, PA: Lippincott Williams and Wilkins 2005.

Riley P, Rooney S, Bonser R, Guest P. Imaging the post-operative thoracic aorta: normal anatomy and pitfalls. Br J Radiol 2001 Dec; 74(888): 1150–8.

Schroeder S, Kopp AF, Baumbach A et al. Noninvasive detection and evaluation of atherosclerotic coronary plaques with multislice computed tomography. J Am Coll Cardiol 2001; 37: 1430–5.

Schroeder S, Kuettner A, Leitritz M et al. J Comput Assist Tomogr 2004; 28: 449–54.

Sebastià C, Pallisa E, Quiroga S, Alvarez-Castells A, Dominguez R, Evangelista A. Aortic dissection: diagnosis and follow-up with helical CT. RadioGraphics 1999; 19: 45–60.

Svensson LG, Labib SB, Eisenhauer AC et al. Intimal tear without hematoma: an important variant of aortic dissection that can elude current imaging techniques. Circulation 1999: 99; 1331–6.

Therasse E, Soulez G, Giroux MF et al. Stent-graft placement for the treatment of thoracic aortic diseases. Radiographics 2005; 25(1): 157–73.

van der Laan MJ, Bartels LW, Viergever MA, Blankensteijn JD. Computed Tomography versus Magnetic Resonance Imaging of Endoleaks after EVAR. Eur J Vasc Endovasc Surg 2006; 32(4): 361–5.

Viles-Gonzales JF, Poon M, Sanz J et al. In vivo 16-slice, multidetector-row computed tomography for the assessment of experimental atherosclerosis: comparison with magnetic resonance imaging and histopathology. Circulation 2004; 110: 1467–72.

Yamada I, Nakagawa T, Himeno Y, Numano F, Shibuya H. Takayasu arteritis: evaluation of the thoracic aorta with CT angiography. Radiology 1998; 209: 103–9.

9

CT angiography of the abdominal aorta and its branches with protocols

Corey Goldman and Javier Sanz

INTRODUCTION

Multi-detector CT (MDCT) has assumed an increasingly important role in abdominal aortic imaging because relevant branches including the renal, mesenteric, and lower extremity arteries can not only be examined with a high degree of accuracy, but also depicted and measured in three dimensions, serving as a resource for interventional planning and clinical management. While 4-detector CT angiography (CTA) may provide adequate excellent assessment of the abdominal aorta alone, comparative assessment of DSA with 4-detector or 16-detector scanners suggests that branch vessel resolution benefits from increasing the number of detectors. To date, there are insufficient studies using 64-detector scanners to determine if there is significant improvement in resolution compared to 16-detector technology for aortic branch vessels. However it is generally assumed that the improvement in temporal resolution and near isotropic resolution will have a positive impact on the visualization of branches of the visceral branches.

INDICATIONS

See Table 9.1.

ANATOMIC CONSIDERATIONS

The abdominal aorta gives rise to splanchnic vessels and the renal arteries before bifurcation into the common iliac arteries.

Table 9.1 Clinical indications for CTA of the abdominal aorta and its branches

Abdominal aorta
- Acute aortic syndrome
  - Aortic dissection
  - Rupturing aneurysm
  - Penetrating ulcer
- Abdominal aneurysm
  - Diagnosis and surveillance
  - Intervention planning
  - Post-intervention monitoring
- Vasculitides

Renal arteries
- Renal artery stenosis (atherosclerosis, dissection, fibromuscular dysplasia)
- Renal transplant evaluation or follow-up

Mesenteric arteries
- Mesenteric ischemia (atherosclerosis, dissection)
- Tumor encasement
- Liver transplant

Anatomic considerations of the mesenteric vasculature are discussed in Chapter 20. The commonest variation of the mesenteric vessels is separate origin of one or more branches of the celiac trunk. The common hepatic artery may sometimes originate from the superior mesenteric artery (SMA) while the left hepatic branch (of the common hepatic artery) may originate from the left gastric artery (a branch of the celiac trunk). The renal arteries originate directly from the aorta. The right renal originates from the anterolateral aspect of the aorta and passes posterior to the IVC as it courses to the renal hilum. The left renal, on the other hand, arises from the posterolateral aspect of the aorta. Two or more renal arteries supply almost 30% of the kidneys. In some of these cases the main renal artery is duplicated, while in others there are accessory renal arteries that arise either superiorly or inferiorly and attach to either the hilum or the poles of the kidney (polar accessory renal arteries). Accessory renal arteries may also arise from the common iliac or other abdominal vessels.

The IVC lies to the right of the aorta and anterior to it in the abdominal cavity. The size varies phasically with respiration, but should not exceed 2.5 cm. Most anomalies of the IVC occur below the level of the renal veins. These include duplication and transposition. In both of these disorders, the IVC is on the left side and then crosses to enter the right side at the level of the left renal vein. Interruption of the IVC with azygos or hemiazygos continuation is not an uncommon condition and can be seen in 0.5–1% of cases. This is due to the intrahepatic portion of the IVC not developing. The azygos and/or the hemiazygos are very large in these cases and should suggest the diagnosis. The renal veins are formed at the hilum of the kidney. The left vein has a tortuous course and travels in a pre-aortic course to enter the left side of the IVC. It receives, after its formation, the left suprarenal vein from above and the left gonadal vein from below. The right renal vein is shorter, enters the IVC directly, and receives no tributaries. The left renal vein can sometimes be circum-aortic (2–8%) or retro-aortic (1–3%). Accessory renal veins are common on the right side and drain directly into the IVC.

IMAGING PROTOCOL

The protocols provided in the following section are meant to be guides, and each site should modify protocols based on image quality or specific individual requirements.

Patient preparation

Abdominal CTA does not generally require specific patient preparation that differs from other contrast-enhanced CT examinations. If the bowel is to be evaluated with the same test, 500–1000 ml of oral water just prior to the procedure helps with its delineation. Barium contrast should not be used. Contrast precautions should be followed and individuals with contrast allergies should be identified prior to the procedure as these may require steroids and antihistamines. Since adverse reaction to intravenous contrast may involve nausea or vomiting, all patients are required to fast (except for water and medications) for a minimum of 4 hours prior to the procedure. Patients with abnormal renal function require treatment with hydration and/or N-acetylcysteine before and after the test. Diabetic patients taking metformin need to discontinue the drug for 2 days after scanning, and in high-risk patients a repeat renal function test is required prior to re-initiating therapy. In cases of concomitant renal dysfunction, metformin is additionally stopped 48 hours before the procedure. In all subjects with documented or suspected reactions to past injections with contrast materials, premedication with steroids and antihistaminic drugs is mandatory.

The patient is instructed about the procedure, including the performance of limited breath holds, as part of the test. In addition, it is useful to warn the patient regarding possible transient effects of the contrast (warm and flushing feeling throughout the body, metallic taste in mouth, initial burning at injection site, etc.). An intravenous access is placed in the arm (either side is acceptable), ideally with an 18–20 gauge cannula. A vein in the hand or forearm is preferable especially if the arms will be placed above the head. However, the antecubital vein is usually employed if the test is performed with the arms at the side of the body or even with raised arms because of easier access. In the latter case, it is important to instruct the patient not to bend the arm as this may result in kinking of the line and possible local complications during the injection. In general, positioning the arms above the head is preferred to avoid streak artifacts arising from the upper extremity bones and remnant contrast related to intravenous access.

After the test, the patient is reminded to drink sufficient fluids in the following hours. Observation for a period of 20–30 minutes post-procedure is required for patients with known allergies or symptoms during the scan.

Intravenous contrast

In patients with normal renal function, regular non-ionic iodinated contrast (iodine concentration 300–400 mgI/ml) can be used. Iodixanol (Visipaque® GE Healthcare Inc.) may be preferable for patients with impaired renal function. Infusion of saline immediately after the contrast with an automated dual injector provides a more compact bolus that may enable reducing contrast concentration and/or volume to some extent. In average-sized patients, 80 ml of iodine-based contrast is typically the lowest dose for reliable abdominal imaging with 16-detector CTA. In individuals with normal renal function, a volume of 120 ml is preferred, whereas for the morbidly obese patient 150 ml should be considered. Some centers with 64-detector scanners have successfully used as little as 50 ml for renal studies. If the scan is also to include either the aortic arch or lower extremities, at least 100 ml of contrast should be used (preferably 150 ml). To obtain optimal intraluminal attenuation, contrast injection rates of 3–4 ml/s are commonly used in adults; in obese patients a rate of 4–5 ml/s is preferred. Additional details on contrast agents are also provided in Chapter 5.

As with any CTA application, adequate timing of image acquisition is crucial to ensure adequate intravascular opacification during the arterial pass of the contrast. Inappropriate timing may result in insufficient luminal attenuation, whereas late image acquisition may additionally be hampered by venous contamination. This is particularly important in the renal circulation, where arteriovenous transit times are typically very short. With current, 16-slice and higher scanners, the speed of acquisition is improved and venous contamination does not generally constitute a significant limitation.

Different methods for scan timing are available. Most contemporary scanners provide automatic triggered image acquisition, and ideally this should be used on a routine basis. A region of interest (ROI) is placed in the diaphragmatic or supraceliac aorta. A trigger value of approximately 150 Hounsfield units (HU) can be used for most patients, although 125 HU units may provide more reliable triggering in obese patients. Alternatively, test bolus injections using 10–15 ml of contrast administered at the same rate of injection as the one used for the main scan can also be employed with the ROI in the supraceliac aorta, acquiring images every 1–2 seconds. A time–density curve is generated and the time corresponding to a 150–200 HU threshold is used as the scan initiation time. Most scanners have a fixed lag time between scan triggering and scan acquisition (approximately 4 s) and this duration should be included when assessing the duration of the bolus. Typically the bolus duration should cover the scan duration in CTA. As a third option for contrast timing, some centers use a fixed time delay. However, because of interindividual variability in contrast transit times, this option is not recommended.

Scanning protocol

The imaging parameters for different scanners are detailed in Table 9.2. The advantage of having multiple detectors is not only faster scans, but also improved resolution. In general, use of the smallest collimation will provide the best resolution for vascular imaging. Section thickness can be increased in the post-processing phase, if images are too grainy, which is common in obese patients. The scanning volume is set so that the upper limit is the 12th rib, and the caudal limit reaches the

Table 9.2 Scanning parameters for CTA of the abdominal, renal, and visceral arteries

	Siemens		General Electric		Philips		Toshiba	
Direction of scan	Cr-Ca	Cr-Ca	Cr-Ca	Cr-Ca	Cr-Ca	Cr-Ca	Cr-Ca	Cr-Ca
Detectors	16	32 × 2	16	64	16	64	16	64
mAs	225	250	380 mA	400 mA	250	250	250	250
kV	120	100	140	120	120	120	120	120
Rotation time (s)	0.5	0.33	0.5	0.4	0.75	0.75	0.75	0.75
Detector collimation (mm)	0.75	0.6	0.625	0.625	0.75	0.625	0.75	0.625
Slice thickness (mm)	0.75	0.75	0.625	0.625	1.0	0.9	1	0.9
Table speed (mm/s)	24	40.72	13.75	110	15	63.0	15	63
Pitch	1.0	0.7	1.375	1.125	0.938	1.175	0.938	1.175
Kernel/filter	B30f	B20f	Standard	Standard	Standard/B	Standard/B, C	Standard/B	Standard/B, C

Philips parameters provided by Don Boshela BS, RT(R) (CT), Senior CT Product Development, Specialist Philips Medical Systems. Cr-Ca = Cranio-caudal.

upper femoral heads (to include the iliac arteries) or the iliac crest (for limited renal or mesenteric segments only). If aortic pathology is known or suspected in the intrathoracic portion, the scanning volume is modified accordingly. Scanning is performed in the cranio-caudal direction. Cardiac gating is not generally needed, unless the ascending thoracic aorta or the arch is included. In patients with isolated abdominal/pelvic studies, diagnostic images can generally be obtained even without breath hold using a 16-detector CT scanner. Improved quality is seen with a breath hold, which will last approximately 10–15 s with a 16-detector scanner and ~10 s with 64-detector scanners.

For many clinical applications a single acquisition during the arterial peak of the contrast is sufficient. A non-contrast study using 2–5 mm sections (low radiation dose) before the contrast acquisition can reveal hemorrhage or aortic hematoma is recommended in the acute setting (trauma or acute aortic syndrome). A repeat (delayed) scan after the contrast is useful to evaluate venous anatomy, organ perfusion (i.e. kidneys), or slow bleeding. Images are reconstructed at submillimeter slice thickness, with 30–50% overlap.

Image post-processing

A variety of post-processing tools (Table 9.3) can be employed for the analysis of abdominal CTA (see also Chapter 4). Several publications have indicated the superiority of one or another specific modality for image reconstruction and post-processing, to generate the most accurate images. Nevertheless, there is agreement that source images should be reviewed in almost all cases for confirmation. Three-dimensional (3D) volume-rendered images provide useful views in evaluation of aorto-iliac and branch vessel angulation. Volume-rendered images are also very useful for identifying accessory renal arteries, celiac artery branching variants, and relative anterior–posterior positions of renal artery ostium. While 3D images can be used for screening for stenosis, filtering artifact can lead to overestimation of apparent stenosis. Frequently, multiple post-processing tools are utilized for a single study, and the user is encouraged to become fluent in all of them.

CLINICAL INDICATIONS
Abdominal aorta

Acute aortic syndrome evaluation (Chapters 8 and 18)

Acute aortic syndromes at the level of the abdominal aorta occur more commonly as a consequence of a ruptured abdominal aortic aneurysm (AAA), or due to the extension of a dissection involving the descending thoracic aorta. Symptomatic, isolated dissection of the abdominal aorta has been reported, although it constitutes a rare finding. Similarly, penetrating, ulcerated plaques tend to occur more commonly in the thoracic segments of the aorta. Abdominal pain in the context of an acute aortic syndrome can be evaluated by ultrasonography, CTA, and/or MR angiography (MRA). Each study type has benefits and limitations, and in practice, the studies are often used in conjunction. In the chest, cardiac-related motion artifact has classically been a limitation to CT imaging of the aortic arch. Some authors have suggested the superiority of MRA or ultrasound; however, these recommendations are based on CTA studies that were not cardiac-gated and did not employ current generation MDCT scanners. Because of its

Table 9.3 Post-processing techniques

	Strengths	Weakness
3D volume rendering	Evaluates vessel angulation Easy to interpret Allows rotation in 3D space	Cannot visualize calcium or stents
Multi-planar reformat (MPR) slabs	Allows visualization of isolated coplanar anatomy	May not visualize vascular structures out of chosen plane
Maximum intensity projection (MIP)	Highlights contrast and readily identifies calcium	Bone interferes with vessel visualization if in same projection line May overestimate and sometimes under-estimate stenosis
Curved multiplanar reconstruction	Allows visualization of tortuous vessels Allows accurate measurements of diameters perpendicular to blood flow	Distortion of anatomy furthest from axis of reconstruction Requires verification of path on orthogonal images

potential diagnostic utility, CTA in the acute setting is considered a preferred imaging tool because it provides angiographic imaging in a facile non-invasive manner and includes as information on soft tissue structures including complications (hemorrhage). Because cardiac-related motion artifacts are not present in the abdominal aorta, gating is generally not required and MDCT constitutes an excellent diagnostic tool.

Performing a non-contrast scan before iodine administration can reveal areas of acute hemorrhage within an aortic dissection plane, peri-aortic or retroperitoneal structures. This study also allows for comparison of subtle changes in thrombus opacification after contrast injection, suggesting a slow bleed. In addition to the initial image acquisition performed during maximum arterial opacification, a delayed acquisition approximately 1–2 minutes after the initial study can also help to identify slow hemorrhage and associated venous abnormalities.

In cases of aortic dissection, several signs may be useful to differentiate the true from the false lumen (also discussed in Chapter 8). Briefly, the false lumen is larger than the former, and it may be partially or totally occupied by thrombus or linear remnants of the media ('cobwebs'). In addition, the angle between the false lumen and the intimal flap is usually acute ('beak sign'). Because atherosclerotic calcification tends to occur in the intima and the dissection plane is usually in the media, flap calcification tends to be located on the side facing the true lumen.

When assessing the abdominal aorta, either in cases of dissection or (AAA), the relationship between aortic branches and the diseased aortic segment should be noted (Figure 9.1), particularly the presence of an occluded branch. This can have a significant impact on patient management, including the decision for surgery vs medical management. Other anatomic features that need to be identified are detailed in the subsequent section regarding AAA, as well as in Chapter 18.

It is important to realize that while CTA is nearly 100% sensitive for detecting AAAs, differentiation of acutely ruptured from non-ruptured aneurysms has a sensitivity that is substantially lower. In a clinical study comparing CTA with open surgery, CTA had only 79% sensitivity in patients with known AAA and suspected rupture on clinical grounds. Thus, clinical presentation should be strongly considered despite a negative CT study in a patient with suspicion of impending rupture of an abdominal aneurysm.

Additional pathology that can be identified with CTA includes ulcerated atherosclerotic plaques with extension through the vessel intima, penetrating ulcers that extend through the media, and pseudoaneurysms that extend to the adventitia and beyond. The latter abnormality appears as an out pouching of the vessel lumen, and can be visualised in volumetric reconstructions. Planar images are also necessary because they allow visualization of the actual vessel wall and serve as a means of differentiating the various types of pathology.

Abdominal aortic aneurysm (see also Chapter 18)

Diagnosis and surveillance of AAA

Abdominal aneurysms are often asymptomatic and are detected incidentally during imaging studies performed for other reasons. Dedicated primary screening is nonetheless indicated for certain subgroups of the population, as specified in Chapter 18. AAAs have a predicable rate of growth based on size and there are published guidelines for frequency of surveillance. Classically, primary surveillance of a documented AAA is performed using ultrasound. In the absence of significant bowel gas, true transverse measurements can be reliably obtained with this technique. Aortic diameter measurements derived from CT scans have classically been taken from axial or transverse images, which can be inaccurate for measuring the true diameter of a tortuous aorta. With the advent of spiral CT and true isotropic spatial resolution, accurate diameter measurements of the aorta can be taken from curved multiplanar reformations, which represent a true diameter of the aorta perpendicular to the flow of blood. Despite this improvement, axial images are commonly used as a source for aortic diameter measurements. Therefore, when reporting aortic diameters, a statement regarding the axis of measurement should be included, i.e. transverse or reconstructed.

In most cases in routine practice, diameter measurements of the vessel lumen are reported, as well as true vessel size. This is important, as the true degree of aortic dilatation may be masked in cases of significant mural thrombosis if only luminal measurements are taken. More recently, studies have suggested that vessel area may be more accurate to assess risk of rupture. Aneurysm volume in particular, seems to be a better measure of aneurysm growth or post-stent graft placement regression. However, these measurements are more time consuming and such practice has not become standard. Assessment of aneurysmal extent, morphology (eccentricity), and branch involvement should also be reported. As mentioned before, mural clot is a common finding in AAA, and its presence and amount can be easily detected with CTA (Figure 9. 2).

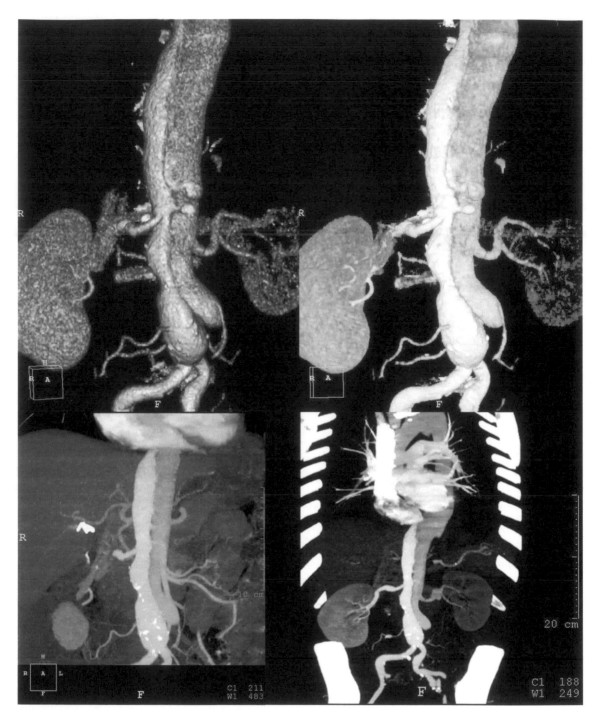

Figure 9.1 An aortic dissection with extension into the abdomen can be appreciated after electronic bone removal (pixels greater than 350 Hounsfield units removed) on 3D volume reconstruction (upper left). Changes in the color scheme with an increase in the median pixel brightness and narrowing of the window better depict the origin of the right renal artery from the true lumen and the left renal artery from the false lumen (upper right). A maximum intensity projection with a 60 mm thickness (slab MIP) demonstrates calcium in the abdominal aorta and reveals segments of the celiac, superior mesenteric, and lumbar arteries in relation to the hepatic parenchyma (bottom left). Attempts to increase the slab thickness resulted in interference from bright projections of the vertebral bodies and overlying mesenteric vessels (not shown). A curved multi-planar reconstruction with a 15 mm thickness from the aortic arch to external iliac arteries has an appearance similar to a standard angiogram (bottom right). There is bright opacification from contrast in the superior vena cava in the upper aspect of the image adjacent to the heart (bottom right).

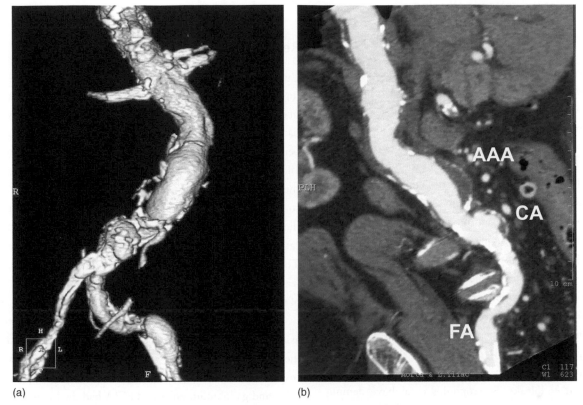

(a)　　　　　　　　　　　　　　　　　　(b)

Figure 9.2　The volume-rendered image (a) of this aorta does not adequately reveal diffuse aneurysmal involvement. A curved multi-planar reconstruction (b) of this tortuous aorta enables electronic linearization of the aorta perpendicular to the flow of blood and provides a more reliable assessment of abdominal aneurysm length. In this image an abdominal aortic aneurysm is adjacent to a common iliac artery aneurysm. A fusiform aneurysm of the left common femoral artery is also demonstrated inferiorly. The relation of the aortic and iliac wall with medial calcifications relative to the contrast-containing lumen allows for differentiation of true aneurysms with mural thrombosis (as shown) from penetrating ulcer or pseudoaneurysm.

CTA is highly reproducible for the quantification of AAA dimensions. However, until there is standardization of reporting that addresses the possibility of taking measurements from curved planar images, and the need for ionizing radiation and potentially nephrotoxic contrast agents, CTA cannot be advocated as the preferred method for routine AAA surveillance.

AAA intervention planning

Surgical intervention can be planned on the basis of CTA findings. Similarly, CT imaging is increasingly employed in the planning of AAA endovascular stenting. Some workstations incorporate dedicated 3D software packages, which can assist in aortic stent planning, and it has been demonstrated that CTA suffices for successful repair of aneurysms without the use of prior standard angiography. This feature is particularly of value in tortuous aneurysms, whereas aortography measurements are less reliable. In a study examining 30 patients with aneurysms, Diehm et al

found that CTA was associated with superior intra- and inter-observer reliability for several aortic aneurysm and iliac artery measurements when compared to standard digital substraction angiography (DSA).

Morphologic features of AAAs that may have an impact on endovascular repair and that need to be reported in a CTA study include:

(1) The proximal neck diameter and length relative to the renal artery origins and superior mesenteric artery.

(2) The diameter and configuration of the aneurysm body.

(3) The distal neck length and diameter relative to the aortic bifurcation.

(4) Common iliac artery involvement and length.

(5) Relation of the hypogastric (internal iliac) arteries to a point of potential distal fixation.

(6) Angulation and diameter of the iliac arteries and common femoral arteries.

Post-aortic stent graft monitoring

Repaired aortic aneurysms, particularly those treated percutaneously, require periodic surveillance because of the risk of stent graft migration and/or endoleak. CTA offers some advantages for the detection of endoleaks and determination of the responsible mechanism (endoleak type; see Chapter 8) over alternative imaging modalities. In the abdominal aorta repaired with an aortic stent graft, the commonest endoleak is type II, or persistent pressurization of the sac owing to a back bleeding vessel. The incidence of endoleak after aortic endovascular grafting can be as high as 10–20%. There have been comparative studies examining the use of ultrasound vs CTA as a means of identifying endoleaks. Although duplex ultrasound is safe and easily performed, it has lower sensitivity for the detection of endoleaks and its routine use for this purpose is not recommended. In general, CTA is also more sensitive than DSA because branch vessels are imaged simultaneously with the aneurysm sac in CTA, whereas a time delay may occur between maximum aortic opacification and branch vessel opacification for DSA. In patients with known endoleaks, Stavropoulos et al have demonstrated 86% agreement between CTA and DSA. Patients incorrectly classified by CTA included 3 out of 36 patients as having a type II leak and 1 out of 36 patients as having a type III leak. All were actually type I leaks. One additional patient was incorrectly labeled as a type 1 endoleak, but was a type II endoleak on DSA. Aneurysm volume after stent repair as measured on CTA has also been demonstrated to be useful in evaluating endoleaks. Lack of volume decrease in the aneurysm of at least 0.3% at 6 month follow-up indicates the need for closer surveillance, and has a higher predictive accuracy for an endoleak than changes in maximum diameter.

Connective tissue disorders and vasculitis

In the abdomen, CTA is useful for visualizing large and medium size vasculitides, including Takayasu's arteritis, polyarteritis nodosa, and Behçet's disease. These disorders may involve the abdominal aorta or its branches, and may be associated with areas of luminal stenosis and/or aneurysmal dilatation. In addition, inflammatory thickening of the arterial wall can be readily depicted. More recently, Crohn's disease small bowel inflammation has been reported to be assessed well because it is accompanied by pronounced hyperemia that is seen on CTA.

Renal arteries

Renal artery stenosis (see also Chapter 19)

Current MDCT scanners offer superb spatial isotropic resolution unsurpassed by other imaging modalities. This results in excellent image quality and the ability to accurately evaluate renal artery anatomy (including the presence and number of accessory branches, Figure 9.3), as well as the presence and severity of significant luminal stenoses. In practice, the use of CTA is somewhat limited in the presence of concomitant renal dysfunction, which may not be uncommon in the setting of renovascular disease constituting a contraindication for the administration of iodinated contrast agents. The presence of calcified plaques may obscure lumen visualization, although this is occasionally overcome with the use of thin, high-resolution reconstructions (see Figure 9.4).

In 2001, a meta-analysis by Vasbinder et al comparatively assessed the accuracy of various non-invasive imaging modalities for diagnosing renal artery stenosis in patients with suspected renovascular hypertension. They demonstrated that CTA and gadolinium-enhanced MRA had the highest diagnostic accuracy compared with duplex ultrasound or captopril scintigraphy. The areas under the receiver operating characteristic curves for the ability to detect hemodynamically significant renal artery stenoses were 0.99 for CTA, 0.99 for gadolinium-enhanced MRA, 0.97 for non-gadolinium-enhanced MRA, 0.93 for ultrasonography, 0.92 for captopril renal scintigraphy, and 0.72 for the captopril test. The CTA studies evaluated in this meta-analysis employed single-slice spiral technology. Using a 4-detector system, Willmann et al demonstrated 92% sensitivity and 99% specificity for renal artery CTA. This diagnostic accuracy was not significantly different from that obtained with MRA. In a subsequent prospective multi-center triple-imaging study in 2004 examining CTA (including both single- and multi-detector row systems), MRA, and DSA, Vasbinder et al published sensitivity for both CTA and MRA as less than 65% as compared with DSA. In this study, a significant proportion of the patients with renal artery stenosis had fibromuscular dysplasia, a disorder more prevalent in children and young adults. Fibromuscular dysplasia is associated with more distal stenoses that are therefore more difficult to detect, whereas most cases of stenosis secondary to atherosclerotic disease are located proximally.

In general terms, the clinical utility and diagnostic ability of CTA in the evaluation of renal artery disease is well documented, and offers the benefits of being a non-invasive study. It is likely that studies using 16- and 64-detector systems

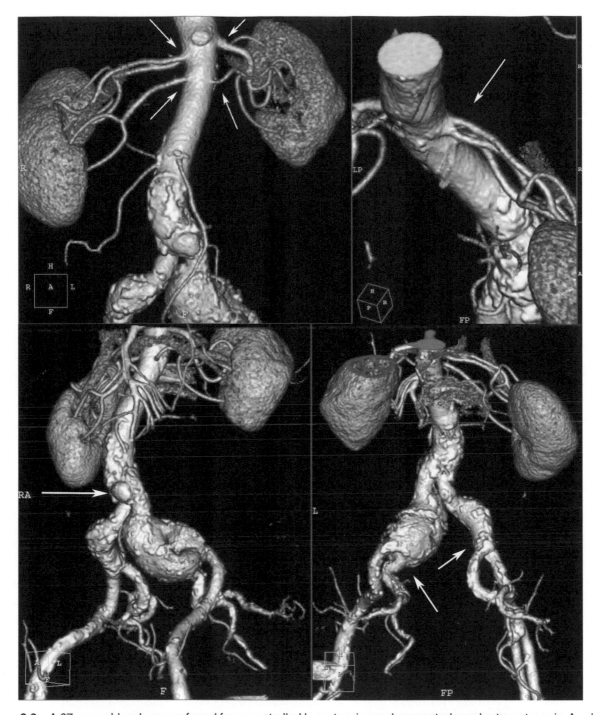

Figure 9.3   A 67-year-old male was referred for uncontrolled hypertension and suspected renal artery stenosis. A volume-rendered image of the abdominal aorta (upper left) demonstrates duplication of the renal arteries bilaterally (arrows). The superior right renal artery is better depicted in a superior-posterior oblique view (upper right, arrow). Incidental findings include a penetrating ulcer at the aortic bifurcation (lower left, arrow) and bilateral common iliac aneurysms (lower left and lower right panels). A posterior view of the aortic bifurcation demonstrates the relation of the internal iliac arteries to the aneurysms (lower right, arrows). This case also demonstrates the extensive aortic calcification (white) that is often common in patients with peripheral arterial disease.

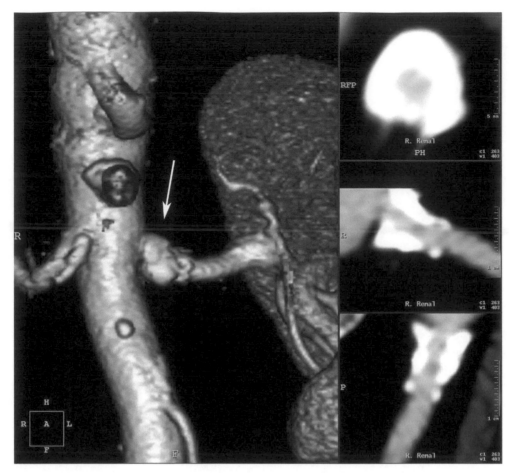

Figure 9.4   Circumferential calcium (arrow) of the left renal ostium in a volume-rendered image (left) of the left renal artery obscures visualization of a stent as well as the lumen of the vessel. Orthogonal curved planar reconstructions (right) demonstrate a patent lumen.

will result in enhanced diagnostic performance in evaluating renal atherosclerotic disease, although such investigations are pending. Similarly, MDCT has also proven to be useful in other clinical scenarios, such as fibromuscular dysplasia, renal artery aneurysms, or dissection, although the comparative accuracy to other imaging modalities has not been fully investigated. In addition, CTA can be useful in the follow-up of patients after renal artery intervention (i.e. stenting; Figure 9.5).

Renal transplant evaluation

CTA is being increasingly utilized in the definition of renal artery and vascular anatomy prior to renal transplant. To date, CTA is the preferred modality for renal donor assessment and allows for higher accuracy than MRA in the identification of multiple renal arteries and veins. A delayed parenchymal view 2 minutes post-injection should be performed to

identify masses and adequately define the collecting system or stones. Specific aspects of vascular anatomy relevant for renal transplant include accessory renal arteries, gonadal and adrenal arteries, accessory renal veins and retro-aortic renal veins (Figures 9.6 and 9.7). Additionally, any pathologic arterial feature including stenosis, plaque, aneurysm, or fibromuscular dysplasia, is relevant.

Mesenteric arteries

Mesenteric ischemia

The celiac and/or superior mesenteric arteries are commonly involved in acute and chronic mesenteric ischemia. Acute mesenteric ischemia is commonly embolic or thrombotic and is often associated with mesenteric vessel occlusion. Branch vessels from the celiac trunk or superior mesenteric artery may be involved. Acute mesenteric ischemia can also occur as

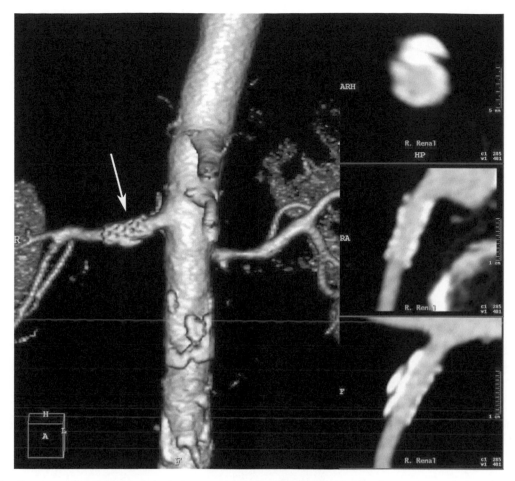

Figure 9.5   One year after right renal stent placement, a patient had decline in blood pressure control, and an abdominal CTA was performed using automated trigger bolus at 125 Hounsfield units with the region of interest in the suprarenal abdominal aorta. A contrast dose of 80 ml (350 mgI/ml) followed by 50 ml of saline, both at a rate of 4 ml/s, were used for arterial opacification. The volume-rendered image (left) confirms the presence of a right renal stent (arrow) in a calcific renal artery, and is also suggestive of mild left renal artery stenosis. Orthogonal curved planar reconstructions (right) examine the right renal artery relative to a reconstructed path in lateral, superior, and anterior projections (1 mm thickness) and demonstrate a patent stent.

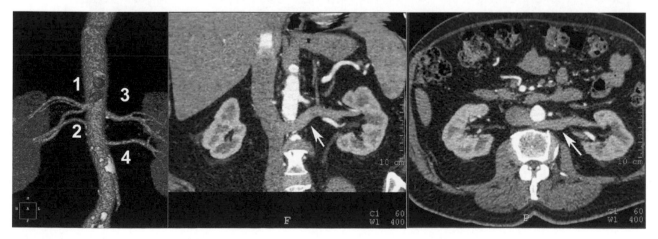

Figure 9.6   A middle-aged man volunteered to be a kidney donor. A CTA was performed using 0.75 collimation, 120 kV and 120 ml of iodinated contrast agent (350 mgI/ml) followed by 50 ml of normal saline at a rate of 4 ml/s. Automated trigger bolus using a threshold of 120 Hounsfield units at the suprarenal abdominal aorta demonstrates the presence of bilateral renal artery duplications (1–4; left). Maximum intensity projections in the frontal (middle) and the transverse plane (right) demonstrate the course of a retro-aortic left renal vein (arrows).

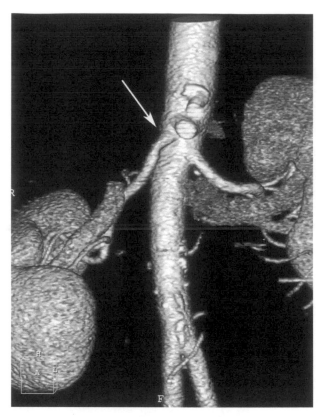

Figure 9.7 An anterolateral origin (arrow) of the right renal artery in a patient with a ptotic kidney is easily appreciated in a volume-rendered image of the abdominal aorta.

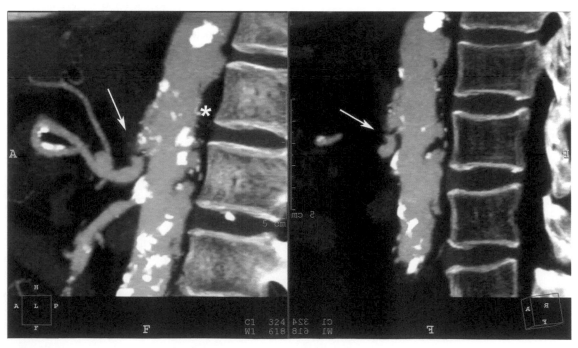

Figure 9.8 A severe celiac artery origin stenosis (arrow) is depicted in this 15 mm lateral MIP projection of the abdominal aorta (left). The origin of the superior mesenteric artery is obscured by calcific plaque and represents a drawback of maximum intensity projections containing vascular calcifications. Extensive posterior aortic plaque with ulceration (*) appears as irregularity in the posterior wall. A tangential view of the celiac artery origin (right) has the appearance of a penetrating ulcer and demonstrates the importance of not relying on a single projection for diagnosis.

a result of small vessel vasospasm. In contrast, chronic mesenteric ischemia or 'abdominal angina' typically has a more insidious onset, and is associated with main celiac trunk and/or superior mesenteric artery occlusion or severe stenosis. Classically, chronic mesenteric ischemia involves obstruction of at least two of the three main mesenteric arteries. However, there are reports indicating single vessel involvement, particularly with median arcuate ligament syndrome. Other disorders that are associated with mesenteric ischemia include dissection or aneurysms (Figure 9.8).

Tumor encasement

Tumor involvement of the main celiac or mesenteric arteries, particularly by pancreatic tumors, can prevent surgical resection. CTA essentially has replaced standard DSA in the pre-operative assessment of pancreatic tumors. Branches of the celiac and superior mesenteric vessels are difficult to assess on axial or transverse sections due to their oblique course. However a slab MIP in the frontal or coronal plane often gives excellent visualization of the first- and second-order celiac artery and superior mesenteric artery branches.

Liver transplant

CTA is ideally suited for identifying arterial and venous anatomy for pre-operative evaluation of hepatic transplant. Aspects of the evaluation include the arterial supply, venous anatomy, portal anatomy, parenchymal assessment, and evaluation of liver volume.

Limitations

The most obvious limitations of CTA for the evaluation of abdominal vascular pathology are the need for ionizing radiation, and the concomitant use of potentially allerg and nephrotoxic contrast agents. The information obtained with CTA is primarily anatomic, in contrast to other techniques such as MRA or ultrasonography that may additionally provide functional information, such as measurements of velocity across a renal stenosis, or cine images of a dissection flap. When evaluating branch stenoses, the presence of severe calcification may hamper adequate estimation of the severity of luminal narrowing (Figure 9.8). As mentioned in the chapter different post-processing techniques have specific advantages and disadvantages, and emphasis must be put on analyzing source images and confirming findings in different reconstructions. Motion artifacts can occur, especially with breathing. Streak artifacts are less common in the abdominal aorta.

CONCLUSIONS

CTA with current multi-detector scanners provides high-resolution images of the abdominal aorta and its branches in a very short examination time. This feature is particularly attractive in the acute setting, where a variety of both vascular and extravascular disorders can be evaluated in a single setting in only a few seconds. In the patient with chronic conditions, CTA provides accurate and reproducible measurements of arterial dimensions, and can detect the presence of dissection, stenosis, or aneurysmal dilatation with high diagnostic accuracy. Due to these advantages, CTA is increasingly employed as the modality of choice for the planning of different types of vascular intervention, including endovascular repair of abdominal aneurysms or renal artery stenting. Besides depicting luminal abnormalities, CT provides concomitant assessment of pathology in the arterial wall (atherosclerotic plaque, calcification, etc.) and of extravascular structures. In clinical practice, these attractive features of CTA must be balanced with the small risk of complications associated with the use of iodinated contrast and ionizing radiation.

PRACTICAL PEARLS

- Always review post-processed images in different orientations, and concomitantly evaluate the source images, for the confirmation of findings.

- Use the thinnest detector collimation to improve longitudinal resolution.

- When evaluating suspected acute aortic syndromes, a precontrast scan may aid in the detection of hemorrhage.

- A repeat scan 1–2 minutes after the arterial CTA acquisition can be useful in some clinical scenarios depicting renal perfusion, venous anatomy, or slow bleeding.

- Post-stent evaluation requires repeating a CTA acquisition 2 minutes after the arterial acquisition. Endoleak is diagnosed when contrast is detected in the aneurysm sac.

- For optimal timing, avoid fixed delays and rely on automated bolus tracking or test bolus techniques.

FURTHER READING

Diehm N, Herrmann P, Dinkel HP. Multidetector CT angiography versus digital subtraction angiography for aortoiliac length measurements prior endovascular AAA repair. J Endovasc Ther 2004; 11(5): 527–34.

Filis KA, Arko FR, Rubin GD, Zarins CK. Three-dimensional CT evaluation for endovascular abdominal aortic aneurysm repair. Quantitative assessment of the infrarenal aortic neck. Acta Chir Belg 2003; 103(1): 81–6.

Frauenfelder T, Wildermuth S, Marincek B, Boehm T. Nontraumatic emergent abdominal vascular conditions: advantages of multi-detector row CT and three-dimensional imaging. Radiographics 2004; 24: 481–96.

LePage MA, Quint LE, Sonnad SS, Deeb GM, Williams DM. Aortic dissection: CT features that distinguish true lumen from false lumen. AJR 2001; 177: 207–11.

Napoli A, Fleischmann D, Chan FP et al. Computed tomography angiography: state-of-the-art imaging using multidetector-row technology. J Comput Assist Tomogr 2004; 28 (Suppl 1): S32–45.

Rubin GD. Techniques for performing multidetector-row computed tomographic angiography. Tech Vasc Interven Radiol 2001; 4(1): 2–14.

Rubin GD. 3-D imaging with MDCT. Eur J Radiol 2003; 45 (Suppl 1): S37–41.

Rubin GD. MDCT imaging of the aorta and peripheral vessels. Eur J Radiol 2003; 45 Suppl 1: S42–9.

Stavropoulos SW, Clark TW, Carpenter JP et al. Use of CT angiography to classify endoleaks after endovascular repair of abdominal aortic aneurysms. J Vasc Interven Radiol 2005; 16(5): 663–7.

Vasbinder GB, Nelemans PJ, Kessels AG et al. Diagnostic tests for renal artery stenosis in patients suspected of having renovascular hypertension: a meta-analysis. Ann Intern Med 2001; 135(6): 401–11.

Vasbinder GB, Nelemans PJ, Kessels AG et al. Accuracy of computed tomographic angiography and magnetic resonance angiography for diagnosing renal artery stenosis. Ann Intern Med 2004; 141(9): 674–82.

Willmann JK, Wildermuth S, Pfammatter T et al. Aortoiliac and renal arteries: prospective intraindividual comparison of contrast-enhanced three-dimensional MR angiography and multidetector row CT angiography. Radiology 2003; 226: 798–811.

Willoteaux S, Lions C, Gaxotte V, Negaiwi Z, Beregi JP. Imaging of aortic dissection by helical computed tomography (CT). Eur Radiol 2004; 14(11): 1999–2008.

Wyers MC, Fillinger MF, Schermerhorn ML et al. Endovascular repair of abdominal aortic aneurysm without preoperative arteriography. J Vasc Surg 2003; 38(4): 730–8.

Yee J, Galdino G, Urban J, Sawhney R. Computed tomographic angiography of endovascular abdominal aortic stent-grafts. Crit Rev Comput Tomogr 2004; 45(1): 17–65.

10

CT angiography of the upper extremities with protocols

Emil I Cohen, Amish Doshi, and Robert A Lookstein

INTRODUCTION

As recently as 10 years ago, computed tomography (CT) angiography (CTA) was first described as a technique to non-invasively evaluate vascular structures via a peripheral injection of contrast.

The first clinical application of this technology for the upper extremities was with single-row helical scanners where the technique was used to evaluate the configuration and patency of the subclavian arteries. With the recent introduction of multi-detector technology including widespread availability of 16- and 64-detector scanners, the use of CTA to evaluate the upper extremity vascular supply is rapidly replacing conventional angiography, not only for diagnosis but also for treatment planning. The recent technologic advancements with multi-detector CT (MDCT) now allow large volume coverage with higher spatial resolution. This chapter reviews the technical factors that must be taken into consideration in planning and interpreting CTA, as well as the applications that are most relevant to arterial pathology of the upper extremity.

INDICATIONS

Table 10.1 lists the indications for CTA of the upper extremity.

Table 10.1 Indications for CT angiography of the upper extremity

- Normal anatomy
- Variant anatomy
- Subclavian artery stenosis
- Subclavian artery aneurysms
- Acute and chronic upper extremity ischemia
- Dialysis graft surveillance
- Surveillance following endovascular therapy

FUNDAMENTALS

The most important step in planning a CTA is determining the area of interest to be imaged. This is most relevant for early generation scanners, whereas with the newer 16- and 64-detector scanners, the speed of the study makes any area of coverage technically feasible in a single acquisition (Chapter 1). Specifically relevant to the evaluation of the upper extremity is the fact that the arterial supply to the upper extremity begins at the aortic arch. Thus any CTA study of the upper extremity must include imaging of the chest. Our institution's protocol is typically to place the patient's arm under evaluation at their side in a comfortable anatomic position. The intravenous access must be in the contralateral arm to diminish the artifact of the injection bolus in the venous system. This arm may be placed above the head or at the side; the latter will allow for simultaneous evaluation of both extremities, although arterial evaluation in the arm with the intravenous line may be hampered due to venous opacification. With the patient's arm at their side, the CTA examination of the upper extremity closely resembles a CTA of the chest, abdomen, and pelvis, with a larger field of view. This allows for visualization of the entire vascular supply to the extremity from the aortic valve to the fingertips in a single acquisition. Although breath holding is not necessary for the evaluation of the upper extremity arterial system, it is advisable to perform the acquisition in apnea to decrease motion artifacts at the level of the arch.

Typical protocols for this study are listed here for a variety of commercially available scanners (Table 10.2).

Contrast is usually injected through a large bore intravenous access (20 gauge or larger) at a rate of 4–5 ml/s. Our clinical experience has been that non-ionic contrast with high iodine concentration is optimal for imaging in the typical patient. The recommended injected dose of iodinated contrast for CTA is 1–1.5 g iodine/s. The total volume of contrast is adjusted based on considerations regarding scanning time, which depends on anatomic coverage, scanner model, and imaging protocol (see Chapter 5).

The data set is usually reconstructed at the minimum collimation width (0.75 mm for 16-slice scanners and 0.6 mm for 64-slice scanners). The modern scanner can easily yield well over a thousand high-resolution images per examination. Fortunately, the vendors from various post-processing companies have many software programs for the quick and accurate assessment of these images. A modern workstation is capable of numerous tasks but the end results for CTA can be grouped into three image formats. These include volume-rendered (VR), maximum intensity projection (MIP), and curved planar reformatted (CPR) images (for detailed information, see Chapter 4).

In our institution, the data set is reviewed on a three-dimensional (3D) workstation where it is reconstructed as both VR and MIP images. Due to the intimate relationship of most vessels of interest with adjacent osseous structures, most workstations offer tools to selectively remove osseous structures while leaving the vessels of interest intact. The osseous structures are removed by a region-growing algorithm, which varies from vendor to vendor. The final reconstructions derived from VR and MIP reformations are generally captured in views that resemble traditional angiographic views (frontal and two oblique orientations) in order to facilitate easy interpretation for referring physicians. These images are then sent to a picture archiving communications system (PACS). Thick slices (2 mm) are also sent to the PACS system for review of the remainder of the chest.

CLINICAL APPLICATIONS

MDCT angiography to assess normal anatomy of the upper extremity

Anatomic assessment may be necessary for planning of surgical intervention or for endovascular access. The arterial

Table 10.2　Scanning protocols for CT angiography of the upper extremity

	Siemens		General Electric		Philips		Toshiba	
Detectors	16	32×2	16	64	16	64	16	64
mAs					250 mAs	250 mAs	200	SureExposure™
kV	120	120	120	120	120	120	120	120
Rotation time (s)	0.5	0.33	0.5	0.4	0.75	0.75	0.5	0.5
Detector collimation (mm)	0.75	0.6	0.625	0.625	0.75	0.625	0.5	0.5
Slice thickness (mm)	0.75	0.75	0.625	0.625	2.0	0.9	0.5	0.5
Translation speed (mm/s)[a]					19	63.0	15	41
Pitch[b]					1.188	1.175	0.938	0.641
Kernel/filter	B30f	B20f	Standard	Standard	Standard/B	Standard/B,C	FC10	FC81

[a]Table speed (Philips).
[b]Pitch = table feed per rotation/total width of the collimated beam.
Philips parameters provided by Don Boshela BS, RT(R) (CT), Senior CT Product Development, Specialist Philips Medical Systems.
Toshiba parameters provided by Toshiba America Medical Systems.
SUREExposure™ adjusts the tube current during scanning. Often reducing total dose by up to 40% per patient.

blood supply to the upper extremity originates from the subclavian arteries. The right subclavian artery arises off the brachiocephalic artery while the left subclavian artery is typically the third branch vessel off the aortic arch. The area from the aortic arch or the bifurcation of the brachiocephalic artery to the lateral aspect of the first rib defines the subclavian artery. The subclavian artery exits the thoracic cage between the anterior and middle scalene muscles and then passes between the clavicle and the first rib. The major branches off the subclavian artery include the internal mammary artery, the thyrocervical trunk, and the costocervical trunk. The subclavian artery becomes the axillary artery as it courses past the lateral aspect of the first rib. The branches of the axillary artery include the superior thoracic artery, the lateral thoracic artery, the thoracoacromial artery, the subscapular artery, and the circumflex humeral artery. Lateral to the teres major muscle, the axillary artery becomes the brachial artery. The first branch off the brachial artery is typically the profunda brachial artery. The terminal branches of the brachial artery include the radial, ulnar, and interosseus arteries (Figure 10.1). A common variant is a high origin of the radial artery off the brachial or axillary artery in up to 15% of cases (Figure 10.2).

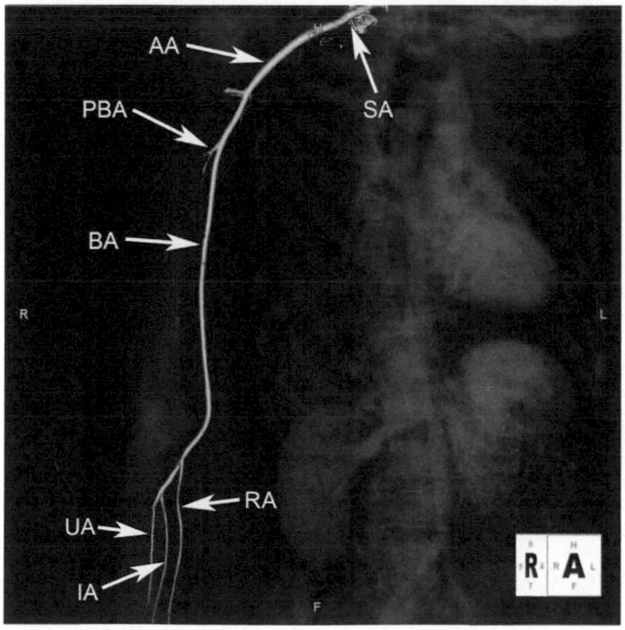

MDCT angiography to diagnose variant subclavian artery anatomy

Anatomic variations may impact clinical management of arterial pathology. CTA is excellent for delineating variant anatomy of the arch vessels including aberrant origins of the subclavian arteries. The most common variant encountered is an aberrant origin of the right subclavian artery in the setting of a normal left aortic arch. This variant is strongly correlated with dilatation of the origin of the aberrant right subclavian artery, also known as a diverticulum of Komerall. Similar abnormal anatomic relationships can be seen for the left subclavian artery (Figure 10.3).

MDCT angiography to diagnose subclavian artery stenosis

CTA can be employed for diagnosis and characterization of narrowing and occlusion of the subclavian artery.

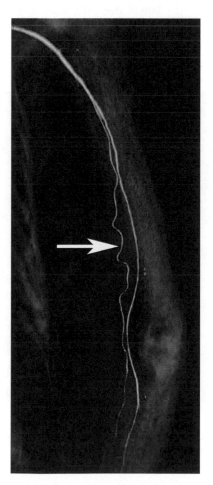

Figure 10.1 Normal anatomy. Three-dimensional CT volume-rendered image (right anterior oblique) shows the normal arterial vascular anatomy of the right upper extremity. SA, subclavian artery; AA, axillary artery; PBA, profunda brachial artery; BA, brachial artery; RA, radial artery; UA, ulnar artery; IA, interosseous artery.

Figure 10.2 Aberrant radial artery. Three-dimensional CT volume-rendered image (right anterior oblique view) shows an aberrant origin of the radial artery (arrow) from the midportion of the brachial artery.

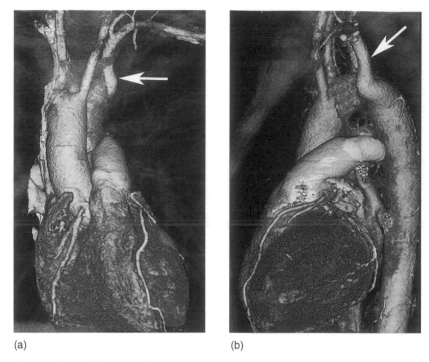

(a)   (b)

Figure 10.3 Right-sided aortic arch with an aberrant left subclavian artery. Three-dimensional CT volume-rendered images, anteroposterior (a) and lateral views (b), show a right-sided aortic arch. An aberrant origin of the left subclavian artery is also seen (arrow).

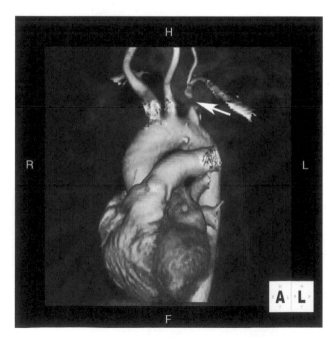

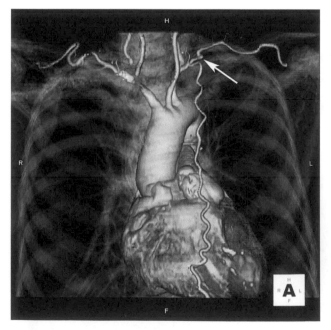

Figure 10.4 Left subclavian artery stenosis. Three-dimensional CT volume-rendered image (left anterior oblique view) shows a focal high-grade stenosis of the left subclavian artery (arrow) just distal to its origin.

Figure 10.5 Takayasu's arteritis. Three-dimensional CT volume-rendered image (anteroposterior view) shows occlusion of the left subclavian artery (arrow) with arterial collateralization.

Subclavian artery narrowing can occur from a number of etiologies. The most common etiology is atherosclerotic disease, which typically is an extension of atheroma from the aortic arch into the origins of the arch vessels (Figure 10.4). Vasculitis can also affect the subclavian artery, especially in young patients. Typical vasculitides that have a predilection for the subclavian artery include Takayasu's disease (Figure 10.5), which typically affects young women from Asia and Central and South America but is increasingly recognized in North America; giant cell arteritis, which typically affects women in their sixth and seventh decades; and radiation arteritis. Another uncommon cause is fibromuscular dysplasia. Most cases of subclavian artery stenosis have an asymptomatic course, and although arm claudication may occur, this is usually rare because of extensive collateral flow (Figure 10.5). A stenosis located proximal to the origin of the vertebral artery may cause flow reversal in the latter (subclavian steal). The combination of retrograde vertebral flow and neurologic symptoms (dizziness, vertigo, visual changes) triggered by exercise of the arm is known as subclavian steal syndrome.

MDCT angiography to diagnose subclavian artery aneurysm

CTA plays a role in the diagnosis and planning for repair of subclavian artery aneurysms. True aneurysms are rare and much less common than pseudoaneurysms. The most common causes are arteriosclerosis (Figure 10.6), thoracic outlet obstruction (a mechanical, post-stenotic dilation), post-traumatic (i.e. gun-shot, blunt trauma) and aberrant (malposition) right or left subclavian arteries, and miscellaneous.

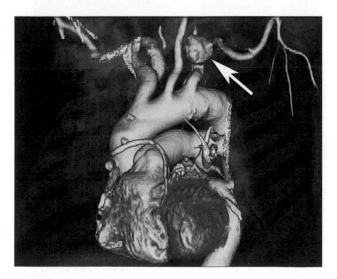

Figure 10.6 Left subclavian artery aneurysm. Three-dimensional CT volume-rendered image (left anterior oblique view) shows a focal aneurysm of the left subclavian artery (arrow).

Rare causes include syphilis, tuberculosis, and abnormalities of the vessel wall (fibromuscular dysplasia). In most cases an asymptomatic pulsatile mass is detected either above or below the clavicle (collar bone). Symptoms such as dysphagia (difficulty swallowing), stridor (difficulty breathing), chest pain, hoarseness, upper extremity fatigue, numbness/tingling, and gangrene or ulceration of the fingers may develop with progressive enlargement of the aneurysm. These result from compression of adjacent structures (i.e. nerves, veins, trachea, or esophagus), thromboembolism (blood clots breaking off from the wall of the aneurysm), or rupture into the soft tissues of the neck. With the relatively recent availability of covered stents to treat subclavian artery aneurysms, diagnosis with CTA has become the test of choice in order to facilitate treatment planning. CTA allows accurate measurements of the diameter and length of the segment to be treated so that the appropriate endograft can be chosen. CTA can also be utilized for post-intervention surveillance to assess for endoleaks or deformity of the device.

MDCT angiography to diagnose upper extremity ischemia

CTA can be readily used to assess the etiology and anatomic location of the ischemic upper extremity. Common causes include atherosclerotic disease (Figure 10.7), embolism, and vasculitis. Atherosclerotic disease can occur anywhere, but typically affects the larger arteries of the upper extremities including the brachial artery, unless the patient is diabetic or on hemodialysis in which case the arteries of the forearm and hand are typically affected. Embolism is another common cause of upper extremity ischemia and occurs typically from a cardiac source in a patient with atrial fibrillation, but also from a venous source in a patient with a right-to-left intracardiac shunt. Another common cause of upper extremity ischemia is embolism from a subclavian artery aneurysm in the setting of thoracic outlet syndrome. The natural progression of this disease is degeneration of the aneurysm, which forms mural thrombus and results in embolic events in the upper extremity. The most common presentation of these patients is a blue hand or finger(s). Other causes include hypercoagulable states due to abnormalities in coagulation pathways and with collagen vascular diseases such as SLE and scleroderma.

MDCT for evaluation of upper extremity trauma

It is estimated that the upper extremity is involved in up to 40% of extremity-penetrating trauma. Symptoms of extremity vascular injury include active arterial hemorrhage,

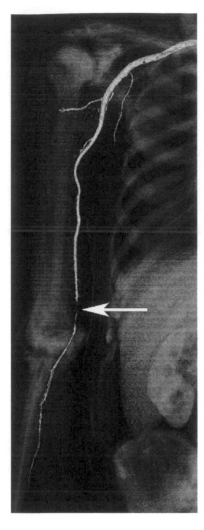

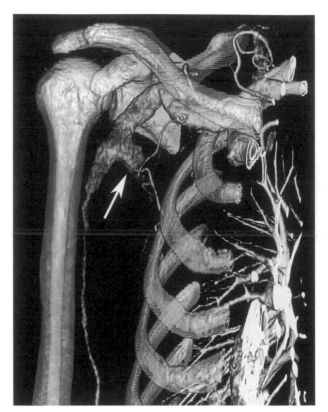

Figure 10.8 Right axillary artery pseudoaneurysm. Three-dimensional CT volume-rendered image (right anterior oblique view) of a 52-year-old male after stab injury to right axilla shows a large focal pseudoaneurysm originating from the right axillary artery (arrow).

Figure 10.7 Brachial artery stenosis. Three-dimensional CT volume-rendered image (anteroposterior view) shows a focal segment of severe narrowing at the distal brachial artery (arrow).

a thrill or bruit in the affected extremity, an expanding hematoma, acute extremity ischemia, or an asymmetric pulse deficit in the injured extremity. Trauma can also result in vascular spasm, an intimal tear, pseudoaneurysm (Figure 10.8), arteriovenous fistula, or occlusion. CTA offers a global non-invasive assessment of the trauma patient that can isolate an injury and help plan treatment.

MDCT angiography assessment for dialysis graft patency surveillance

A promising application for MDCT angiography is in the surveillance of hemodialysis access (fistulae or graft). Because the study is very rapid and there is no concern for the administration of iodinated contrast to this patient population, this modality offers a rapid, high spatial resolution study to assess for graft patency. The arterial inflow and

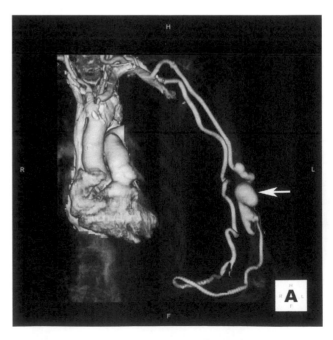

Figure 10.9 Arteriovenous graft pseudoaneurysm. Three-dimensional volume-rendered image (anteroposterior view) shows a large pseudoaneurysm (arrow) involving the venous anastomotic site.

venous outflow of the graft can be rapidly assessed in a matter of seconds and localize areas of stenosis (Figure 10.9). This surveillance can improve the safety of any surgical or endovascular revision, by assessing the entire graft and directing therapy at the area of abnormality, thus sparing the remainder of the graft from an invasive interrogation.

MDCT for surveillance following endovascular therapy

With the recent widespread application of endovascular therapy for arterial pathology, including atherosclerotic

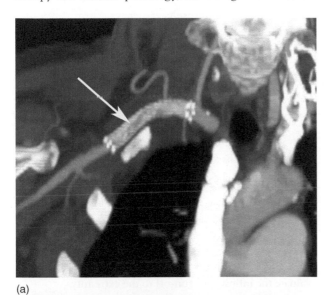

(a)

and aneurysmal disease, there is an increasing need to follow up these patients to assess for the durability of the repair. CTA offers an excellent option to monitor for the continued success of the procedure and can be used to assess for in-stent stenosis following bare metal stent therapy for atherosclerotic stenosis or occlusion (Figure 10.10). The areas of recurrent disease or intimal hyperplasia in the acute period following therapy appear as areas of low attenuation within the confines of the high attenuation metallic stent. An important technical issue to keep in mind is the metallic composition of the stent. Most commercially available stents are made of stainless steel and nitinol, which create minimal artifacts during CTA and allow for in-stent visualization. New stent designs include cobalt–chromium and platinum alloys, which are more radiopaque and may create more artifacts and prevent in-stent visualization.

The use of CTA is also helpful for the surveillance of patients following stent graft repair of peripheral aneurysms (Figure 10.11). CTA is very accurate at detecting endoleaks or incomplete exclusion of flow to the aneurysm sac (Figure 10.12). CTA can also detect deformity of the stent graft, which can lead to device failure in the future. Most importantly, CTA can assess for shrinkage of the aneurysm sac, which typically indicates successful treatment.

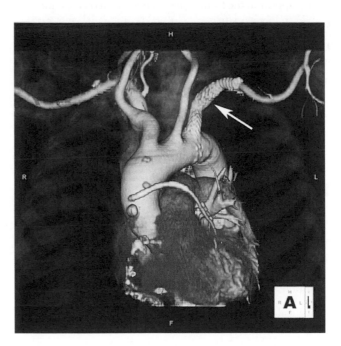

(b)

Figure 10.10 In-stent restenosis. (a) A slab MIP image shows a right subclavian artery stent with intraluminal low-density material (arrow). (b) Magnified thin section MIP image more clearly demonstrates the filling defect (arrow) within the mid-portion of the stent compatible with in-stent stenosis.

Figure 10.11 Left subclavian artery stent graft. Three-dimensional CT volume-rendered image (left anterior oblique view) shows a stent graft extending from the origin to the mid-portion of the left subclavian artery (arrow).

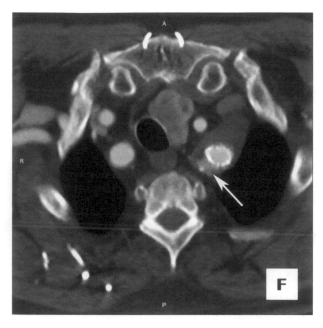

Figure 10.12 Endoleak. Conventional CT angiogram axial image shows a left subclavian artery stent graft with contrast seen outside the lumen of the stent (arrow) and within the subclavian aneurysm representing an endoleak.

PERFORMANCE

Unfortunately the clinical use of MDCT angiography for the evaluation of the upper extremity has been only recently reported. As a result there is a paucity of reported data, most of which appear in the form of abstracts presented at scientific meetings. In 2005, Hellinger et al reported on a single center experience in the use of MDCT angiography for the evaluation of upper extremity ischemia in 40 patients. Their group found the study to be diagnostic in all cases and to help guide treatment in over 80% of cases. With respect to the evaluation of trauma, CTA has similarly been shown to be highly accurate when compared to conventional angiography.

LIMITATIONS

The major limitations to this imaging modality for the evaluation of the arterial supply for the upper extremities are limitations in the performance of CTA in general. These include:

1. Motion artifacts related to patient motion.

2. Surgical or other foreign material resulting in artifact in the area of interest.

3. Inadequate vascular enhancement due to improper timing bolus or poor cardiac output.

4. Inadequate radiation penetration secondary to enlarged body habitus in incorrect scanner settings.

CONCLUSIONS

With the recent introduction of MDCT angiography for the evaluation of the peripheral circulation, there is no vascular territory that cannot be imaged. This has been extended to the upper extremity with a broad set of accepted clinical indications. While there is currently a paucity of reported data to validate the use of this modality, it is being used ever increasingly with excellent results.

PRACTICAL PEARLS

- To image the upper extremity, place the extremity of interest in a comfortable anatomic position at the patient's side. This allows for an acquisition that is similar to a standard chest, abdomen, and pelvis scan.

- Remember to place the intravenous access in the extremity that is not of clinical interest to prevent artifact from the injection bolus.

- Always image from the aortic arch to the fingertips to evaluate the inflow and run-off to the extremity.

FURTHER READING

Fleischmann D, Hallett RL, Rubin GD. CT angiography of peripheral arterial disease. J Vasc Interven Radiol 2006; 17(1): 3–26.

Hellinger JC, Frisoli JK, Sze DYH et al. Hemodialysis access evaluation: early experience with upper extremity multidetector-Row CT angiography. Society of Interventional Radiology, Phoenix, Arizona, 25–30, Mar 2004. J Vasc Interven Radiol 2004; 15(2): S252.

Hellinger JC, Napoli A, Schraedley-Desmond P et al. Multi-detector-row CT angiography of the upper extremity: comparison with digital subtraction angiography. Chicago, Illinois: Radiologic Society of North America, 1 Dec 2004.

Hellinger JC, Fleischmann D, Rubin GD. Evaluating upper extremity arterial disease with multidetector-row CT angiography. Experience in 40 examinations. Society of Interventional Radiology, New Orleans, Louisiana, 4, April 2005. J Vasc Interven Radiol 2005; 16(2): S59.

Soto JA, Munera F, Morales C et al. Focal arterial injuries of the proximal extremities: helical CT arteriography as the initial method of diagnosis. Radiology 2001; 218(1): 188–94.

11

CT angiography of the lower extremity circulation with protocols

Emil I Cohen, Amish Doshi, and Robert A Lookstein

INTRODUCTION

Invasive digital subtraction angiography is the traditional method by which disease of the lower extremities has been assessed, but it is an expensive and time-consuming procedure with a complication rate of approximately 2–3%. To avoid unnecessary invasive diagnostic procedures and to evaluate possible therapeutic options before an intervention, a non-invasive examination assessing the extent of disease in a patient presenting with lower extremity pathology is often indicated.

The introduction of 4-slice CT scanners in 1998 with a temporal resolution of 0.5 s enabled the use of multi-detector CT for vascular applications. Further advances in detector and gantry design led to the introduction of 8-, 16-, and 64-slice units into the clinical environment, with corresponding improvements in gantry rotation times and temporal resolution. The extended array of detectors in the z-axis has enabled rapid volume acquisition while improved x–y resolution in conjunction with thin collimation has enabled acquisition of images with submillimeter isotropic resolution.

The incremental gains in acquisition speed and spatial resolution have enabled the establishment of CT angiography (CTA) as a modality of choice in angiographic assessment of the lower extremities. Currently, CTA is invaluable in providing high-resolution visualization of the peripheral vessels including the capability to assess distal vessel disease. However, CTA is still limited in its ability to compensate for motion and beam hardening artifacts from densely calcified vessels.

The goal of this chapter is to provide the reader with a practical approach to perform quality CTA examinations of the lower extremity along with specific approaches to optimize imaging for the various clinical indications (Table 11.1). Additionally, the relative advantages and disadvantages of CTA and pearls and pitfalls for this specific clinical application will be discussed.

ANATOMIC CONSIDERATIONS

Figure 11.1 illustrates the normal anatomy of the lower extremity vessels. Typically, the anatomic area covered by most CTA studies in patients presenting with lower extremity

Table 11.1 Principal indications to lower extremity CTA

- Acute and chronic peripheral arterial disease
- Vasculitis
- Aneurysmal disease
- Post-intervention follow-up (e.g., graft, stent, prosthsis, etc.)
- Other indications (e.g., congenital abnormalities, trauma, arterio-venous malformations, neoplastic disorders, etc.)

symptoms includes the abdominal aorta, branches, pelvic vessels, and lower extremity vessels. The aorta and iliac arteries are also referred to as inflow vessels. The femoral and popliteal arteries are referred to as outflow vessels. The distal vessels include the tibial (anterior and posterior) and peroneal arteries.

Femoral arteries

The external iliac artery continues as the common femoral artery below the level of the inguinal ligament. The common femoral artery bifurcates into the superficial femoral and the profunda femoris (deep femoral). The profunda is an important source of collaterals to the lower extremity in the event of occlusion of the common or superficial arteries. The profunda has two important branches, the medial circumflex and the lateral circumflex branches. The medial branch, by anastomosing with the obturator and internal pudendal arteries of the internal iliac in the pelvis, may represent an important collateral source in the event of a common femoral occlusion. The lateral circumflex branch divides into the ascending and descending branches. The descending branch of the lateral circumflex often supplies collaterals to the thigh in the event of occlusion of the superficial femoral artery and anastomoses with the geniculate vessels.

Popliteal trifurcation

In most cases (>90%) the popliteal artery gives rise to the anterior tibial branch and the tibio-peroneal trunk below the level of the popliteus muscle, located well below the level of the knee joint. The tibio-peroneal trunk bifurcates into the common peroneal and the posterior tibial branch after traveling a short course. In the remaining cases anatomic variations such as absence of a tibio-peroneal trunk (true trifurcation), a short tibio-peroneal trunk, or high take-off of the anterior tibial or posterior tibial branches (at or above the level of the knee joint) may be seen. These variations, although not clinically relevant, may occasionally be significant in the event of revascularization procedures or surgery in the knee joint region.

Distal vessels in the lower extremities

In the normal adult, the anterior and posterior tibial arteries are the dominant vessels supplying the foot. The peroneal, although subject to much anatomic variation, is rarely

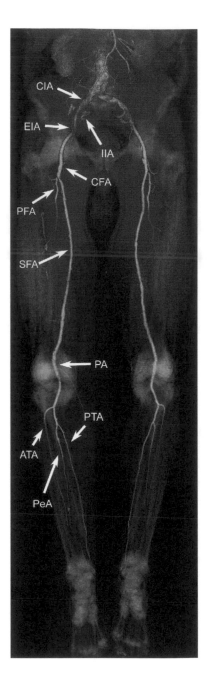

Figure 11.1 Vessels of the abdomen, pelvis, thighs, and legs. Three-dimensional CTA volume-rendered image (anteroposterior view) shows the normal arterial vascular anatomy. CIA, common iliac artery; EIA, external iliac artery; IIA, internal iliac artery; CFA, common femoral artery; PFA, profunda femoris artery; SFA, superficial femoral artery; PA, popliteal artery; PTA, posterior tibial artery; ATA, anterior tibial artery; PeA, peroneal artery.

absent and represents an important source of collaterals in the event of an arterial occlusion. The anterior tibial and posterior tibial may be absent or terminate early in about 2% and 5% of cases, respectively. The peroneal artery ends by giving rise to the anterior and posterior perforating branches (4–6 cm above the level of the ankle) and supplies collaterals in the event of occlusion of the other vessels. The posterior tibial ends by dividing into the lateral and medial plantar branches while the anterior tibial ends by dividing into the arcuate and the deep plantar branches. The arcuate branch gives rise to the dorsal metatarsal branches while the deep plantar branch joins the lateral plantar branch of the posterior tibial to constitute the plantar arch.

CLINICAL PRESENTATION OF LOWER EXTREMITY ARTERIAL DISEASE

Peripheral arterial disease (PAD), which is caused by atherosclerotic stenosis of the arteries to the legs, is an important manifestation of systemic atherosclerosis. With a prevalence in North America and Europe estimated at approximately 27 million people (16% of the population 55 years and older), it is an important public health issue. Advanced age, smoking, and diabetes are the atherosclerotic risk factors with the strongest association with PAD, and intermittent claudication, defined as pain in the muscles of the calf or thigh with ambulation, is the earliest and the most frequent presenting symptom. As the disease evolves in severity, patients might have pain at rest and, in the late stages, the hypoperfusion of the skin and the skeletal muscles progresses to ischemic ulceration and gangrene. Major amputation is a concrete risk for this last category of patients, but in the general PAD population the risk of limb loss is overshadowed by the risk of cardiovascular and cerebrovascular events (including myocardial infarction, stroke, and death). However, signs of chronic PAD can be frequently subtle and may only include diminished pulses in the lower extremity. For the diagnosis, the measurement of the Doppler ankle brachial index (ABI) is a simple, non-invasive method used to rule out the presence of PAD (ABI < 0.9). To assess the functional involvement in patients with PAD, one of the most standardized tests is the 6-minute walk test measuring the distance traveled. If necessary, CTA (or MR angiography, MRA) may then be obtained to better elucidate the extent and severity of the vascular disease burden and to plan treatment.

Acute limb ischemia has a typical clinical presentation constituted by the '5Ps' (pallor, pain, pulselessness, paresthesias, and paralysis). In individuals without prior history of PAD, the etiologies usually include embolism, trauma, and dissection. In individuals with prior surgical intervention, graft or stent occlusion due to thrombosis may present with symptoms of acute limb ischemia. In this case, usually the severity of the clinical presentation guides the physician to the diagnosis and invasive catheterization of the lower extremity arteries is directly indicated in the majority of cases.

PROTOCOL CONSIDERATIONS

Although there are numerous multi-detector CT scanners available on the market, to obtain a study capable of adequately assessing the distal vessels in the lower extremities, which are on the order of 1–3 mm in diameter, a minimal detector collimation of 1–2 mm is necessary. Typically, ≥ 8-detector scanners are used, but 4-slice CT scanners are also able to produce images of sufficient quality. On the current scanners, a submillimeter in-plane resolution for peripheral CTA may be obtained in most patients of normal stature.

The patient is placed feet first and supine on the scanner table, with feet and ankle joints in neutral position. The typical field-of-view (FOV) extends from the lower thorax (diaphragm) to the toes, with an average scan length of 110–130 cm. A scanning protocol for peripheral CTA should always include (1) a scout image, (2) a test bolus or bolus triggering acquisition (based on the operator's preference), and (3) CTA acquisition during the arterial contrast phase. A second late CTA acquisition of the distal territories may be prescribed in case of inadequate pedal opacification during the arterial CTA. An entire peripheral CTA study may be easily performed in 10–15 minutes.

Acquisition parameters

The selection of the specific acquisition parameters depends on the employed scanner model. In general, acquisition parameters for peripheral CTA are not significantly different from the ones used for abdominal CTA (Table 11.2). A tube voltage of 120 kV and a tube amperage of 200–250 mAs (milli Ampere seconds) adjustable based on the patient's body size, are generally used. Breath holding is requested only for the first segment (abdomen/pelvis) of the image acquisition.

In multi-detector CT spiral scans, the volume coverage speed (v, cm/s) can be estimated by the following formula:

$$v = \frac{M s_{coll} p}{t_{rot}}$$

where M = number of simultaneous acquired slices, s_{coll} = collimated slice width, p = pitch, and t_{rot} = gantry rotation time.

Table 11.2 Scanning protocols for the lower extremities

	Siemens		General Electric		Philips		Toshiba	
Detectors	16	32×2	16	64	16	64	16	64
mAs	150	250	380 mA	Smart mA	250 mAs	250 mAs	350 mA	250 mA
kV	120	120	140	140	120	120	120	120
Rotation time (s)	0.5	0.33	0.5	0.5	0.75	1.0	0.5	0.5
Detector collimation (mm)	0.75	0.6	1.25	0.625	0.75	0.625	0.5	0.5
Slice thickness (mm)	1	0.75	1.25	0.625	2.0	1.0	0.5	0.5, 1.0
Translation speed (mm/s)			27.5		19	47.0	23	53
Table speed (Philips)								
Pitch[a]	1	0.6	1.375	1.375	1.188	1.175	1.438	0.828
Kernel/filter	B30f	B30f	Standard	Standard	Standard/B	Standard/C	FC10	FC30

[a] Pitch=table feed per rotation/total width of the collimated beam.
Philips parameters provided by Don Boshela BS, RT(R) (CT), Senior CT Product Development Specialist, Philips Medical Systems.
Toshiba parameters provided by Toshiba America Medical Systems.

By considering the formula reported above, it is evident that volume coverage can be increased by singularly or concomitantly changing the various scanner parameters (i.e., wider s_{coll}, shorter$_{rot}$, higher p and larger M). With current multi-slice CT, volume coverage speed may be too fast for an adequate visualization of contrast in the entire lower extremity vascular tree, especially in patients with significant stenotic lesions. For instance, a 64-slice scanner ($M=64$), with 0.625 mm collimation, pitch of 1.375, and gantry rotation time of 0.5, scan be as fast as 110 mm/s. Such a coverage speed poses a considerable danger of 'out running' the bolus when the table moves faster than the contrast medium bolus. It has been shown that consistently good results in peripheral CTA can be achieved if maximum acquisition speed does not exceed 30 mm/s. With a 4-slice scanner, a beam collimation of 4 × 2.5 mm, a pitch of 1.5, and 0.5 s gantry rotation time would provide a volume coverage speed of 30 mm/s. With a 16-slice scanner, a volume coverage speed of 28.8 mm/s is obtained with 16 × 0.75 mm beam collimation at 0.5 s gantry rotation time and pitch of 1.2. The 64-slice scanners (64 × 0.6 mm detector configuration with Siemens scanners) have to be slowed down even more by choosing longer rotation times or by reducing the pitch to values below 1. A suitable protocol for a 64-slice CT scanner includes 0.5 s gantry rotation time and pitch 0.8 for a volume coverage speed of 30.7 mm/s. A system with 64 × 0.625 mm collimation (GE scanners) has to be operated at a slower gantry rotation time of 0.7 s and a pitch of 0.5625 to achieve a volume coverage speed of 32 mm/s.

Contrast injection

Intravenous contrast medium is injected by using a power injection into an antecubital vein (20–22 gauge cannula). The time the contrast takes to travel from the injection site to the aorta (transit time) is variable between patients. The individual transit time may be measured in the single patient by using a small test bolus injection, or it may be estimated by using an automated bolus triggering technique. In addition, the transit time of intravenous contrast agents traveling from the aorta to the popliteal artery has also been shown to vary significantly between patients in relation to the severity of atherosclerotic disease. Empirically, a contrast bolus length of at least 30 s should be used to enable all patients to be imaged.

In our institute, we utilize a protocol in which the patient is scanned from the dome of the diaphragm to the feet, with the scan parameters being adjusted so that the scan duration is approximately 35 s. Obviously, the use of a 64-detector system should be preferred whenever possible to achieve a higher slice resolution.

When the bolus chase technique is employed, 100–120 ml of contrast (with an iodine concentration between 320 and 370 mg/ml) are administered at a rate of 4 ml/s. When an automated bolus detection algorithm is used, the region of interest is set up in the aorta immediately below the level of the diaphragm. A repetitive monitor acquisition (120 kV, 10 mAs, 1 s interscan delay) is started

10 s after contrast injection begins. The actual peripheral CTA acquisition is then started when the contrast enhancement reaches a prespecified level (typically set between 150 and 200 Hounsfield units (HU). In general, the use of 370 mg/ml contrast agents yields excellent results. Several authors have utilized lower iodine concentrations with equally good results, but some of them have utilized a higher flow rate to compensate for the lower iodine concentration. The use of a higher iodine concentration also allows for a lower injection rate when a standard 20 gauge IV access cannot be obtained. In this case, the flow rate has to be decreased to 3–3.5 ml/s, but the higher iodine concentration will continue to yield good results.

Reconstruction parameters

With peripheral CTA, the modern scanners can easily yield well over a thousand high-resolution images per examination. A modern workstation is capable of numerous tasks, but the most common is to provide post-processed images that fulfill the purpose of rapid and accurate image review.

A medium-to-soft reconstruction kernel is generally applied for image reconstruction in peripheral CTA. The image formats most favored for assessment of peripheral vessels are no different from other applications and include transverse source images, volume rendering (VR), shaded surface rendering (SSR), maximum intensity projection (MIP), multi-planar reformation (MPR), and curved planar reformatted (CPR) images. Chapter 4 provides additional details on these various image formats.

Review of transverse CT images is always mandatory for the assessment of extravascular processes. For this purpose, contiguous 5 mm slices may be reconstructed to allow a rapid review of the entire scanned image volume.

MIP images are formed by projecting the highest pixel values in a slab of data onto a two-dimensional (2D) image. This technique resembles digital subtraction angiography except that calcified plaques are also visualized and can obscure images. In VR images, trapezoids are used to convey the complete data set of 3D information by utilizing shading of the pixels. Due to the intimate relation of most vessels of interest with adjacent osseous structures most workstations offer tools to selectively remove these structures while leaving the vessels of interest intact. The osseous structures are removed by a region-growing algorithm, which varies from vendor to vendor. The final product from VR and MIP images is generally captured to resemble a traditional angiographic examination by displaying each region (abdomen, pelvis, thigh, and distal vessels) in a frontal and two oblique orientations. VR and MIP images have unique advantages and disadvantages. VR images are more pleasing to the eye and provide a 3D representation of anatomy. MIP images lack a 3D quality, but allow differentiation of calcified plaques and stents from the adjacent dense contrast, which can be hard to separate on a VR image. Unfortunately, vessel calcification and stents completely obscure the vessel lumen in both VR and MIP images.

MPR and CPR images can partially help to overcome these issues by further elucidating the anatomy of a tortuous vessel or a complex stenosis (especially in the presence of calcification or stent) and aid in quantification of the area of narrowing. In a busy practice, it is advisable to hire dedicated imaging technicians, who aid in the reconstruction of raw data. These technicians must have a firm knowledge of anatomy and be aware of common therapeutic options.

Reporting and archiving

Considering the large number of images produced by a lower extremity CTA, data from submillimeter acquisitions are frequently used to reconstruct data sets with an increased section thickness. Generally, two data sets are obtained from each CTA examination, a set of 'thick' slices for the general assessment of organs and osseous structures (5.0 mm section thickness) and a set of 'thin' images for post-processing (0.6–0.75 mm section thickness). The high-resolution slices should contain at least a 25% overlap for improved end results subsequent to processing.

A systematic approach is required for a comprehensive yet easily comprehensible report. At our institution, evaluation is commenced with careful attention to the organs and viscera of the abdomen and pelvis. Comments about the presence or absence of a normal appearance to the abdominal organs which are completely visualized on a CT examination are necessary, as incidental findings are routinely present and may have serious implications. The vessels are assessed with respect to the direction of arterial flow. Stenoses, when present, are commented on and described in terms of location, extension, and severity. Additional findings including the presence of aneurysm, dissection, thrombus, calcification, or ulceration are noted.

The storage of the large amount of data generated by these studies is an ongoing problem. While at our institution we store all data generated by our scans except for the raw data, other institutions primarily store the reconstructed images from the higher resolution images and the thicker reconstructions to alleviate storage demands. Fortunately, this issue is less of a problem in the current market where storage prices continue to decrease.

CLINICAL APPLICATIONS

Acute and chronic atherosclerotic disease

Atherosclerotic PAD is the commonest indication for CTA evaluation. PAD (defined as abnormal ABI < 0.9) is present in up to 25% of individuals above the age of 70 years. There is a strong predilection to affect older individuals. Other risk factors include smoking, diabetes mellitus, and hypercholesterolemia. Several conditions other than atherosclerosis may present with symptoms that mimic the latter. These include congenital and acquired coarctation of the aorta, endovascular fibrosis of the external iliac artery (iliac artery syndrome in cyclists), fibromuscular dysplasia, popliteal cyst, cystic medial disease, popliteal entrapment, collagen vascular disease (pseudoxanthoma elasticum and Marfans's syndrome), and inflammatory arteritis (Taka-yasu's disease and thromboangioitis obliterans – Buerger's disease). All these entities need to be identified and differentiated from atherosclerosis for appropriate therapeutic planning.

The goal of CTA in PAD is to determine the length, number, severity, and location of stenoses. In conjunction with the patient's manifestations, activity status, and goals, findings on CTA may help determine choice of therapy (conservative, interventional, or surgical). Data from a CTA can help plan the percutaneous access route as well as the equipment that will be necessary for endovascular repair. CTA is equally useful for surgical planning as it can define proximal and distal anastomotic sites, concomitant disease processes (e.g., aneurysm, dissection, etc.) and sizing of prostheses/stents. Atherosclerotic disease affecting the inflow vessels (Figure 11.2) will often be treated by catheter-based therapy, with good results and little morbidity. Often the success of therapy, whether surgical or endovascular, depends on the extent of disease in the vessels distal to the area of disease and/or the presence of diabetes. The diabetic patient will often have more severe distal disease and may require bypass grafting. CTA assessment of the degree of stenosis in the distal vessels in this group is often limited if dense calcifications are present (Figure 11.3).

CTA may also be employed in the setting of acute lower extremity ischemia. Thromboembolic disease typically presents as an acute condition and must be treated on an emergency basis. Judicious use of CTA is required, as a delay in therapy can have serious consequences for the patient. In general, if the lower extremity is clinically deemed viable, CTA can aid in the assessment of the degree and extent of occlusion as well as elucidate possible embolic sources. In general, the presence of collateral vessels can aid in differentiating an acute versus chronic occlusion (Figure 11.4). However, unnecessary delay related to the performance of any diagnostic test should be avoided in the attempt to increase the chances of successfully re-establishing perfusion to the affected leg.

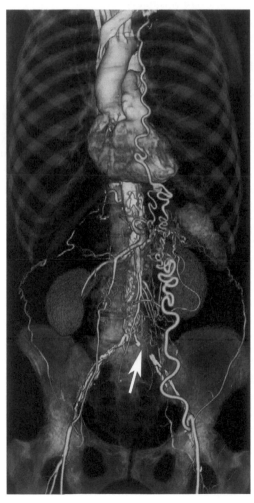

Figure 11.2 Left common iliac artery occlusive disease. Three-dimensional CTA volume-rendered image (antero-posterior view) shows complete occlusion of the left common iliac artery (arrow). Severe narrowing of the right common iliac artery is also noted. There is reconstitution of the bilateral common femoral arteries via collateral arterial pathways.

Vasculitis

Takayasu's arteritis generally affects the aorta and visceral vessels. The disease predominantly involves the media and it is rare for the disease to extend to the iliac vessels and the lower

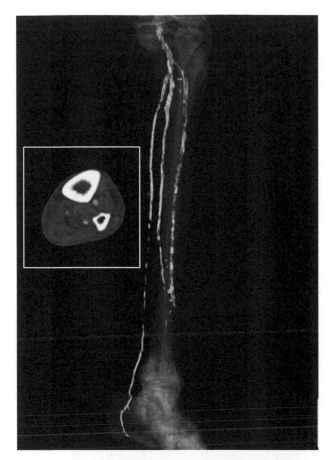

Figure 11.3 Distal lower extremity atherosclerotic disease. Three-dimensional CTA volume-rendered image (right anterior oblique) shows severe three-vessel atherosclerotic disease of the leg. Axial CTA image (inset) shows calcification within the walls of the anterior tibial, posterior tibial, and peroneal arteries with poor luminal visualization.

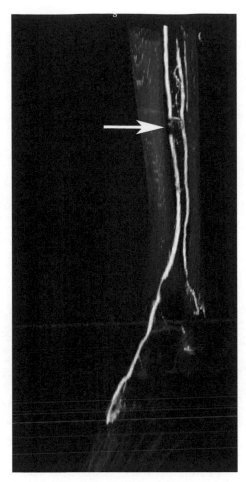

Figure 11.4 Occlusive disease. Three-dimensional CTA volume-rendered image (left anterior oblique view) shows a segmental occlusion of the anterior tibial artery (arrow) with small bridging collateral arteries.

extremities. It affects young female patients and manifests as wall thickening of the aorta, with associated narrowing, stenosis, and occlusions (Figure 11.5). The extent of contrast enhancement of the thickened wall has been correlated with the degree of acute inflammation although this could represent a non-specific finding.

Buerger's disease typically affects the small-to-medium sized arteries of the extremities. It manifests angiographically as a 'corkscrew' appearance in the distal arteries (this is, however, not typical for this disorder) and, clinically, the patient can present with claudication (predominantly foot or calf claudication), with or without ulcerations of the digits. Buerger's disease is strongly associated with smoking and a smoking cessation program has been shown to halt or dramatically slow down the progression of the disease.

Giant cell arteritis presents in older patients and classically affects medium sized vessels. It can involve the great vessels off the arch as well as the lower extremity vessels. It can present in a fashion similar to Takayasu's arteritis, but

the patient's age and the pattern of the diseased vessels will aid in differentiation (Figure 11.6).

Polyarteritis nodosa typically presents with non-specific vascular symptoms and is strongly associated with hepatitis B infection. When vascular involvement is present it is usually restricted to the visceral vessels, but clinically the patient can present with microvascular PAD and bilaterally symmetric gangrene.

Drug-induced vasculitis is often seen in patients engaged in recreational drug use as well as patients on clinically indicated therapy. The drugs most often associated with vasculitis are amfetamine derivatives and cocaine. Vasculitis can also be a side-effect of some drugs including ephedrine and L-dopa. These patients usually present with vascular stenosis without significant atherosclerotic plaque burden and are often of a younger age. The small-to-medium sized vessels are typically affected. CTA is particularly useful in this patient group as it allows for accurate assessment of vessel wall thickness and inflammation.

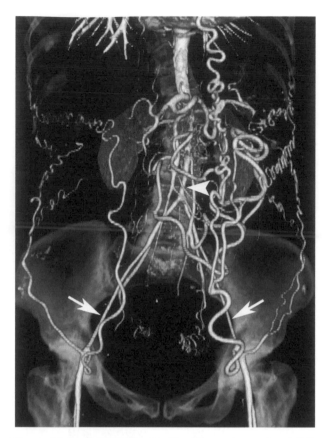

Figure 11.5 Takayasu's arteritis. Three-dimensional CTA volume-rendered image (anteroposterior view) shows circumferential severe narrowing of the distal abdominal aorta (arrowhead), and the common iliac and external iliac arteries bilaterally (arrows). Multiple collateral vessels can be appreciated.

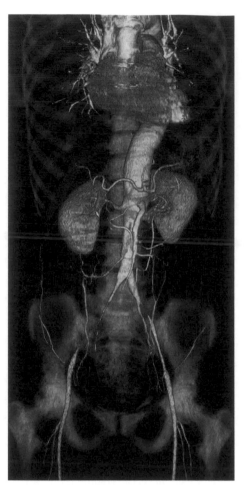

Figure 11.6 Giant cell arteritis. Three-dimensional CTA volume-rendered image (anteroposterior view) shows occlusion of the bilateral common iliac arteries and the proximal portion of the right external iliac artery.

Aneurysms

CTA may be indicated for the detection as well as the follow-up of patients with peripheral aneurysms, being useful in the assessment of aneurysm location, number, size, and complications (e.g., thrombosis, rupture, distal embolization, etc.). Aneurysms of the lower extremity vasculature are a frequent complication of atherosclerotic or inflammatory disease. The most frequent site of extra-aortic aneurysms is in the popliteal region (Figure 11.7), but they can also involve other vascular territories (Figure 11.8) and are frequently bilateral (Figure 11.9).

Therapy is usually indicated if the aneurysm exceeds 2 cm and/or there is mural thrombus. As the popliteal region is difficult to dissect without significant damage to adjacent structures, the usual course of therapy is to bypass the affected region, usually with a saphenous vein graft. Preventive measures may also be pursued if the vessels distal to the aneurysm are diseased and thereby increase the risk of eventual thrombosis.

Bypass graft and endovascular stent evaluation

There is a high rate of graft failure of up to 30% in the first 2 years, which in part is dependent on graft type (vein or artificial material) and/or length and status of distal run-off vessels. In general, autologous venous grafting yields far better results than synthetic grafts and above the knee grafts perform better than below knee locations. Surveillance of grafts is important and is primarily performed by sonographic evaluation. In the event of questionable graft failures or stenosis a peripheral CTA may add significant additional information (Figures 11.10 and 11.11). Graft complications also include aneurysms (frequently involving the anastomotic segment) and pseudoaneurysm formations, which can also be diagnosed using CTA.

Endovascular therapy with stent placement needs frequent follow-up to assure proper patency. While this can usually be performed with ultrasound, evaluation for in-stent

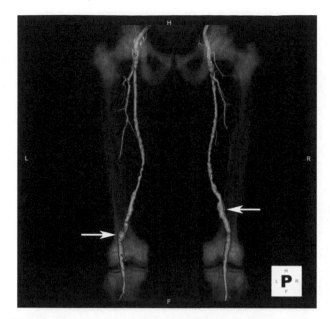

Figure 11.7 Bilateral popliteal artery aneurysms. Three-dimensional CTA volume-rendered image (posteroanterior view) shows focal aneurysmal dilatation of the bilateral popliteal arteries (arrows).

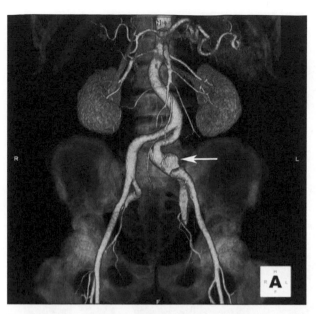

Figure 11.8 Left common iliac artery aneurysm. Three-dimensional CTA volume-rendered image (anteroposterior view) shows a focal aneurysmal dilatation of the distal portion of the left common iliac artery (arrow).

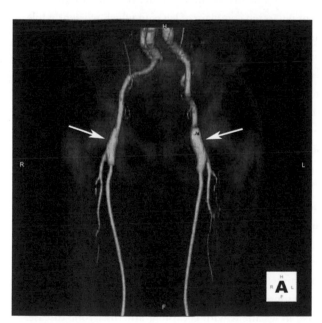

Figure 11.9 Bilateral common femoral artery aneurysms. Three-dimensional CTA volume-rendered image (antero-posterior view) shows aneurysms of the common femoral arteries bilaterally, extending to the origins of the superficial femoral arteries (arrows).

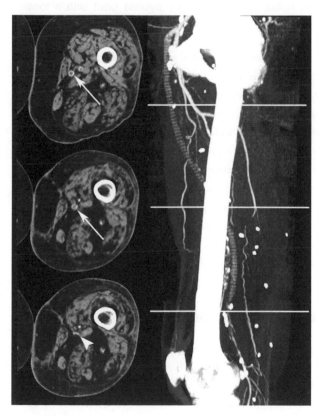

Figure 11.10 Femoral popliteal arterial bypass graft failure with collapse at distal anastomosis. Maximum-intensity projection (MIP) image with corresponding contrast-enhanced axial CT images shows the course of an occluded femoral popliteal artery bypass graft. Collapse of the bypass graft (arrowshead) is visualized.

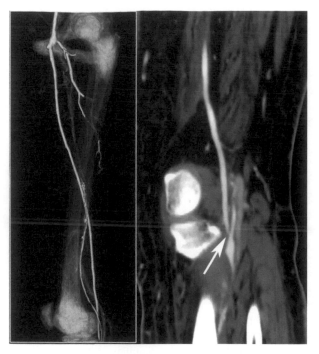

Figure 11.11 Femoral popliteal artery bypass graft with distal anastomotic stenosis. Three-dimensional CTA volume-rendered image (right image, lateral view) and curved plane reformatted (CPR) image (left image) show a patent femoral popliteal artery bypass graft with a focal high-grade stenosis seen at the distal anastomosis (arrow).

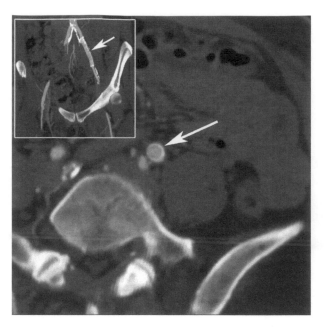

Figure 11.12 Evaluation of stent graft repair. Axial and curved planar reformatted (CPR, inset) images from a peripheral CTA show a left common iliac artery stent (arrows). Axial image allows for evaluation of the in-stent lumen.

stenosis is sometimes required in areas which are difficult to assess. There is little literature on this topic, but recent research has indicated that stents composed of nitinol demonstrate less artifactual luminal narrowing than their stainless steel counterparts. Additionally, stents with wider diameters also lead to less artifactual narrowing (Figure 11.12). There is currently no prospective or accumulated retrospective published experience evaluating peripheral stents. From clinical experience, CTA has a good negative predictive value for in-stent stenosis, but its specificity for the degree of narrowing is lacking. When the radiation dose is not prohibitive, increasing the tube current can reduce the metallic artifact.

Other indications

A variety of other conditions may represent less common indications for a peripheral CTA. For instance, arterio-venous malformations and fistulas may be well delineated by acquiring CTA images during the arterial phase and, later, during the venous phase. In other cases, CTA may help in the delineation of the arterial supply and degree of hypervascularity of soft tissue or osseous neoplasms involving the lower extremities.

CTA imaging may significantly contribute to the characterization of congenital abnormalities with direct or indirect

involvement of the peripheral vessels. The persistent sciatic artery, for instance, represents a rare congenital disorder in which the thigh and popliteal arteries derive their blood supply predominantly from the internal iliac artery (Figure 11.13). The native superficial femoral artery, although present, will frequently occlude within the mid thigh. The patient will often complain of leg pain which worsens while sitting. Another congenital condition may lead to the popliteal entrapment syndrome. The presence of occlusive disease in a young patient with no significant past medical history of vascular disease, particularly with symptoms in the calf region, should alert the clinician to the possible presence of a congenital abnormality of migration of the medial head of the gastrocnemius muscle and the subsequent deviation and/or occlusion of the popliteal artery (Figure 11.14).

Vascularized free flaps are increasingly utilized in reconstructive surgery since their introduction in the mid 1970s. A common site of harvesting is the lower extremity in which the peroneal artery is removed along with a fibular flap. Knowledge of the presence of disease in the lower extremity before surgery is critical since the peroneal artery is not a significant source of blood supply in the normal population, but can be, in a patient with coexistent atherosclerotic disease. In general, a lower extremity is chosen for harvesting if removal of the peroneal artery does not compromise the blood supply to the foot. A recent study demonstrated that CTA is well suited for this assessment.

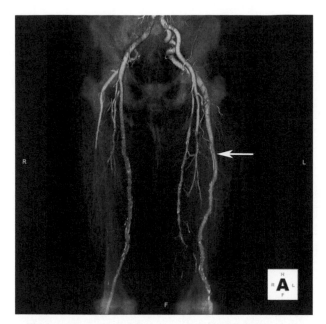

Figure 11.13 Persistent sciatic artery. Three-dimensional CTA volume-rendered image (anteroposterior view) shows occlusion of the distal left superficial femoral artery. The left popliteal artery is supplied by a persistent left sciatic artery fed by the internal iliac artery (arrow).

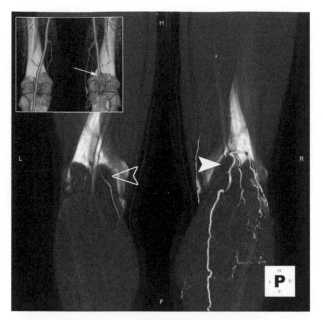

Figure 11.14 Popliteal artery entrapment. Three-dimensional CTA volume-rendered image (posteroanterior view) of a young patient with right calf pain on exertion. The medial head of the right gastrocnemius muscle demonstrates an abnormal origin lateral to the popliteal artery (closed arrowhead). Inset image shows complete occlusion of the right popliteal artery (arrow) with multiple superficial collateral arteries originating just proximal to this level. The normal origin of the medial head of the left gastrocnemius medial to the popliteal artery (open arrowhead) is shown for comparison.

PERFORMANCE OF CTA IN CLINICAL PRACTICE

Peripheral CTA is widely employed for the evaluation of patients with suspected vascular disease of the lower extremity vessels. This modality is broadly available and allows the generation of high-resolution images in a quick scanning session.

The introduction of CTA for peripheral vessel imaging is relatively recent and only a few studies have been devoted to the evaluation of its diagnostic accuracy and the majority of them are based on the use of 4-slice CT scanners. Nevertheless, when compared to invasive angiography, CTA has excellent overall sensitivity and specificity in detecting significant stenotic lesions involving the peripheral arteries. Generally, better results both in terms of accuracy and reproducibility have been reported in the evaluation of iliac and femoro-popliteal arteries compared with the more distal territories. The use of faster scanners (16- and 64-slice) seems to provide a more homogeneous performance throughout the lower extremity arterial tree.

Peripheral CTA is able to provide similar diagnostic performance when compared to MRA and, in general the use of these modalities may depend on institutional preferences and/or availability of these modalities. The preference for one modality over the other in the single patient, if both were available would have to be based on the consideration of respective advantages and disadvantages (Table 11.3).

PITFALLS

When interpreting peripheral CTA images it is crucial to evaluate the images, while keeping in mind the corresponding clinical context and the potential therapeutic options.

The most frequent pitfall encountered during the interpretation of CTA images is represented by the difficulty in the evaluation of vascular segments affected by moderate-to-severe calcification or occupied by a stent. Selection of an adequate windowing set (~1500 window width) may help to reduce the unavoidable blooming effect produced by structures with high signal attenuation. Cross-sectional MPR images of the vessel of interest are very helpful in visualizing, at least in part, the underlying lumen in the presence of intense calcification or stent.

Other interpretation pitfalls such as pseudostenoses or pseudo-occlusions may potentially be generated by inadequate image post-processing (e.g., partial or total vessel removal during MIP image editing, inaccurate centerline definition in CPR images, etc.).

Table 11.3 Relative advantages and disadvantages of CTA and MR angiography (MRA) for the evaluation of peripheral arteries

CTA	MRA
Advantages	Advantages
• Short scanning time	• Good contrast safety profile
• Low operator dependency	• Optimal delineation of vessel wall
• Widespread availability	• Dynamic flow information (phase-contrast, time-resolved imaging)
Disadvantages	Disadvantages
• Radiation exposure	• Technically challenging
• Contrast nephrotoxicity	• Contraindication in patients with metallic implants
• Reduced accuracy in calcified vessels	• Tendency to overestimate stenosis severity

CONCLUSIONS

The continued evolution of CT technology and its application for the diagnosis of diseases of the lower extremities is gaining stature, with publications of clinical studies documenting its accuracy when compared with other modalities. CTA is routinely used in clinical practice and rivals MRA for the non-invasive evaluation of vascular disease. The high in-plane and z-axis spatial resolution of CTA in conjunction with rapid throughput and easy standardizability has enabled its widespread incorporation. Continued areas of limitation include assessment of severely calcified segments and evaluation of in-stent stenosis.

PRACTICAL PEARLS

- Complete the examination in 35 s whenever possible to maintain arterial enhancement and to avoid venous contamination.

- Use a narrow field-of-view to better assess diseased areas.

- Use contrast dosing at between 1 and 1.5 g iodine/s, based on contrast iodine concentration.

- Always examine the source data to increase diagnostic sensitivity.

FURTHER READING

Bron KM. Femoral arteriography In: Abrams HL eds. Abrams Angiography: Vascular and Interventional Radiology 3rd ed. Boston, MA: Little Brown 1983; 1835–76.

Chow LC, Napoli A, Klein MB, Chang J, Rubin GD. Vascular mapping of the leg with multi-detector row CT angiography prior to free-flap transplantation. Radiology 2005 Oct; 237(1): 353–60.

Edwards AJ, Wells IP, Roobottom CA. Multi-detector row CT angiography of the lower limb arteries: a prospective comparison of volume-rendered techniques and intra-arterial digital subtraction angiography. Clin Radiol 2005 Jan; 60(1): 85–95.

Fleischmann D, Rubin GD. Quantification of intravenously administered contrast medium transit through the peripheral arteries: implications for CT angiography. Radiology 2005 Sep; 236(3): 1076–82.

Fleischmann D, Hallett RL, Rubin GD. CT angiography of peripheral arterial disease. J Vasc Interven Radiol 2006; 17(1): 3–26.

Herzog C, Grebe C, Mahnken A et al. Peripheral artery stent visualization and in-stent stenosis analysis in 16-row computed tomography: an in-vitro evaluation. Eur Radiol 2005 Nov; 15(11): 2276–83.

Lawrence JA, Kim D, Kent KC et al. Lower extremity spiral CT angiography versus catheter angiography. Radiology 1995; 194(3): 903–8.

Martin ML, Tay KH, Flak B et al. Multi-detector CT angiography of the aortoiliac system and lower extremities: a prospective comparison with digital subtraction angiography. AJR 2003; 180(4): 1085–91.

Mesurolle B, Qanadli SD, El Hajjam M, Goeau-Brissonniere OA, Mignon F, Lacombe P. Occlusive arterial disease of abdominal aorta and lower extremities: comparison of helical CT angiography with transcatheter angiography. Clin Imag 2004; 28(4): 252–60.

Ofer A, Nitecki SS, Linn S et al. Multidetector CT angiography of peripheral vascular disease: a prospective comparison with intraarterial digital subtraction angiography. AJR 2003; 180: 719–24.

Ota H, Takase K, Igarashi K et al. MDCT compared with digital subtraction angiography for assessment of lower extremity arterial occlusive disease: importance of reviewing cross-sectional images. AJR 2004; 182: 201–9.

Ouwendijk R, de Vries M, Pattynama PM et al. Imaging peripheral arterial disease: a randomized controlled trial comparing contrast-enhanced MR angiography and multi-detector row CT angiography. Radiology 2005 Sep; 236(3): 1094–103.

Rubin GD, Shiau MC, Leung AN, Kee ST, Logan LJ, Sofilos MC. Aorta and iliac arteries: single versus multiple detector-row helical CT angiography. Radiology 2000 Jun; 215(3): 670–6.

Rubin GD, Schmidt AJ, Logan LJ, Sofilos MC. Multi-detector row CT angiography of lower extremity arterial inflow and runoff: initial experience. Radiology 2001 Oct; 221(1): 146–58.

Willmann JK, Mayer D, Banyai M et al. Evaluation of peripheral arterial bypass grafts with multi-detector row CT angiography: comparison with duplex US and digital subtraction angiography. Radiology 2003 Nov; 229(2): 465–74.

Willmann JK, Baumert B, Schertler T et al. Aortoiliac and lower extremity arteries assessed with 16-detector row CT angiography: prospective comparison with digital subtraction angiography. Radiology 2005; 236: 1083–93.

Wright LB, Matchett WJ, Cruz CP et al. Popliteal artery disease: diagnosis and treatment. Radiographics 2004; 24(2): 467–79.

12

Fundamental principles of MR imaging

Santo Dellegrottaglie and Sanjay Rajagopalan

INTRODUCTION

Magnetic resonance (MR) imaging allows the generation of high-quality images of body structures enabling a plethora of clinical applications. A basic understanding of the physical principles of MR is mandatory to fully appreciate the potential of this versatile imaging modality. The familiarity with some of these fundamental concepts allows the operator to interact with the scanner and workstation during an MR examination (i.e., image planning, acquisition, and interpretation) and to make appropriate modifications if necessary to acquire the best possible images.

The following sections provide some of the basic concepts in MR imaging. For a more comprehensive discussion of MR principles, the interested readers are referred to dedicated texts.

PHYSICAL BASE OF MR IMAGING

Nuclear magnetic resonance

The term *MR imaging* refers to the production of images based on process of absorption and emission of energy induced in atomic nuclei exposed to a magnetic field. The original term *nuclear magnetic resonance* (NMR) was dropped in favor of MR imaging in order to dissociate the imaging technique from other radioactive methodologies. In general, NMR exploits the magnetic properties of nuclei with an odd number of protons, neutrons, or both (a spin quantum number (I) of zero indicates equal protons and neutrons while $I > 0$ indicates an unbalanced number of neutrons and protons) to generate an MR signal. Because of the imbalance in charges, the nucleus of these elements has an *intrinsic nuclear spin* that is associated with an angular moment. The nucleus of hydrogen, besides being the most abundant element in the body, is comprised of a single proton and, thus, has a net magnetic moment. For these reasons, protons are typically used for signal generation in MR imaging. However, certain isotopes of many other elements (e.g., carbon-13, sodium-23, fluorine-19, phosphorus-31, etc.) can also produce an MR signal and may be used for spectroscopic applications.

Hardware for MR imaging

A typical MR system consists of: a *superconducting magnet*, responsible for the generation of a constant (static) magnetic field; a *transmitter coil*, which produces the radiofrequency (RF) pulses applied to obtain proton excitation; *gradient coils*, used to generate magnetic field gradients in the three spatial directions and responsible for the process of spatial localization of the generated signal; and *receiver coils*, that are able to record and measure the produced signal. For general clinical applications, volume coils such as the body coil may be used as a receiver coil. In cardiovascular imaging, better results are obtained by using surface phased-array coils. These coil systems are constituted by multiple (up to 36) independent elements and can be placed really close to the imaged structure, optimizing the transmission and reception of RF pulses.

MR SIGNAL FORMATION

Proton magnetic properties

As mentioned above, *hydrogen* has a nucleus consisting of a single proton and behaves as a tiny bar magnet. In basal conditions, the magnetic moment of each single proton is pointed in a different direction and they null each other. When placed in an external magnetic field (1.0–3.0 Tesla (T) with common clinical MR scanners), protons will tend to align with it, creating a *net magnetic moment* (Figure 12.1). With the patient inside the scanner, the resulting net magnetization from the body protons is aligned with the *main external field* (B_0) and, thus, with the main direction of the scanner bore (Figure 12.2). By convention, the magnetization along the scanner is commonly referred to as *longitudinal magnetization* (M_z), while the magnetization perpendicular to it is called *transverse magnetization* (M_{xy}). As will be discussed in the following paragraphs, it is important to keep in mind that only the component M_{xy} of proton magnetization can be registered and measured by the receiver coil.

A coordinated manipulation of proton magnetization represents the basis for the generation of the MR signal. Initially, the basal condition of equilibrium (with the protons aligned to B_0) is perturbed by the application of radiofrequency (RF) pulses leading to *proton excitation*. In brief, certain RF pulses may induce proton excitation by tipping the net magnetization from the longitudinal to the transverse plane. With the interruption of the RF pulse, the immediate return of the protons to their original state (*proton relaxation*) is associated with release of energy and the generation of an MR signal.

Proton excitation

In reality, with the body protons exposed to B_0, the nuclear magnetic moment of the single proton is not perfectly aligned to B_0, but is characterized by a movement around it similar to that of a gyroscope. This wobbling movement around B_0 is called *precession* and, when constant conditions are maintained, protons will process with a characteristic frequency (*Larmor precession frequency, f*). The frequency *f* is directly proportional to the strength of the magnetic field (*B*) with a relationship expressed by the *Larmor equation* (*f* = γ*B*, where γ refers to a characteristic property of each nucleus, called the gyromagnetic ratio). The frequency of precession for hydrogen is 42.58 MHz/T, which corresponds to 63 MHz at field strength of 1.5 T and 128 mHz at 3T, and is in the radiofrequency (RF) range. Of note, *f* values may slightly vary for protons in relationship to the molecular environments that they are in and protons in water precess 220 Hz faster than protons in fat.

By applying brief RF pulses at the Larmor frequency, it is possible to transiently change the energy state of the protons. However, only RF pulses having a frequency corresponding to the precession frequency of the protons are able to interfere with their energy status (*resonance phenomenon*).

Before the application of an RF pulse, the net magnetization comprises only longitudinal magnetization (M_z) that, in a standard MR system, cannot be measured. In this condition, no net transverse magnetization (M_{xy}) is generated

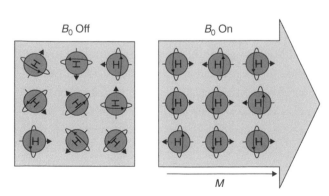

Figure 12.1 Behavior of hydrogen (H) protons exposed to an external magnetic field (B_0). In the basal condition (B_0 Off), the small magnetic moments of the single body protons cancel each other. When exposed to B_0 (B_0 On), the protons' alignment to B_0 leads to the generation of a net body magnetization (*M*).

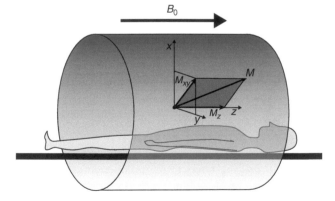

Figure 12.2 Schematic representation of the patient's body positioned inside an MR scanner. The longitudinal magnetization (M_z) is aligned with the external main field (B_0) and the long direction of the scanner bore. The transverse magnetization (M_{xy}) is oriented on a plane perpendicular to B_0.

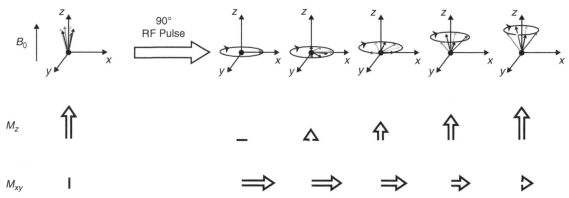

Figure 12.3 Effects of the application of a radiofrequency (RF) pulse on proton magnetization. Initially, the protons precess around the direction of the net external magnetic field (B_0). All protons precess at the same velocity (defined by the Larmor equation), but they are not in phase. As a result, in these conditions the longitudinal magnetization (M_z) is maximal, but no transverse magnetization (M_{xy}) is present. Immediately after the application of an RF pulse ($\alpha = 90°$ in the example), the proton magnetization is completely flipped into the xy-plane (proton excitation) and protons begin to precess all together (in phase). At this time point, proton magnetization is completely constituted by M_{xy}, with M_z reduced to zero. When the RF pulse is switched off, the protons immediately start to realign with B_0 (increasing M_z) and to lose the coherence of phase (decreasing M_{xy}). The result of the sum of these simultaneous events, representing the process of proton relaxation, is the production of an MR signal.

by the precessing protons because each proton precesses independently from the others (they are not in phase).

The process of *proton excitation* is represented by the creation of M_{xy} through the application of an appropriate RF pulse. The RF pulse is produced by the transmitter coil and its principal effects are (1) to tilt the net magnetization away from the z-axis by a certain angle, and (2) to make all the protons precess together (in phase) (Figure 12.3). As a result of application of the RF pulse, M_z decreases while M_{xy} increases by a proportional amount. This transverse magnetization (M_{xy}) will then generate a detectable signal.

The stronger the RF energy applied to the protons the greater the angle of deflection (*flip angle*, α) of the magnetization from the longitudinal to the transverse plane. For instance, a 90° RF pulse will completely flip the magnetization into the x–y plane, while a 180° RF pulse will flip the magnetization to the opposite direction of B_0. The magnitude of α is directly proportional to the strength of the RF magnetic field (B_1) and to the RF duration ($\alpha = \gamma B_1 t$, where γ is the gyromagnetic ratio and t is the duration of the RF pulse).

Proton relaxation

When the transmitter coil is turned off and the RF pulse is terminated, B_0 returns to being the only magnetic field affecting the precessing protons. Immediately, protons begin to return to the original orientation and energy level, in a

process called *proton relaxation*. This is constituted by two simultaneous yet independent processes: (1) protons realign to B_0 with a progressive recovery of M_z or longitudinal magnetization (*longitudinal relaxation*); and, at the same time, (2) protons lose phase coherence and M_{xy} or transverse magnetization disappears (*transverse relaxation or decay*) (Figure 12.3).

The processes of longitudinal and transverse relaxation are regulated by the abilities of protons to exchange energy. Longitudinal relaxation is represented as a positive exponential function describing the time-dependent recovery of M_z (Figure 12.4). This process is based on the net transfer of energy from single excited protons (spins) to the molecules of the surrounding tissue environment (lattice) and is also referred to as *T1 relaxation or spin-lattice relaxation*. The exchange of energy can occur efficiently only when a proton experiences another magnetic field (produced by contiguous molecules) fluctuating near the Larmor frequency. Molecules such as pure water are characterized by elevated rates of molecular motion, which produce fluctuating magnetic fields at a frequency far from the Larmor frequency. This makes the energy exchange with the surrounding lattice less efficient and produces long T1 values. In body tissues, water is partially bound to various macromolecules and, compared to free water, the magnetic field fluctuation is at a slower rate (closer to the Larmor frequency). Thus, in tissue circumstances (in fat, for example) the exchange of energy between protons and surrounding lattice is favored and leads to correspondingly shorter T1 values.

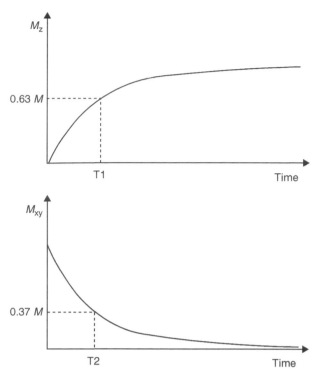

Figure 12.4 The recovery in longitudinal magnetization (M_z) is described by a positive exponential function where the time constant T1 expresses the time needed for M_z to recover 63% of its initial value. Similarly, the decay in transversal magnetization (M_{xy}) is described by a negative exponential curve and the time constant T2 refers to the time needed for 63% of the original M_{xy} to decay. For simplicity, the two curves are graphically represented using comparable time units. In reality, the T1 recovery is a slower process (500–1500 ms) in comparison to the fast T2 decay (10–100 ms).

In a similar way, the transverse decay is represented as a negative exponential function describing the loss of M_{xy} over time (Figure 12.4). This process is mainly dependent on the exchange of energy between adjacent protons (or spins) within the tissue and is also called *T2 relaxation or spin-spin relaxation*. T2 relaxation results from any process that causes protons to lose their phase coherence (spin dephasing). In many cases, this is generated by the small local magnetic field variations related to the interaction between protons within the tissue itself. Because of the fast molecular motion, spin-spin interaction is not efficient in pure water and this produces long T2 values. In tissues with large macromolecules, such as fat, water is partially bound to these macromolecules and the resulting slow molecular motion makes spin-spin interaction very efficient (short T2 values).

In most cases, the loss of phase coherence of the protons is not only related to the spin-spin interaction and cannot be simply described by the T2 relaxation curve. Magnetic field inhomogeneity may contribute significantly to accelerate the process of spin dephasing that, in this case, is defined as *T2* relaxation*. Compared to the T2 relaxation, the T2* curve depicts a similar but faster phenomenon and, in this case, T2* is the time constant describing the exponential loss of transverse magnetization.

Generating an MR signal

In the previous paragraphs, the events following the application of an RF pulse have been described. An adequate RF pulse is able to flip the proton magnetization from the longitudinal to the transverse plane. The generation of an MR signal is based on the fact that a precessing transverse magnetization (M_{xy}) results in the induction of a current in the receiver coil. In case of protons precessing in phase, the generated signal will be proportional to the sum of the single proton magnetizations. In reality, the rapid loss of phase coherence of the precessing protons causes an exponential decline in the amplitude of the recorded signal with time. The MR signal is therefore typically represented as an oscillating signal, called *free induction decay* (FID), characterized by an exponential decay of its amplitude with a time constant corresponding to T2* (Figure 12.5).

The FID signal is extremely transient and cannot be directly and immediately detected by the receiver coil. Particular manipulations of the FID signal are able to generate a reflection of the signal itself, called an *echo*. The time interval between the RF pulse and the detected echo is referred to as *echo time* (TE) (Figure 12.6). More than one RF pulse needs to be applied to obtain the multiple signals that are used to generate an entire MR image. The time interval between two consecutive RF pulses is defined as *repetition time* (TR).

SPATIAL LOCALIZATION

To produce a clinically meaningful image, the signal coming from protons in the different areas of the body needs to be spatially differentiated. Spatial localization in MR exploits the direct relationship existing between frequency of precession (f) and strength of the applied magnetic field as described by the Larmor equation.

Linear magnetic field gradients, generated by three pairs of gradient coils (in the x-, y- and z-direction), are used for the MR signal localization in space. These gradients add to

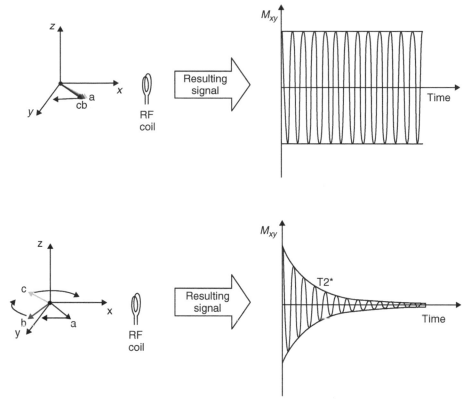

Figure 12.5 Generation of the MR signal. In the presence of multiple protons (a, b, and c in the example) precessing in phase, a single cumulative signal is recorded by the radiofrequency (RF) coil. In reality, because of spin–spin interactions and magnetic field inhomogeneity, the protons precess with slightly different frequencies and quickly lose the phase coherence. The resulting signal (free induction decay, FID) decreases exponentially over time with a time constant T2*.

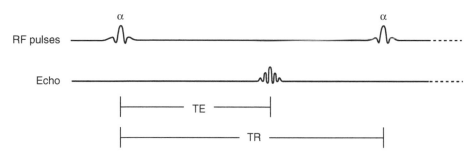

Figure 12.6 Diagram representing the time relationship between the radiofrequency (RF) pulse and the generated echo signal. The time interval between each RF pulse and the following echo (TE) is a fraction of the longer time interval between two consecutive RF pulses (TR).

or subtract from the main B_0 field as a function of distance. Since the frequency of precession (f) is proportional to field strength, f becomes a linear function of position when a linear magnetic field gradient is applied and the precise Larmor frequency of the RF pulse needed to excite a spatially distinct location can be determined a priori. Typically, the effect obtained on protons with the application of a linear gradient needs to be only transitory and well limited in time. For this reason, each application is actually composed of a pair of opposite gradient pulses: the first gradient pro-

duces proton dephasing and the second rephases the protons at the same location (Figure 12.7). After the interruption of the gradients, the net result on the final spin magnetization is negligible, at least for stationary protons.

Spatial localization in MR imaging is a process that, at least for two-dimensional (2D) imaging, includes three steps: (1) *slice selection*, (2) *frequency encoding*, and (3) *phase encoding*. By convention slice selection is performed in the z-direction, frequency encoding in the x-direction and phase encoding in the y-direction. However, it is important

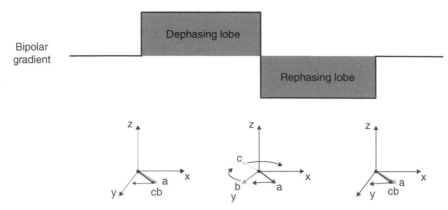

Figure 12.7 Effect of the application of a biphasing gradient on proton precession. By modifying the frequency of precession, the application of a linear magnetic field gradient causes proton dephasing (along the direction of the applied gradient). In the majority of applications, proton dephasing produced by a linear gradient needs to be effective only for a limited period of time. In the example, three protons (a, b, and c) are located in different positions along the direction of the applied gradient. The initial dephasing lobe of the gradient produces proton dephasing, but this may be (completely or partially) compensated by the application of a compensatory lobe (rephasing lobe).

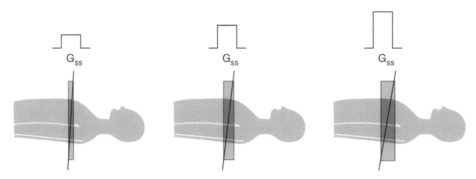

Figure 12.8 Effects of the slice-select gradient (G_{SS}) on image slice thickness. Assuming a constant transmitter bandwidth, a stronger G_{SS} produces thinner slices, and vice versa.

to keep in mind that, in practice, the three orthogonal directions may be interchanged.

Slice selection

During the acquisition of an MR image, only tissues within the selected slice are excited by the RF pulse and contribute to the signal generation. To image a certain slice, RF excitation is performed during the application of a magnetic field gradient (*slice-select gradient*, G_{SS}).

The RF pulse generated by a transmitter coil is characterized not just by a single frequency, but by a range of frequencies and is commonly referred as the *transmit* bandwidth (tBW). An RF pulse with a certain tBW will be able to excite all the protons with a frequency of precession within the range of the tBW. The slice thickness of an acquired image may be selected by modifying either the

strength of G_{SS} or the tBW. For example, to obtain a thinner slice either a stronger G_{SS} or a smaller tBW can be used (Figure 12.8).

Frequency encoding

Once a tissue slice has been selected, additional steps are needed to localize the source of signal within that specific slice (in-plane localization). In the absence of further manipulation, all the protons included in a slice will precess at the same frequency with no possibility for spatial differentiation. Frequency encoding represents a practical way to resolve this issue.

A linear field gradient (*frequency-encoding or readout gradient*, G_{RO}) is applied along the x-direction at the moment of signal sampling. In this way, protons already excited are made to emit signals of different frequencies based on their location along the x-direction. The different frequency of signal emission is used to derive spatial localization along one of the in-plane directions (frequency encoding).

One important consequence of the application of G_{RO} is that the produced signal will be composed of a range of frequencies (Figure 12.9). At the time of analysis, a Fourier transform of the signal will be necessary to obtain a map of its frequency components.

The range of frequencies collected by the receiver coil is defined as the *receiver* bandwidth (rBW, expressed in kHz/image or Hz/voxel). It is important to avoid any confusion between the rBW and the transmit band width (tBW) mentioned in the previous section which refers to the frequency composition of the RF excitation pulse. The rBW is directly proportional to the strength of G_{RO} and, thus, the stronger G_{RO} the wider is the range of frequencies of the produced signal, and vice versa. During the application of G_{RO}, the MR signal is sampled by the receiver coil (*echo sampling*) and the rBW defines the range of frequencies to be sampled. The process of echo sampling is crucial to guarantee the correct signal interpretation and image representation. The ratio between sampling rate and the number of samples of the signal is defined as *sampling frequency* (Figure 12.10). For an accurate image representation, the sampling frequency must be at

least twice the value of the highest frequency component of the signal (*Nyquist theorem*). In case of signal undersampling, the result will be an inappropriate interpretation of the high-frequency components of the signal (*aliasing*) with imperfect representation of the imaged structures (Figure 12.10).

Phase encoding

Spatial localization in the second in-plane direction (y-direction) is achieved by applying a *phase encoding gradient* (G_{PE}). Phase encoding is the most time-consuming step of the entire process of spatial localization as each measurement requires application of repeated gradients.

With the application of G_{RO}, protons in different locations on the x-direction will precess with different frequency, but in phase. The G_{PE} introduces a phase shift that varies linearly with position along the y-direction. In this manner, by accounting for differences in both frequency and phase, in-plane spatial localization can be obtained. Typically, G_{PE} is applied at some time-point between the RF excitation and the echo sampling. Phase encoding is time-consuming because this step has to be repeated multiple times using G_{PE} of different strength to achieve different phase shifts each time. The number of repetitions is equal to the number of image voxels in the y-direction (*number of phase-encoding steps*, N_{PE}).

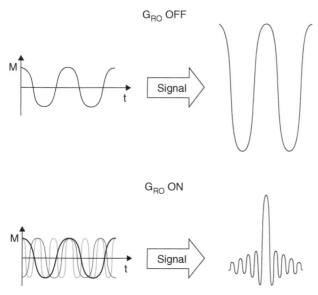

Figure 12.9 Effects of the application of a frequency-encoding or read-out gradient (G_{RO}) on MR signal composition. In the absence of G_{RO}, the sum of all the protons precessing in the imaged slice produces a simple sinusoidal signal (G_{RO} OFF). When G_{RO} is applied, multiple frequencies contribute to generate the cumulative signal (G_{RO} ON). The mathematical representation of this signal (echo) is a sync function.

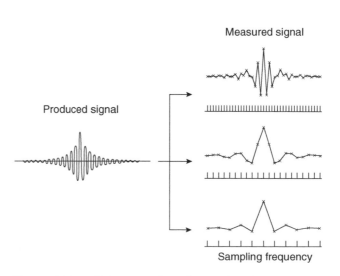

Figure 12.10 Echo sampling of a produced signal. The information contained in the measured signal is progressively compromised by decreasing the sampling frequency (from top to bottom).

In three-dimensionsal (3D) imaging, RF excitation is obtained by applying a non-selective pulse and two sets of phase-encoding steps (N_{PE1} and N_{PE2}) are employed to obtain spatial localization in the slice-encoding and phase-encoding planes.

After each application of G_{PE}, a signal (or echo) is collected. Each echo contains information from the entire imaged slice and is used to fill a line of the 2D (or 3D) data space called k-space (Figure 12.11). When all the gradient coils for spatial localization are operative, each echo will be constituted by a composition of single signals (with different amplitude, phase, and frequency) produced by the excited protons.

A *Fourier transformation* step is involved in the data processing required to fill k-space with the information provided by the measured signal. In very simple terms, Fourier transformation analysis consists in deriving amplitude and phase (over time) of each single frequency-component included in a complex signal. A fundamental characteristic of k-space is that it represents not only the Fourier transformation of the imaged tissue slice, but also the Fourier transformation of the corresponding MR image. In fact, the MR image is derived by applying a Fourier transformation to k-space data, which assigns a numeric value, subsequently converted in signal intensity, to each element (pixel or voxel) of the MR image.

k-SPACE

An MR signal derived from a tissue slice is constituted by numerous RF waves combined to generate a single composite waveform (echo). After its collection, this signal is processed to produce digital data that consist of a set of numbers corresponding to points along the waves (*analog-to-digital conversion*). These numbers may be represented as a grid of points called *k-space*. It is crucial to understand that each point in the k-space is not related to a single image point, but contains information from all the portions of the imaged tissue slice.

k-Space composition

As described above, the multiple echoes acquired to derive an MR image are obtained using phase-encoding gradients (G_{PE}) of variable strengths (Figure 12.11). Each acquired MR echo is stored to fill a line of k-space, where both image contrast and image details are incorporated.

Echoes obtained by applying strong G_{PE} are used to fill the superior and inferior edges of k-space. In contrast, the center of k-space is composed of echoes obtained by applying weak or no G_{PE}. Anatomic structures which are located very close to each other in the imaged slice typically produce signals with relatively similar frequency and may not be resolved when weak G_{PE} are used. On the other hand, strong G_{PE} may be able to induce a detectable phase shift even between really close protons, allowing for the identification of contiguous anatomic structures in the imaged slice. For these reasons, echoes stored in the periphery of k-space are able to provide information on fine details, although the more intense signal dephasing also results in reduced signal intensity. The weak G_{PE} used to generate the echoes stored in the center of k-space induce minimal or no dephasing and the resulting echoes tend to be rich in signal (amplitude), but poor in resolving ability. Thus, tissue contrast is principally determined by the information stored in the center of k-space, while the periphery of k-space encodes image details (Figure 12.12).

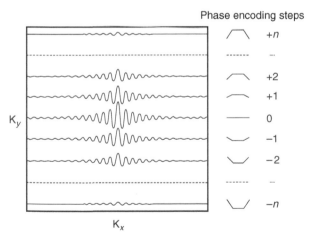

Phase encoding steps

+n

+2

+1

0

−1

−2

−n

K_y

K_x

Figure 12.11 Phase-encoding steps and k-space filling. An echo is measured after each application of the phase-encoding gradient (G_{PE}) and is used to fill a single line of k-space. When no phase encoding is applied ($G_{PE}=0$), the protons are in phase and the maximal signal amplitude is obtained (this echo is stored at the center of k-space). With the application of G_{PE}, the phase encoding creates proton dephasing and the net signal measured is proportionally reduced. K, spatial frequency in the x and y direction.

k-Space filling schemes

The k-space constitutes a grid of numbers and the data to fill this grid can be collected in many different ways. The scheme used for the k-space filling can follow many different

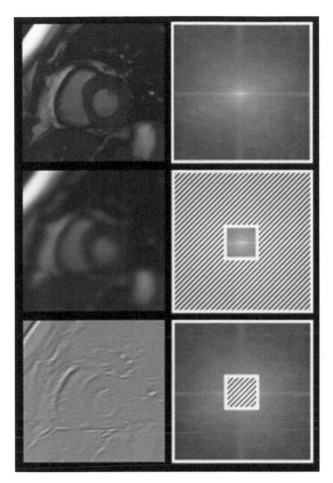

Figure 12.12 Differential value of the center and periphery of k-space in determining image characteristics. Cardiovascular MR images (left) and the corresponding k-space representation (right) are presented. The full utilization of k-space leads to a complete MR image (top panels). By removing data from the periphery of k-space, the resulting image will maintain full contrast, but loosing fine details (mid panels). By removing the center of k-space, information related to details and edges are preserved, but the absence of image contrast significantly reduces the overall information content of the image (bottom panels).

geometric trajectories (linear or non-linear). By applying linear trajectories, horizontal lines of k-space are collected. With a common *linear sequential scheme*, the echo filling starts from one side of the k-space and moves to the other side, passing through the k-space center (Figure 12.13). In a *linear centric scheme*, the central portion of k-space is filled first, followed by the periphery. Since the center of k-space contributes disproportionately to image contrast, efficient sampling of information in this area may be warranted in applications where image contrast plays a dominant role in analysis of structures (e.g. in contrast angiography). Thus, better and more efficient approaches have been developed to

sample the center of k-space. For example, non-Cartesian trajectories (e.g., radial, spiral, etc.) may be employed to obtain rapid and efficient filling of the center in comparison to the periphery of k-space. The choice of the specific k-space filling scheme to be used in each clinical application is based on multiple technical, methodologic, and clinical considerations.

Partial k-space acquisition

Some of the properties of k-space have been exploited to generate techniques based on a partial acquisition of the information needed to generate an MR image (*partial k-space acquisition*) to enable fast MR imaging.

A fundamental property of k-space is its *symmetry* (conjugate symmetry or Hermetian symmetry). One half of k-space is identical to the other half. Several techniques to allow fast MR imaging take advantage of this characteristic of k-space and the fact that at least theoretically, an entire MR image may be reconstructed by acquiring only half of the k-space data (*partial Fourier imaging*). A good example of this approach is represented by the HASTE (Half-fourier Acquisition Single-shot Turbo spin Echo) sequence, in which a few more than half of the entire phase-encoding lines (N_{PE}) are collected and the remaining are calculated assuming k-space symmetry (Chapter 13).

Another derivation for acquiring k-space information selectively takes advantage of the differential composition of k-space, with information pertaining to image contrast in the center and information pertaining to image details at the periphery. Thus, it is possible to sacrifice part of the data stored in the periphery of k-space, in order to speed up MR imaging. In one of these approaches, called *truncated k-space filling,* only the center of k-space is filled with actual data, while the information pertaining to the k-space periphery is not collected. In this case, in order to maintain constant, the final number of phase encode lines (N_{PE}) unchanged, the missing data in the k-space are not calculated (like in partial Fourier imaging), but are simply replaced by zeroes (*zero filling* or *zero interpolation*). The result is that the real spatial resolution of the image is actually reduced, but the apparent spatial resolution remains unchanged.

When applicable, the methods of partial k-space acquisition allow substantial reduction in scan time duration. Unfortunately, the feasibility of these approaches may be limited in some applications by the significant decline in the signal-to-noise ratio of the image, which is mainly a consequence of the saving in scan time duration by the reduction

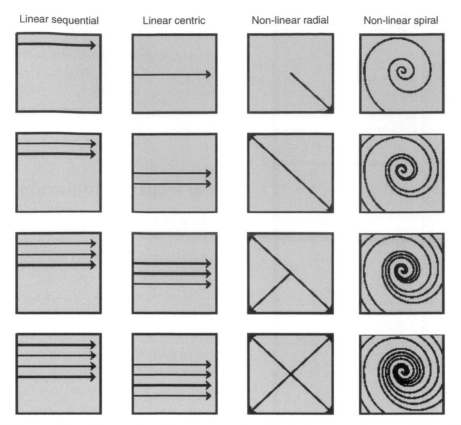

Figure 12.13   K-Space filling schemes. Graphic representation of the initial steps of k-space filling with some of the most common filling schemes (trajectories).

on phase encode steps (see next section). Furthermore, the presence of magnetic field inhomogeneities may invalidate the assumptions that allow partial k-space acquisitions (i.e. that one half of k-space is identical to the other) and compromise the fidelity of data acquisition.

IMAGE QUALITY AND SCAN TIME DURATION

Fast image acquisition is frequently required in cardiovascular MR imaging. In most cases, a complete set of images needs to be acquired in a single breath hold or within the circulation time of a tight contrast bolus and, frequently, scan time duration can be reduced only through a sacrifice in image quality.

Determinants of image quality

In medical imaging, the term *image quality* typically refers to the ability of the obtained image to provide an adequate answer to one or more clinical questions (diagnostic or clinical image quality). Technically, image quality refers to the fidelity of representation of the imaged structures and is the composite of multiple elements, including spatial resolution, image contrast, and occurrence of image artifacts.

MR images are constituted by multiple 3D units (*voxels*) organized in a spatial grid. Based on the signal collected by the receiver channels and stored in k-space, the computer assigns (after a Fourier transformation of the k-space data) a particular numeric value to each of these voxels. The numbers are subsequently converted to a grayscale of signal intensities, leading to image formation.

Multiple parameters are typically used to define the characteristics of an MR image.

Dimensions. In MR imaging, data acquisition may result in either 2D or 3D images. With 2D MR imaging, a tissue slice with a certain thickness (typically 3–10 mm in the z-dimension) is acquired. Usually, multiple 2D images need to be obtained to completely cover an anatomic structure of interest. 3D MR images allow the representation of an entire image volume, with the possibility of reformatting the images into any space plane during the post-processing evaluation.

Field of view (FOV). The FOV defines the size (expressed in mm or cm) of the region being imaged on the two or three dimensions. In current MR systems, the typical FOV is between 350 and 500 mm.

Matrix. The matrix expresses the number of digitized units (voxels) included in the image and is described as the product of two numbers for 2D images (e.g., 256 × 256, 512 × 256, 256 × 128, etc.) or three numbers for 3D images. For the reasons discussed above (i.e., the phase-encoding steps are time-consuming), it is much more efficient to perform frequency encoding than phase encoding and thus, the bigger number always refers to the frequency-encoding direction.

Spatial resolution. The spatial resolution of an image in the *x–y* plane is reflected by the voxel size (Vox) in that plane (unless zero interpolation has been used). Vox may be obtained by the ratio of the field-of-view and the matrix size (Vox = FOV/N, where FOV and N refer to the field-of-view and matrix size in the *x*- or *y*-direction). It is evident that a higher spatial resolution can be obtained either by increasing the matrix size or by decreasing the FOV. Any increase in spatial resolution, however, is paralleled by a decrease in signal-to-noise ratio (see below). Frequently, Vox is not equal in the different directions of a 3D image. Isotropic voxels (with the same value of spatial resolution in the three directions) are desirable in 3D imaging to allow multi-planar image reformatting.

Signal-to-noise ratio (SNR). MR signal measurements are always affected by a certain amount of noise, represented by random signal perturbations originating from the body of the patient, the scanner, and the surrounding environment. All the images contain noise and this is usually expressed in relative terms as SNR. Many image parameters (variable in relation to the employed scan sequence) contribute to determine the final SNR. The following simplified formula accounts for the major parameters involved in the determination of SNR:

$$SNR \propto (B_0 \times Vox \times N_{PE} \times N_{EX})/\sqrt{rBW}$$

where B_0 is the main magnetic field, Vox is the voxel size (which is reciprocal to spatial resolution), N_{PE} is the number of phase-encoding lines, N_{EX} is the number of excitations, and rBW is the receiver bandwidth. Obviously, an increased SNR may be obtained by using an MR scanner able to generate higher B_0 (3 T versus 1.5 T). Decreasing BW will also increase SNR.

Contrast-to-noise ratio (CNR). When analyzing an image, it is essential to be able to distinguish between different anatomic structures (e.g., blood versus vessel wall). This ability is significantly affected by the level of noise. The CNR for the structures A and B can be calculated as the difference between the signal of the structures divided by noise (CNR=[signal A – signal B]/noise).

Strategies to manipulate scan time duration

Imaging scan time (T_{SCAN}) for a 2D image may be derived by the following equation:

$$T_{SCAN} = (TR \times N_{PE} \times N_{EX})/N_{ECHO}$$

where TR is the repetition time, N_{PE} is the number of phase-encoding steps, N_{EX} is the number of times the RF excitation is repeated or number of signal averages, and N_{ECHO} is the number of signals or echoes produced after each excitation. In the equation describing the imaging scan time for a 3D image, the parameter N_{PE} is substituted by the product $N_{PE1} \times N_{PE2}$ where the latter referred to as the two phase-encoding directions.

Multiple approaches may be applied to reduce T_{SCAN} by acting (directly or indirectly) on one or more of the elements included in the equation reported above.

Reducing TR. A practical way to reduce TR is by decreasing the TE, which is a major determinant of the total TR duration (Figure 12.6). For this reason, the TE values are minimized as much as possible during an MR angiographic study that depends on short imaging times. The period devoted to signal sampling is an important determinant of TE duration and, thus, of TR duration. TE can be shortened by increasing the sampling frequency and this is obtained by increasing the receiver band width (rBW) (Figure 12.10). However, the consequence of reducing sample time by increasing rBW is that there is a loss of SNR.

Reducing N_{PE}. A powerful way to contain T_{SCAN} is by reducing N_{PE}. However, reducing N_{PE} will lead to a decrease in spatial resolution (assuming a constant imaging FOV) and SNR. This can be avoided with the use of a *rectangular FOV*. A contemporaneous decrease in FOV dimension in the phase-encoding direction (keeping constant the dimensions in the frequency-encoding direction) proportional to the N_{PE} reduction will maintain the spatial resolution at the same level, while accomplishing a reduction in T_{SCAN}. The use of rectangular FOV finds convenient applications in thoracic or abdominal imaging, as at this level the body size is significantly smaller in one dimension (anterior-posterior). Furthermore, a significant reduction in the N_{PE} required to generate an MR image may be possible when techniques of *partial k-space acquisition* are employed, with a consequent saving in T_{SCAN}. The use of *parallel imaging techniques* also presents another opportunity to dramatically shorten T_{SCAN} by a factor of 2, 4, or more (see the section on Parallel imaging).

Reducing N_{EX}. To contain the T_{SCAN}, a single RF excitation ($N_{EX} = 1$) is used in most cases. In circumstances when T_{SCAN} duration is not a concern (i.e., free breathing imaging), multiple N_{EX} can be employed with the intention to obtain increased image SNR.

Increasing N_{ECHO}. The T_{SCAN} may be reduced by increasing the N_{ECHO} (referred to as *echo train length* in spin-echo imaging and *lines per segment* in gradient-echo imaging). With most of the MR imaging techniques commonly employed, multiple echoes are produced after a single RF excitation. Thus, multiple signals are collected during a single TR interval. In some applications (*single-shot imaging*), the entire image matrix information can be derived after a single RF pulse by acquiring a large portion of k-space and employing partial Fourier methods to derive the reminder (i.e. HASTE imaging).

The various approaches reported above may be implemented separately or in combination to reduce T_{SCAN}. Particular attention needs to be paid to preserving spatial resolution while trying to contain the duration of image acquisition. Furthermore, it is important to keep in mind that, reduction in T_{SCAN} is accomplished through a proportional decrease in image SNR. Thus, one of the most challenging aspects of MR imaging is maintaining an adequate balance between duration of image acquisition, image resolution, and signal.

SIGNAL UNDERSAMPLING AND IMAGE WRAPPING

The wraparound artifacts may occur whenever the dimensions of the object cannot be contained within the specified field of view (FOV). This may occur along any axes, but almost exclusively in the phase, or slice-encoding directions and is a consequence of *aliasing* (Figure 12.14). Aliasing occurs because structures outside the FOV are exposed to the applied linear gradients and contribute to the composition of the final signal. These structures, are usually exposed to the edges of the gradients and consequently produce high-frequency signals. Aliasing in the frequency-encoding direction is a consequence of the fact that an undersized frequency-encoding dimension of the FOV translates into a sub-optimal sampling frequency (as expressed by the rBW) that is adequate to sample the high frequency in the measured echo. Similarly, when a rectangular FOV is used, it implies k-space undersampling in the phase-encoding direction. As a result, the FOV may be too small in the phase-encoding direction to include all the structures present in the imaged slice. Whether the FOV is undersized in the frequency-encoding direction or in the phase-encoding direction, in both cases the undersampling of the high-frequency signals produced by the structures outside the FOV will result in their misrepresentation in the reconstructed image (wrapping).

PARALLEL IMAGING

Parallel imaging represents an important strategy for fast cardiovascular MR imaging. Parallel imaging techniques are based on the optimization of the information provided by a phased-array coil with multiple receiver elements with the objective to obtain a reduction in scan time duration

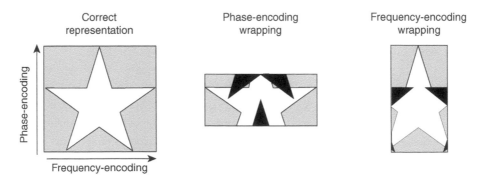

Figure 12.14 The correct representation of an imaged element is dependent on the selection of an adequate FOV size. Wraparound artifacts occur when an undersized FOV is selected, in the phase-encoding, frequency-encoding or slice encoding direction, in relation to the dimensions of the imaged structure. With an undersized FOV, the portions of the imaged element extending beyond the defined FOV are incorrectly reproduced on the opposite side of the reconstructed image (wrapping).

(T_{SCAN}). Parallel imaging is highly flexible and it can be integrated into virtually any pulse sequence and combined with other fast imaging methods. In brief, the reduction in T_{SCAN} with parallel imaging is based on a significant reduction in the number of phase-encoding steps (N_{PE}). As described before, reducing N_{PE} represents one of the most efficient ways to reduce T_{SCAN}. However, if one were to keep image resolution or voxel size constant, the consequent shrinking in FOV results in wraparound artifacts (see the section on image wrapping). If anatomic structures contained in the imaged slice are excluded from the FOV, this will result in an incorrect mapping of these structures within the obtained image. Wraparound artifacts are particularly undesirable because, by projecting peripheral anatomic structures at the center of the reconstructed image, they can compromise visualization of the structures of interest.

Principles of parallel imaging

The great advantage with parallel imaging is that it allows a dramatic reduction in the acquired N_{PE} and a consequent containment of T_{SCAN} with no deterioration in the final spatial resolution of the acquired image. Parallel imaging permits a reduction of N_{PE} without the occurrence of wraparound artifacts by providing a clever system to resolve this inconvenience.

As discussed above, a significant T_{SCAN} shortening may be obtained by using rectangular FOV. At the k-space level, a reduction in the FOV size corresponds to a reduction in the N_{PE}. For instance, a 50% reduction in the FOV size may be achieved by sampling every other line of k-space with a consequent 50% shortening in T_{SCAN}. In most cases, the T_{SCAN} saving is paid for by the occurrence of wrap-around artifact (Figure 12.15).

Parallel imaging techniques are based on the independent measurement of signal from multiple element coils. The factor by which N_{PE} can be reduced depends on the quantity of element coils aligned along the phase-encoding direction (usually 2 or 4). Correspondingly, the T_{SCAN} is typically shortened by a factor of 2 or 4 with parallel imaging while further accelerations, although possible, are generally limited by the associated SNR reduction.

Multiple different approaches have been developed for parallel imaging and they can be grouped in two main categories called SENSE (SENSitivity Encoding) and SMASH (SiMultaneous Acquisition of Spatial Harmonics). In general, the characteristics of the same signal as detected by each coil element of a phased-array multi-element coil are compared and are used to resolve image wrapping. With SENSE and SENSE-like techniques, the process of correction of the wraparound artifacts is operated directly at the level of the image. The comparison of the signal measured by each coil leads to the unwrapping of the acquired image. With SMASH and SMASH-like techniques, the k-space undersampling is resolved by calculating the missing lines of k-space and reconstituting an entire set of N_{PE}. In any case, a full-size FOV is derived from a rectangular FOV obtained in a shorter T_{SCAN} while maintaining the spatial resolution.

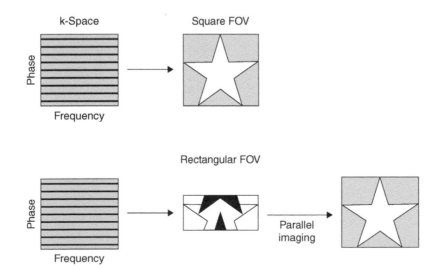

Figure 12.15 Parallel imaging effects on field-of-view (FOV) size. The phase-encoding undersampling associated with the generation of a rectangular FOV may lead to an undersized FOV compared to the imaged element (image wrapping). With parallel imaging techniques, a full square FOV may be reconstructed by exploiting the different characteristics of the same signal as measured by each of the element coils in a phased-array coil with multiple receiver elements.

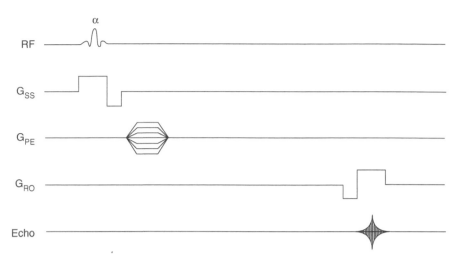

Figure 12.16   Pulse sequence diagram. In the example, a radiofrequency (RF) pulse is sent with a certain flip angle (α) to induce proton excitation. Spatial localization is obtained by applying magnetic field gradients in the x- (G_{RO}), y- (G_{PE}), and z-directions (G_{SS}). The result is a signal (echo) detected by the receiver coil. The diagram highlights the specific timing of the different events: G_{RO} is applied in coincidence with the emission of the echo (during the echo sampling or read-out); the graphic representation of G_{PE} emphasizes the repetitive application of multiple alternate gradients with increasing strength; G_{SS} is applied in coincidence with the RF pulse.

MR PULSE SEQUENCES

The sequence of events comprising of sending the RF pulse (transmitter coil), creating the gradients for spatial localization (gradient coils), and collecting the signal (receiver coil) is globally defined as the *pulse sequence*. The composition of a pulse sequence may be graphically represented with conventional diagrams (Figure 12.16).

Pulse sequences commonly used in cardiovascular MR imaging can be classified into two main categories: *gradient-echo sequences* and *spin-echo sequences*. Both approaches are based on the concept that the free induction decay (FID) signal generated immediately after the application of an RF pulse is too close to the pulse itself to be detected by the receiver coil (frequently working, alternatively, as transmitting and receiver coil and also called transceiver coil). A solution to this problem is through the deliberate delay of the original signal to generate a so-called echo. Gradient-echo and spin-echo techniques fundamentally differ in the modalities used to create an echo of the original FID signal.

Gradient-echo imaging

In gradient-echo imaging the initial RF pulse is followed by the application of a couple of gradients: the first gradient accelerates the proton dephasing starting at the interruption of the RF pulse and the second gradient produces a quick proton

rephasing. The result is the generation of an echo of the original signal and the collection of this echo is used to fill one line of k-space. The process can be repeated multiple times to collect all the information required to complete an MR image. More practically, in fast gradient-echo techniques, multiple echoes may be produced after each RF pulse through the application of a series of gradients (Figure 12.17). The number of echoes (k-space lines) obtained after each RF pulse is commonly expressed as *lines per segment*. In single-shot gradient-echo techniques such as *echo planar imaging*, all the lines required to fill the entire k-space are collected after the application of a single RF pulse. The amplitude of each echo as well as the number of echoes that can be generated after each RF pulse is governed by the T2* decay phenomenon.

Gradient-echo imaging typically employs an RF pulse with a partial flip angle ($<90°$). The advantage of using a partial flip angle is in the residual longitudinal magnetization (M_z) left after the application of the RF pulse. In these conditions, there is no need to wait a long time to allow a sufficient recovery of M_z before applying the following pulse. Really short TR times may be used with these sequences, resulting in fast MR imaging.

On the other hand, by using short TR times in some circumstancs the transverse magnetization (M_{xy}) may not have fully decayed before the next RF pulse is applied. This may be the source of image artifacts and different ways to handle this issue have been developed: in *spoiled gradient-echo* techniques such as FLASH (Fast Low Angle SHot), FFE (Fast

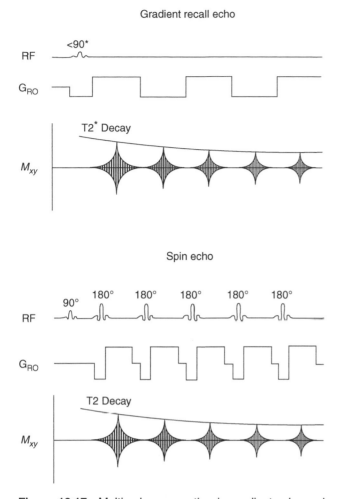

Gradient recall echo

Spin echo

Figure 12.17 Multi-echo generation in gradient-echo and spin-echo sequences. In a gradient-echo sequence, a single radiofrequency (RF) pulse with partial flip angle ($\alpha < 90°$) is followed by multiple echoes when a series of read-out gradients (G_{RO}) is applied. The intensity of each echo decreases based on T2* decay. Of note, G_{RO} are used in gradient-echo imaging to obtain the frequency encoding of the image, but also to generate the echo itself. In a spin-echo sequence, multiple echoes are generated by applying, after the initial 90° RF pulse, a series of 180° RF pulses. In this case, the intensity of the echoes decreases over time according to the T2 decay curve (the effect of magnetic field inhomogeneity is cancelled by the 180° RF pulses).

Field Echo), or SPGR (SPoiled GRass), special modifications are added to the image sequence to eliminate any residual M_{xy} (spoiling); in the *steady-state gradient-echo*, including True-FISP (Fast Imaging with Steady state Precession), Balanced-FFE, and FIESTA (Fast Imaging Employing STeady-state Acquisition), the residual M_{xy} is not eliminated but is used to increase the final signal intensity. Fast T1 weighted gradient-echo sequences (FLASH, SPGR, or FFE) are typically applied for contrast-enhanced MRA and flow-sensitive imaging.

Spin-echo imaging

Spin-echo imaging is based on the application of an initial 90° RF pulse immediately followed by a 180° RF pulse. In these sequences, the 180° RF pulse has a similar role to the gradients applied in gradient-echo imaging. Immediately after the cessation of the 90° RF pulse, protons start to dephase, but the direction of the dephasing is inverted by the application of the 180° RF pulse. The result is that, by going back to the original position, at a certain time point, protons will return in phase. This will generate an echo of the original signal occurring at the time point TE (echo time). By acting as a refocusing pulse, the 180° RF pulse occurs at a time point that is exactly mid-way between the initial 90° RF pulse and the generated echo (so it corresponds to TE/2).

The generated echo is used to fill one line of k-space. In fast spin-echo techniques (or turbo spin-echo techniques), multiple lines of k-space may be collected by the application of a series of 180° RF pulses after a single 90° RF pulse (Figure 12.17). The number of echoes produced after each 90° RF pulse is called the *echo train length* (ETL). In the single-shot spin-echo techniques such as *HASTE*, all the echoes needed to obtain an entire MR image (by using the short-cut of a partial Fourier reconstruction) are collected after a single 90° RF pulse.

The 180° RF pulses used in the spin-echo sequences eliminate the effect of local magnetic field inhomogeneity on proton dephasing. Thus, the decrease in the signal amplitude observed when multiple echoes are produced is governed by the T2 decay (and not by the T2* decay). Consequently, these sequences are less susceptible to local field inhomogeneities. Compared to gradient-echo imaging, moreover, true T2 weighted images may be produced by using spin-echo sequences. In addition, scanning time is typically longer in these sequences (longer TR times), but this results in higher image SNR. MR images obtained by spin-echo imaging provide excellent anatomic evaluation of body structures, including vessels.

MR IMAGE CONTRAST

In MR imaging, the signal produced by body tissues is principally a result of the intrinsic properties of each specific tissue based on its biochemical composition. Again, based on differences in the physical and chemical properties, the MR signal may be selectively enhanced or suppressed by introducing specific modifications to the imaging scan sequence. Finally,

MR tissue contrast may also be modified by using specific contrast media.

Intrinsic tissue contrast mechanisms

In general, the signal intensity of each voxel in an MR image is proportional to the amount of signal attributed to that particular spatial location at the end of the complex process of signal production, collection, and interpretation.

Since protons are responsible for generation of MR signal, the measured signal is certainly representative of the total *proton density* (PD) of the tissue (proton number per unit volume). A tissue with a higher amount of protons available to interact with RF pulses will generate a more intense MR signal compared to a tissue with a low PD. Longitudinal relaxation and transverse relaxation are also factors that influence the signal intensity and, therefore, image contrast. T1 and T2 relaxations represent inherent properties of the tissues, mostly defined by the ability of the tissue protons to exchange energy.

A way to obtain tissue contrast in MR imaging is by taking advantage of differences in PD, T1 recovery, and T2 decay of various tissues. In clinical MR imaging, image contrast can be modified by the operator to generate PD-, T1- and T2-weighted images, by adjusting specific image parameters (TR and TE) in a manner that is variable for the different pulse sequences (Table 12.1).

Image contrast in gradient-echo imaging. Fast imaging with spoiled gradient-echo sequences is based on the use of ultra-short TR times. Image contrast cannot be influenced by differences in T1 relaxivity (speed of longitudinal magnetization recovery) when very short TR times are employed.

A short TR combined with appropriate TE, by emphasizing T2* tissue differences, will generate T2*-weighted images. It is important to note that, in gradient-echo imaging, T2-weighted images are really T2*-weighted. T1-weighted images, in which differences in signal amplitude are based on different tissue T1 times, can only be obtained by using relatively longer TR times. Finally, short TR and short TE will avoid any T1 and T2* effects, and the resulting image will be PD-weighted.

Image contrast in spin-echo imaging. In spin-echo imaging, by using short TR only tissues with short T1 can recover longitudinal magnetization before the next 90° RF pulse is applied, and the resulting image will be T1-weighted. With long TR, all the tissues have time to recover (regardless of the T1 properties) and the effect of T1 on image contrast will be minimized. When long TE times are used, signal amplitude will be higher for tissues with a slow decay in transverse magnetization (long T2) and the image will be T2 weighted. In contrast, usage of short TE will minimize the effect of T2 decay and, therefore, the T2 weighting. To summarize, with spin-echo imaging, T1-weighted images are obtained by selecting short TR (maximizes the T1 contrast) and short TE (minimizes the T2 contrast), T2 weighting is obtained with long TR (minimizes T1 contrast) and long TE (maximizes T2 contrast) and, finally, PD weighting is obtained using long TR (minimizes T1 contrast) and short TE (minimizes T2 contrast).

Preparatory pulses

Image contrast may also be modified by applying additional RF pulses (*preparatory pulses or prepulses*) to the regular imaging scan sequence. These prepulses modify in a selective or

Table 12.1 Determination of image contrast by different combinations of repetition time (TR) and echo time (TE) in gradient-echo and spin-echo imaging. The reported parameters to obtain T1, T2, and proton density (PD)-weighted imaging are referred to as generic spoiled gradient-echo and spin-echo sequences

	Sequence	
Image contrast	Gradient-echo	Spin-echo
T1-weighted	Long TR – short TE	Short TR – short TE
T2-weighted	Short TR – long TE[a]	Long TR – long TE
PD-weighted	Short TR – short TE	Long TR – short TE

[a] This combination of parameters in spoiled gradient-echo imaging produces T2*-weighted images.

non-selective way the MR signal produced by the body tissues.

Inversion recovery. Image contrast strongly dependent on T1 relaxation time may be obtained by introducing a 180° RF prepulse (*inversion pulse*) in the imaging sequence. The application of an inversion pulse completely inverts longitudinal magnetization (M_z) which will start to recover immediately after the interruption of the pulse. The rate of M_z recovery is determined by the T1 time of each tissue. At a certain characteristic time point during the recovery of T1 (that is specific for each tissue) there will be no residual M_z to flip into the transverse plane (Figure 12.18). Thus, application of an excitation RF pulse at this characteristic time point (*null point*) will have no effect on the production of transverse magnetization (M_{xy}). In this case, the tissue will not produce any detectable signal and, consequently, will appear dark or 'nulled' on the produced image. The time interval between the inversion pulse and the excitation pulse is referred as inversion time (TI). If the excitation RF pulse is applied with a TI corresponding to the null point of a certain tissue, that tissue will not contribute to the generated echo (tissue suppression). The time at which a specific tissue appears nulled can be identified depending on the T1 of the tissue for a specific B_0 and can be approximated by the formula TI = 0.67 × T1 of tissue at 1.5 T. Based on the clinical application, inversion pulses can be non-slice-selective (where an entire volume is subjected to a 180° pulse) or may be slice-selective (where the 180° pulse is directed only to a prespecified slice).

Selective signal saturation. An additional approach to obtain tissue suppression is based on *signal saturation*. Techniques for selective signal saturation rely on the application of a 90° RF pulse (*saturation pulse*) immediately followed by a *dephasing gradient*. The saturation prepulse excites the tissue protons, generating measurable M_{xy}. The subsequent application of the dephasing gradient produces fast dephasing of the protons, precluding their involvement in the generation of the MR signal following the next excitation RF pulse. Signal saturation may be either selective for specific tissue slices (*spatially selective saturation*) or for particular tissues (*frequency-selective or chemically selective saturation*). Spatially selective saturation may be useful in cases when the signal from a certain region of the FOV is not desired (i.e., to reduce wraparound artifacts and motion artifacts). In these cases, a slice-selective saturation prepulse is applied to affect only a defined region (*saturation band*) that will

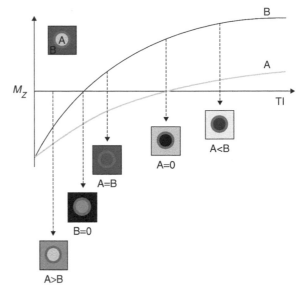

Figure 12.18 Tissue suppression with inversion recovery technique. The reported example is referred to a hypothetical blood vessel. Tissue A (blood) has a longer T1 time than tissue B (perivascular tissue), testified by a slower recovery in longitudinal relaxation (M_z). After the application of an inversion pulse (180° radiofrequency pulse), various image contrasts may be obtained by changing the inversion time (TI) of the imaging sequence. With a short TI, the faster recovery of tissue B leads to lower signal intensity compared to tissue A (A > B). A really long TI generates the opposite situation, with greater signal produced by tissue B compared to tissue A (A < B). The TI time may be selected to correspond to the null point of one of the imaged tissues (the null point occurs earlier for tissue B than for tissue A). In the resulting images, a complete suppression of the signal corresponding to the nulled tissue is obtained (A = 0 and B = 0). Of note, a particular value of TI (intermediate between the null points for the two tissues) corresponds to a condition where the positive value of M_z for tissue B is equal to the negative value of M_z for tissue A (A = B). In this particular circumstance, the signal produced by the two tissues will be isointense (the magnitude and not the phase of M_z determines the resulting signal).

not contribute to the final signal production. Chemically selected saturation is based on the difference in precession frequency between fat and water protons. The precessing frequency of water and fat protons is slightly different (220 Hz in a 1.5 T scanner, with water protons precessing faster than fat protons). This approach may be exploited in circumstances where the signal produced by fat needs to be removed from the acquired image (fat suppression). In this case, a non-slice-selective saturation prepulse centered on the fat frequency is applied at the beginning of the sequence, followed by a dephasing gradient. The result is a complete suppression of signal from fat protons

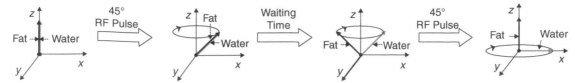

Figure 12.19 Selective water excitation. After the application of a non-selective RF prepulse ($\alpha=45°$ in the example), fat and water spins will precess with a slightly different precession frequency. After waiting a certain time, fat and water spins will be in the opposite phase. At this point, the application of a second prepulse ($\alpha=45°$) centered on water frequency will result in a transverse magnetization equal to zero for fat (fat suppression) and maximal for water.

(saturation), with the water protons participating solely in the generation of the image.

Alternative techniques for fat suppression. Fat suppression may also be obtained as an indirect consequence of a *selective excitation* of water protons. The difference in fat and water precession frequency results, after waiting a short time interval, in a difference in precession phase. By adequately timing the application of a second RF prepulse selective water excitation may be achieved with concomitant fat suppression (Figure 12.19). However, field inhomogeneity can dramatically decrease the efficiency of this approach. Less demanding in terms of requirement for field homogeneity is fat suppression based on the use of STIR (short tau inversion recovery) sequences. STIR employs a non-slice-selective 180° inversion pulse with an inversion time (TI) specifically selected to null fat (typically, TI=160 ms at 1.5 T). The STIR sequence provides excellent fat suppression, but is not highly specific for fat considering that other tissues with short T1 may also be suppressed.

Contrast agents

Specific contrast agents may be utilized to alter the intrinsic contrast of tissues on MR images. The most commonly used agents are chelates of *gadolinium* (Gd^{3+}), a heavy metal ion belonging to the lanthanide family with strong paramagnetic properties. Gadolinium chelates alter the magnetic properties of adjacent protons by shortening the T1 and T2 relaxation times. At the concentrations used for clinical imaging, T1 shortening represents the dominant effect and this is used, in MR angiographic techniques, for example, to increase the signal intensity from blood vessels. When the concentration of gadolinium chelates exceeds a certain level, the T2 shortening becomes more prominent, leading to a dramatic reduction of the resulting signal intensity

with possible artifactual images (pseudostenosis) (also see Chapter 14).

The gadolinium-based contrast media currently employed for clinical cardiovascular applications are extracellular, with an extremely favorable safety profile. Chapter 14 provides a more extensive discussion about the contrast agents used for MR imaging.

MR ARTIFACTS

Many types of artifacts may occur in MR imaging and may variably affect the information content of clinical images. Artifacts can be induced by factors related to the patient, to the hardware system, or to the process of signal production and collection. Some of the most common of these artifacts are discussed in this section.

Motion artifacts

Patient motion during the image acquisition is a frequent source of artifacts in MR imaging. These artifacts may be generated by voluntary or involuntary movements (e.g., respiration, cardiac motion, arterial pulsatility, etc.).

The appearance of the artifacts may vary depending on the time of occurrence of the movement in relation to the k-space filling process. In general, motion occurring in the middle of the imaging acquisition will produce replication of the imaged structures (ghosting), while motion occurring at the end of the scan, when the periphery of k-space is generally filled, will result in image blurring.

Respiration and cardiac motion consist of repetitive low-frequency events and they usually produce ghosting artifacts occurring in the phase-encoding direction as the duration of time required for phase encoding is at least an order of magnitude higher than the time required for frequency encoding. The intensity of the ghosting artifact is related to the amplitude of the periodic motion and the signal intensity of the moving tissue.

Motion artifacts may be reduced by trying to obtain adequate patient cooperation and by applying all the approaches valuable for the containment of scan time duration (i.e., fast scan techniques). Specific techniques may be implemented to contain motion artifacts produced by involuntary motion (e.g., respiratory navigator, EKG gating, pulsing, etc.). In some cases, spatially selective preparatory pulses (saturation bands) may be applied to specifically null the signal from the structures producing the motion artifact.

Wraparound artifacts

The phenomenon of aliasing as a cause of wraparound artifacts has been discussed elsewhere in this chapter (see also the section on parallel imaging).

Several different approaches may be applied (separately or in combination) to limit the occurrence of image wrapping. Whenever possible, it is important to adjust FOV position and size to include all the structures included in the imaged slice. The FOV size may be conveniently expanded in the frequency-encoding direction without any increase in the scan time. To avoid the reduction in space resolution consequent to FOV expansion, however, signal oversampling is usually applied. This consists of doubling the sampling frequency of the collected signal (by doubling the receiver bandwidth).

As discussed before, parallel imaging based on the use of phased-array, multi-element receiver coils represents an optimal solution to the problem of wraparound artifact without any sacrifice in spatial resolution and scan time duration.

Finally, the application of saturation pulses, by preventing signal production from undesired tissues, can help in reducing image wrapping.

Chemical shift artifacts

Body protons may have slightly different precession frequencies in relation to the diverse molecular environment in which they are included (chemical shift). For example, even if placed at the same location in the body, fat protons precess slower than water protons. By remembering that differences in precession frequency are used to obtain spatial localization

in MR imaging, it is easy to understand that the chemical shift may be responsible for proton mismapping (in the frequency-encoding direction) at the moment of converting the MR signal from the frequency to the spatial domain. The actual intensity of the proton mismapping will be dependent on the main magnetic field and gradient strength.

Chemical shift artifacts are generally observed at the level of the interface between an organ and the surrounding fat. The resulting artifact is generally represented by a dark (or bright) band at the fat–water interface in the frequency-encoding direction.

The use of higher receiver bandwidth or the application of fat suppression techniques may help in reducing chemical shift artifacts.

Straight line artifacts

RF interference may occur when radio waves from various sources outside the MR scanner (e.g., electronic equipment, flickering light bulbs, etc.) contaminate the k-space sampling process during MR imaging. This is seen as a single or multiple stripes in the frequency encode direction. A spike in k-space may cause a 'zebra' pattern artifact. A common cause of spike is electrical discharges from blankets that commonly occur with low humidity. These can be prevented by increasing the humidity inside the MR suite.

Field inhomogeneity and susceptibility artifacts

Minimal imperfections in the main magnetic field homogeneity are more common at the periphery of the magnetic field and may generate a significant degradation in the overall image quality. For this reason, the imaged region should always be at the center of the coil. The homogeneity of the main magnetic field should be periodically verified and specific corrections for local field inhomogeneities may be prescribed by the operator at the level of the imaged region (volume shimming).

The homogeneity of the main magnetic field may be significantly disturbed by the presence of metallic implants in the patient's body. The presence of paramagnetic/ferromagnetic implants may be responsible for image distortion and signal loss (susceptibility artifacts). In general, spin-echo sequences should be preferred in these circumstances, considering that gradient-echo sequences are more sensitive to the occurrence of susceptibility artifacts (although this may also be exploited in some circumstances, to obtain relevant clinical information). The use of high receiver bandwidth and short TE also helps to limit these artifacts.

Truncation or Gibbs artifacts

The complex signal produced during MRI imaging would be adequately represented only by sampling for an infinite time duration. However, signal sampling has to be limited in time and, therefore, the collected signal is always a truncated version of the produced signal. This technical issue is generally corrected through the application of post-processing smoothing filters but, in some circumstances, it may not be sufficient to avoid the appearance of specific artifacts (truncation or Gibbs artifacts). These artifacts typically produce images characterized by blurring of the edges of the imaged structures and, in some cases, edge ringing (i.e., appearance of multiple dark lines immediately adjacent and parallel to high contrast interfaces).

CONCLUSIONS

The enormous clinical versatility of MR imaging together with the ability to obtain high-quality 2D and 3D images using fast scanning sequences, represent the main reason for the current widespread utilization of this imaging modality. To obtain an MR image, the process of signal generation is repeated many times and the collected data are used to fill a digital data space (k-space). Some of the inherent properties of k-space are exploited while designing fast scan sequences.

Image quality and time efficiency of data collection are inversely related in MR imaging, and multiple parameters related to the scan sequence (e.g., echo time [TE], repetition time [TR], inversion time [TI], flip angle, receiver bandwidth, etc.) or the produced image (e.g., field-of-view [FOV], matrix, slice thickness, etc.) may be adjusted to optimize the balance between these two factors.

In MR imaging, the intensity and characteristics of the signal are determined by tissue-specific properties such as proton density (PD), T1, and T2 relaxation. Image contrast may be modulated by the operator by modifying specific scanning parameters (i.e., TE, TR, and flip angle). The signal produced by certain tissues may be suppressed or enhanced in a (more or less) selective way by adding specific modifications to the standard scan sequences or by using contrast agents for MR imaging.

Various imaging artifacts may significantly affect image quality, but multiple strategies have been developed to reduce or avoid their occurrence.

PRACTICAL PEARLS

- MR imaging allows the generation of high-quality images of body structures, enabling a plethora of clinical applications.

- The RF pulse generated by a transmit coil is characterized by a range of frequencies referred to as *transmit bandwidth* (tBW). This is distinct from receiver bandwidth.

- The ratio between sampling rate and number of samples of signal is defined as *sampling frequency*. Sampling frequency must be at least twice the value of the highest-frequency component of the signal to avoid aliasing. Wrap artifact is a consequence of aliasing and can occur in the slice-encoding and phase-encoding direction.

- Voxel size may be obtained by the ratio of the field-of-view and the matrix size (Vox=FOV/N, where FOV and N refer to the field-of-view and matrix size in the *x*- or *y*-direction). Any increase in spatial resolution, however, is paralleled by a decrease in signal-to-noise ratio.

- Fast T1-weighted gradient-echo sequences [i.e., fast low angle shot (FLASH), spoiled gradient acquisition in the steady state (SPGR), or fast field echo (FFE)] are used in contrast-enhanced MRA.

- Spin-echo sequences are rich in signal and less susceptible to artifacts. In fast SE imaging, multiple 180° RF pulses are repeatedly used (echo train). The image contrast is determined by the echo train length (ETL) and the effective TE (TEeff).

- Echo time (TE) is the time from the RF excitation to the center of the echo being received. Shorter TEs allow less signal decay.

- Increasing rBW allows one to decrease TE which then allows one to lower TR and hence scan time.

- A practical way to reduce scan time is to reduce phase encoding steps. Another way to reduce TE is to reduce TR. TE can be shortened by increasing sampling frequency (by increasing receiver bandwidth [rBW]). However, the consequence of increasing rBW is that there is loss of SNR. Specific contrast agents may be utilized to alter the intrinsic contrast of tissues on MR images, the most commonly used agents are chelates of *gadolinium*. Image quality refers to the fidelity of representation of the imaged structures and is the composite of multiple elements, including spatial resolution, image contrast, and occurrence of image artifacts.

- The degree of chemical shift can be readily calculated if one knows the rBW and the FOV. If an image has 256 pixels in the frequency-encoding direction and a rBW of 32 kHz, the rBW/pixel is 32 000/256 = 125 Hz/pixel. At 1.5 T the chemical shift is 225 Hz.

- Truncation artifacts are characterized by blurring of the edges of the imaged structures and, in some cases, ringing (i.e., the appearance of multiple dark lines immediately adjacent and parallel to high-contrast interfaces).

FURTHER READING

Elster A, Burdette JH. Questions and Answers in Magnetic Resonance Imaging. St Louis, MO: Mosby, 2001.

Higgins CB, de Roos A, eds. MRI and CT of the Cardiovascular System. Philadelphia, PA: Lippincott Williams and Wilkins, 2006.

Lee VS. Cardiovascular MRI: Physical Principles to Practical Protocols. Philadelphia, PA: Lippincott Williams and Wilkins, 2006.

MR Pulse Sequences: What Every Radiologist Wants to Know but Is Afraid to Ask. RadioGraphics 2006; 26: 513–37.

13

MR techniques for vascular imaging

Santo Dellegrottaglie and Sanjay Rajagopalan

Multiple MR techniques have been developed to allow the study of vessel lumen and/or vessel wall with a combination of approaches being frequently used in the clinical setting. MR techniques for vascular imaging may be broadly classified as 'black-blood' or 'bright-blood' modalities, based on the appearance of the vascular lumen following application of a certain pulse sequence (Table 13.1). Black-blood imaging is typically obtained using spin-echo (SE) sequences, while bright-blood images are obtained by gradient-recall-echo (GRE) sequences in which flowing blood creates intraluminal signal (spontaneously or through the injection of a contrast agent).

BLACK-BLOOD IMAGING

Black-blood imaging is useful for the characterization of pathologies affecting the blood vessel wall (e.g., atherosclerosis, aneurysms, dissection, intramural hematoma, etc.). MR signal from flowing blood is frequently absent in images

---

Table 13.1 MR techniques for vascular imaging

- **Black-blood imaging**
- **Bright-blood imaging**
  - Time-of-flight imaging
  - Phase-contrast imaging
  - Morphologic imaging
  - Contrast-enhanced imaging

---

obtained with generic SE sequences, however additional modifications may be required to further optimize blood nulling with this technique.

Blood nulling in SE imaging

As described in Chapter 12, the generation of a signal (echo) on SE is based on the application of two sequential radio-frequency (RF) pulses (a 90° pulse followed by a 180° pulse). Only stationary protons lying in the imaged slice are subjected to the effects of these sequential RF pulses (*slice-selective pulses*). Flowing blood that moves into the slice is not exposed to either of these pulses and will not contribute to signal generation. As a consequence, the vessel lumen will appear as an area of *signal void*.

In an SE sequence echo time (TE) is defined as the time interval between the 90° RF pulse and the produced echo. The 180° RF pulse occurs at a time point that is exactly mid-way between the first pulse and the echo (corresponding to TE/2).

Optimal blood nulling is mainly related to two specific image parameters: (1) the distance the blood has to travel during the image acquisition (equal to the slice thickness) and (2) the time interval between the 90° RF pulse and the 180° RF pulse (i.e., TE/2). With a scanning plane perfectly perpendicular to the imaged vessels, a complete intraluminal signal void will be obtained only when the velocity of the blood in the vessel is higher than the ratio between slice thickness and TE/2 (Figure 13.1). In general, the use of a

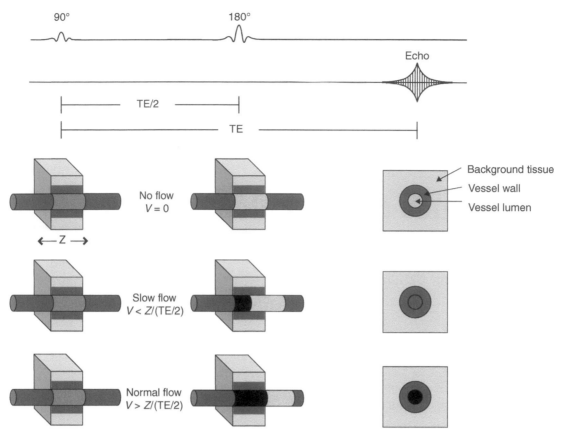

Figure 13.1   Black-blood imaging. Schematic representation of a blood vessel exposed to a 90° radiofrequency (RF) pulse and a 180° RF pulse, followed by the generation of the corresponding signal (echo), as part of an SE sequence. The role of the relationship between slice thickness (Z) and time interval between the two pulses (TE/2) on the resulting signal from blood flowing at a certain velocity (V) is outlined.

thin slice and high TE, helps to achieve complete intra-luminal signal void (good blood nulling).

Inversion recovery sequences

The signal produced by the flowing blood may also be excluded by modifications in the pulse sequence that specifically nulls blood signal.

Inversion recovery (IR) imaging is based on the application of a 180° RF prepulse (*inversion pulse*) to completely invert longitudinal magnetization of the protons. The use of *preparatory pulses* to obtain MR signal suppression has been outlined in Chapter 12. Any tissue may be 'nulled' by timing the application of the excitation RF pulse, to correspond with the time point at which the recovering longitudinal magnetization for that tissue, is passing through the transverse magnetization plane (null point). The time interval between the inversion pulse and the excitation pulse is defined as *inversion time* (TI). By selecting a TI value corresponding to the null point for the tissue, the latter will not contribute to the generation of signal.

Double IR imaging is obtained through a modification of fast SE sequences with the inclusion of two sequential 180° RF inversion pulses applied in rapid succession (Figure 13.2). The first inversion pulse is non-slice-selective and inverts the longitudinal magnetization of all the protons in the field. The second inversion pulse is slice-selective and brings longitudinal magnetization of the protons included in the imaged slice back to the original position. Thus, longitudinal magnetization of stationary protons (such as those in the vessel wall) is completely unaffected. In contrast, protons in the blood pool that are in the slice, are continually replenished by fresh protons that have only been subjected to the first (non-slice-selective) inversion pulse. As a result, the longitudinal magnetization in these flowing protons will be inverted and blood nulling may be obtained by applying an excitation RF pulse at an appropriate TI value. A long TI value needs to be selected to obtain blood nulling (around 650 ms with a 60 bpm heart rate and at 1.5 T). With the administration of gadolinium, the TI is shortened substantially (<150 ms) and thus it may not be possible to select an appropriately short TI to adequately null blood. Thus, it is recommended that double IR prepared fast SE sequences be

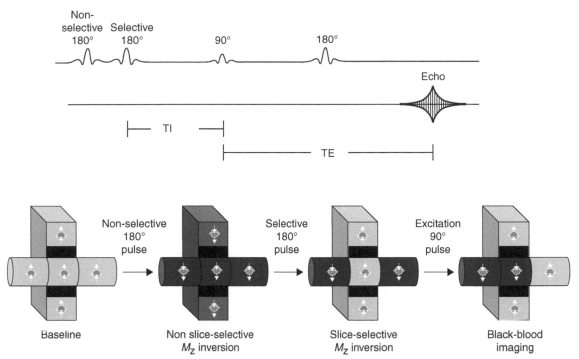

Figure 13.2 Double inversion recovery black-blood imaging. On the top, diagram showing a SE sequence constituted by a 90° radiofrequency (RF) pulse followed by a 180° RF pulse and modified with the introduction of two preparatory inversion pulses represented by a non-slice-selective 180° RF pulse and a slice-selective 180° RF pulse. The 90° RF excitation pulse follows the preparatory pulses after a time interval defined as inversion time (TI) and is then followed by the generation of a signal (echo) at the echo time (TE). On the bottom, schematic representation of a blood vessel demonstrating the effect of the preparatory pulses on the longitudinal magnetization (M_z) of stationary and moving protons. The first non-slice-selective RF pulse induces M_z inversion in all the exposed body protons (stationary and moving). The second preparatory RF pulse is slice-selective and brings M_z orientation of protons included in the selected slice back to the original orientation. By the time the excitation RF pulse is applied, the blood in the imaged slice will be replaced by fresh blood containing protons, which have experienced only the first non-slice-selective inversion pulse. The recovering M_z in blood will follow the TI recovery curve and will cross the zero line at a certain time point. By modifying the TI, the time of application of the excitation RF pulse may be made to coincide with the blood null point, resulting in black-blood imaging.

performed before contrast administration. The TI also needs to be adjusted with heart rate as TI is dependent on TR (time interval between successive 90° RF pulses).

A third inversion pulse may be included in the sequence to obtain fat saturation. The result is a combination of a double IR and a short-tau inversion recovery (STIR) sequence (frequently used for fat suppression, see Chapter 12) that is also referred to as *triple IR sequence*. Triple IR sequences have also been used for coronary MR imaging.

Double IR and triple IR imaging are typically implemented with EKG gating, with a period in diastole being chosen for phase encoding to avoid artifact related to flow variation and pulsatility.

TIME-OF-FLIGHT IMAGING

Time-of-flight (TOF) techniques have the ability to depict arterial or venous vessels without the need for contrast

injection. The clinical utilization of TOF-MRA has been reduced with the advent of contrast-enhanced MRA techniques by virtue of the long acquisition time and susceptibility to artifacts with the former technique. It is, however, a useful back-up modality in the event contrast-enhanced MRA cannot be performed and is still widely used for the evaluation of intracranial arteries and in MR venography (Chapters 15 and 23).

Principles of TOF imaging

TOF-MRA is obtained by employing a GRE sequence optimized to maximize the phenomenon of *'flow-related enhancement'*.

In multi-echo GRE imaging, multiple RF pulses with partial flip angle ($\alpha < 90°$) are applied in rapid succession (short repetition time [TR]) to a selected slice. Doing so, allows little time for complete recovery of longitudinal magnetization before the next pulse is applied, and consequently results in a progressive decline in transverse magnetization over the first several RF pulses, after which steady-state equilibrium is reached (*signal saturation*). This technique results in non-selective signal saturation of stationary protons with a consequent low signal from the selected slice. In contrast, fresh blood moving into the slice will not be exposed to any of these pulses and will be fully magnetized or unsaturated (high MR signal). As a result, in TOF imaging, flowing blood appears bright compared to the dark stationary tissue (flow-related enhancement). Any incoming blood, irrespective of direction and whether arterial or venous, will produce a bright signal in the imaged slice. To obtain images that are specific for arterial flow, a saturation band (spatially selective saturation) can be proximally distally to the imaged slice, in order to suppress signal from undesired venous flow. In contrast, to obtain an MR venogram, the saturation band is applied proximally, to suppress arterial inflow into the imaged slice.

TOF-MRA may be implemented as a two-dimensional (2D) or three-dimensional (3D) technique. 2D TOF-MRA is based on slice-by-slice coverage of a volume of tissue, in which background is adequately saturated and blood appears bright. Multiple contiguous slices are acquired with image overlap to facilitate image reconstruction. Alternatively, acquisition of an entire imaging volume into which blood is flowing is obtained with 3D TOF imaging. The major advantage of 3D TOF techniques is a higher signal-to-noise ratio (SNR), but this comes at the expense of longer scan time compared to 2D imaging. 3D TOF-MRA is particularly helpful in vessels with rapid steady blood flow without respiratory motion (e.g., intracranial vessels).

Imaging parameters

There are several parameters that can dictate optimal TOF imaging.

Relationship between repetition time (TR) and slice thickness. Adequate flow-related enhancement with TOF fundamentally depends on the complete replacement of blood already in the imaging slice with fresh blood ('unsaturated') during the time interval between two consecutive pulses (TR) (Figure 13.3). With a scanning plane perfectly perpendicular to the imaged vessels, complete flow-related enhancement is obtained when the velocity of the blood in the vessel is

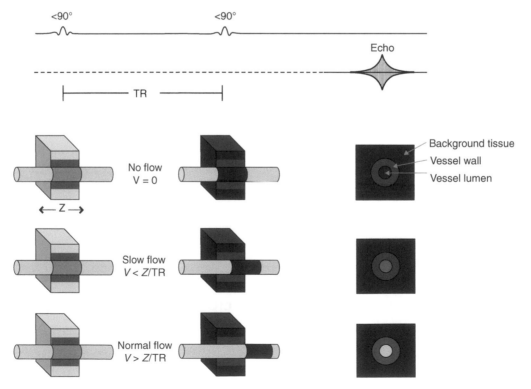

Figure 13.3   Time-of-flight (TOF) imaging. Schematic representation of a blood vessel exposed to a series of radiofrequency pulses with partial flip angle ($\alpha < 90°$) followed by the generation of the corresponding signal (echo) as part of a GRE sequence. The role of the relationship between slice thickness (Z) and time interval between two consecutive pulses (TR) on the resulting signal produced by the flowing blood at a certain velocity (V) is outlined. In general, the use of a thin slice and high TR helps to achieve good flow-related enhancement.

higher than the ratio between slice thickness and TR. In general, better TOF images may be obtained when thin slices and relatively long TR (typically 20–50 ms) are used. The sections should be thin enough to allow for sufficient inflow between RF pulse repetitions, but thick enough to ensure adequate SNR and anatomic coverage. Generally, section thickness from 1.5–2 mm (in small vessels) to 3–4 mm (in larger vessels) may be used. Similarly, TR should be long enough to allow sufficient inflow of unsaturated blood, but short enough to ensure adequate background saturation and to limit scan time duration.

Echo time (TE). TE should be as short as possible (typically, 8–9 ms). The use of short TE limits the occurrence of dephasing artifacts related to flowing blood and flow turbulence.

Flip angle. The use of short TR allows a very limited time for longitudinal magnetization recovery before the next excitation pulse. Thus, with recurrent high flip angle (α) excitations, there will be very little transverse magnetization to generate a signal. On the other hand, the use of RF pulses with high flip angle will produce better suppression of the stationary tissue and greater signal from the unsaturated blood. The α used in TOF balances these two objectives and typically varies between 30° and 60°.

Pitfalls and artifacts

Some important limitations significantly affect the clinical applicability of TOF imaging and these limitations should be kept in mind when using the technique.

Stenosis overestimation. Flow-related dephasing may occur with any GRE sequence when TE is too long. Keeping TE times short, and maintaining high spatial resolution may decrease the effects of flow-related dephasing. Furthermore turbulent blood flow in areas of stenosis may induce dephasing due to intravoxel signal loss (a consequence of loss of phase due to variable velocities in an area of turbulence).

Long scan time. As discussed previously, TOF imaging relies on relatively long TR times. The slice orientation must be perpendicular to the flow direction to avoid artifacts related to in-plane saturation. To minimize artifacts related to vessel pulsatility (*pulsation or ghosting artifacts*), image acquisition is frequently synchronized with EKG. When EKG gating is used, image acquisition occurs only during a limited period

of the cardiac cycle with consequent increase in scan time. The use of long TR and EKG gating, and the need to set the scan slice perpendicular to the imaged vessel (as opposed to longitudinally), may lead to excessively long scan times (several minutes). Long scan times expose TOF images to increased occurrence of breathing artifacts and motion artifacts.

Miscellaneous issues. Blood in vessels which are not truly perpendicular to the acquired section plane or are tortuous may be exposed to unintended repetitive excitation pulses (*in-plane saturation*). This may result in low signal intensity areas that can mimic stenoses. Finally, inappropriate nulling of the retrograde arterial flow in patients with occluded vessels may result through the use of saturation bands to prevent venous signal (spatially selective saturation), which may then inadvertently prevent the visualization of collaterals and reconstituted vessels.

PHASE CONTRAST IMAGING

Phase contrast (PC) imaging is a technique employed to generate MRA images or to obtain velocity-encoded flow images. It is generally used for flow quantification or in the evaluation of the severity of luminal stenoses, particularly in the cerebral and renal arteries. PC imaging can also be used as localizers to plan contrast-enhanced sequences.

Flow-encoding gradients

PC imaging makes use of velocity-induced phase shifts to distinguish flowing blood from stationary tissue. It is commonly performed using GRE techniques incorporating bipolar 'flow-encoding gradients'.

A flow-encoding gradient is composed of a pair of gradients that are equal in magnitude, but with opposite polarity (bipolar gradient). The first lobe causes spin dephasing, while the second lobe (of equal amplitude but opposite sign) induces spin rephasing. A bipolar gradient, thus, causes no net phase shift in stationary tissues. However, protons moving along the direction of the gradients will not be exposed to the two lobes of the gradient at the same intensity and will accrue a net phase shift, proportional to the velocity of movement (Figure 13.4). After the application of the first lobe of the bipolar gradient, the protons will have moved along the gradient direction and will be in a different position by the time the second lobe is applied. The moving protons will experience a magnetic field of a different intensity (stronger or weaker, based on the movement direction) compared to the one produced by the

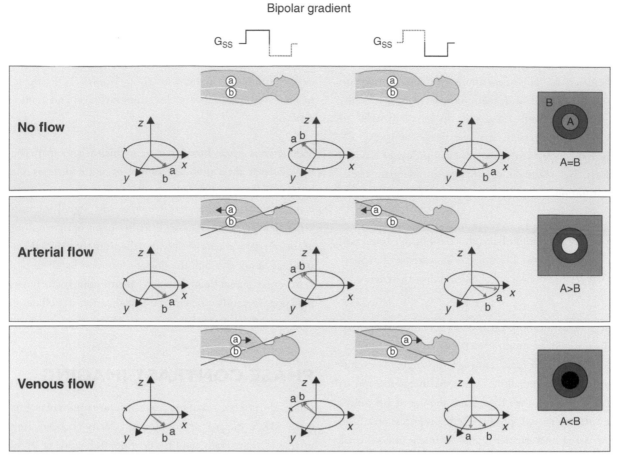

Figure 13.4 Differential effects of a bipolar gradient on stationary and moving protons. A blood vessel is schematically represented with the lumen (A) and the surrounding tissue (B) separated by the vessel wall. The behavior of a hypothetical moving proton (a) corresponding to the flowing blood and of a stationary proton (b) corresponding to the perivascular tissue is depicted in different flow conditions. The top panel illustrates the 'no flow' situation. In these circumstances, the application of a bipolar gradient along the slice-selective direction (G_{SS}) results in no net phase shift for both proton a (intraluminal) and proton b (perivascular). The effect of the positive lobe is perfectly counterbalanced by the negative lobe. In the resulting image, no flow-related enhancement differentiation is obtained (A=B). In the middle panel (simulates arterial flow), proton a is moving along the z-direction (head-to-feet). With the application of the positive lobe of the gradient, proton a will experience a magnetic field with a certain strength, but by the time the gradient is reversed it will be in a different position and exposed to a stronger magnetic field compared to the stationary proton b. In this case, proton a, accumulates a positive phase shift relative to proton b, and this may be used to generate an image with positive intravascular contrast (A > B). The intensity of signal produced is directly proportional to the velocity and direction of the moving proton. The bottom panel (simulates venous flow) illustrates the effects of the application of a bipolar gradient in the situation where proton a is moving with the same velocity, but in the opposite direction (feet-to-head) compared to the previous simulation. In this case, proton a accumulates a negative phase shift relative to proton b, with a corresponding image characterized by a negative intravascular contrast (A < B).

first lobe. Thus, with moving protons (flowing blood), the dephasing will not equal the rephasing, and protons will accumulate a net phase shift relative to stationary protons. The magnitude of the phase shift is dependent on the direction of the moving protons and proportional to their velocity.

To generate MR images with this technique, flow-encoding gradients are applied in the three directions producing three separate data sets (2 directions for 2d imaging). An additional data set is obtained without the application of flow-encoded gradients (mask data set). The four data sets are then combined to reconstruct both magnitude and phase images.

Magnitude and phase images

The different effects of flow-encoded gradients on stationary versus moving tissues may be used to generate image contrast between background structures and blood vessels (*magnitude images*) as well as to derive a flow–velocity map (*phase images*). In the first case, anatomic images are obtained by assigning a specific value of signal intensity to each image voxel, based on the magnitude of the measured velocity. In the second case, a flow–velocity map is generated from the derived net phase shift. In phase images, signal intensity in each voxel is directly proportional to flow velocity (phase shift), but is also related to the directionality of flow. Compared to stationary tissue, a brighter signal is attributed to positive phase shift and a darker signal to negative phase shift.

Velocity encoding

As described above, the amplitude of phase shift is proportional to the velocity of moving protons. Thus, flow velocity may be derived by measuring the phase shift (ranging from $-180°$ to $+180°$). The maximum proton velocity that can be measured (corresponding to a $180°$ phase shift) is referred to as *Venc* (or encoding velocity). The operator defines this parameter at the time of image acquisition. When a certain value of Venc is selected, the MR system modifies the strength of the flow-encoding gradients, so that a proton moving at a velocity corresponding to Venc will generate a $180°$ phase shift. If protons move faster than the selected Venc, the phase shift will be greater than $180°$ and this will be misinterpreted as flow in the opposite direction (*aliasing*). Thus, aliasing will occur for blood flow velocities that are much higher than the preset Venc. On the other hand, inaccurate velocity measurements are obtained when the selected Venc is too high in relation to the flow velocity being measured. Accurate measurements using PC techniques are dependent on selection of the appropriate Venc (slightly higher than the actual maximum velocity) and an acquisition plane perpendicular to the imaged vessel (Table 13.2).

Table 13.2 Typical setting for velocity encoding (Venc) in phase contrast (PC) imaging at various vascular beds

Vessel	Venc (cm/s)
Aorta	150
Pulmonary artery	75
Carotid artery	150
Renal artery	150
Femoral artery	150
Veins	25

Flow quantification

Flow quantification with PC imaging is based on EKG-gated acquisition of multiple 2D images in a single plane. The images can be viewed as a cine loop and may also be referred to as cine PC-MRA. In this manner, *in-plane flow* (imaging plane parallel to the vessel flow) or *through-plane flow* (imaging plane perpendicular to the vessel flow) may be visualized and quantified. With in-plane flow imaging, flow-encoding gradients are applied in the phase and frequency-encoding directions, and an image along the long axis of the vessel is obtained. With through-plane flow imaging, velocity-encoding gradients are applied in the slice-selecting direction and an image along the transverse axis of the vessel is obtained.

Using EKG gating, the series of images can reveal the temporal variation of blood flow over the cardiac cycle. Blood flow velocity and volume may be measured from the flow/time curves. Peak flow velocity across a stenosis may also be measured and the peak pressure gradient can be obtained using the modified Bernoulli equation (pressure gradient $= 4 \times V_{max}^2$) to define the hemodynamic significance of a stenosis.

With 3D PC techniques, flow encoding is simultaneously obtained in the three directions. This approach is able to provide 3D vessel flow, but suffers from some important disadvantages. A long scan time is required to apply the gradients in the three directions. Turbulent flow may induce intravoxel dephasing and consequent signal dropout. This phenomenon may cause overestimation of the severity of a stenosis. On the other hand, in some clinical applications such as renal MRA, the signal dephasing observed on 3D PC images is used to confirm the functional significance of a stenosis (Chapter 19).

CONTRAST-ENHANCED MR IMAGING

Contrast-enhanced (CE)-MRA represents the MR technique of choice for most clinical vascular applications. MR images with this technique are obtained by applying a rapid pulse sequence (typically a spoiled GRE sequence) during the intravenous administration of a contrast agent. Compared to other MRA techniques (i.e., TOF and PC imaging), intravascular signal in CE-MRA is not dependent on flow characteristics (flow-independent), but on the effect of a gadolinium-based contrast agent on blood magnetization (T1-shortening). For this reason, precise timing of image acquisition relative to contrast opacification is extremely important. In light of the requirement for rapid imaging, fast pulse sequences (using ultra-short TR and TE) must be used for CE-MRA.

Spoiled GRE sequence

In CE-MRA, images are generally obtained by applying a 3D *GRE pulse sequence* that uses small flip angles. The general concepts regarding GRE imaging have been discussed in Chapter 12. The application of a partial flip angle RF pulse allows the use of short TR values in GRE imaging with consequent reduction in scan time. This is because a significant amount of longitudinal relaxation (M_z) is left after the application of an RF pulse with a partial flip angle. Thus, there is no need to wait a long time to allow sufficient recovery in M_z before applying the next RF pulse. However, short TR values also may not allow complete decay in transverse magnetization (M_{xy}) between one RF pulse and the other, and a significant level of M_{xy} may still be present at the moment the next RF pulse is applied. To avoid the production of image artifacts due to residual M_{xy} with short TR sequences, different strategies have been developed. One such method is through the application of a spoiler or crusher gradient. This has the effect of dephasing any residual M_{xy} in the selected slice or volume.

Scan parameters

With CE-MRA, TR values in the order of 2–5 ms are typically used. TR is one of the major contributors to the final scan time duration and the use of short TR allows shorter acquisition times. Since TE occupies almost 50% of TR duration in fast GRE techniques, a reduction in TR can be easily accomplished by further shortening the TE (from 2–3 to 1–2 ms). The most efficient way to reduce TE in GRE is by the shortening of the gradient duration. The use of a stronger gradient when applied over a shorter duration, has the same effect on spin precession as a weaker gradient applied for a longer duration (Figure 13.5). The use of small flip angles (10–25°) allows a larger residual M_z, permitting shorter TR intervals. The presence of gadolinium-based contrast agent in blood permits rapid TI recovery of blood over background tissue with two consequences. The first is that rapid TI recovery of gadolinium-enhanced blood allows the use of larger than normal flip angles (25–40°) in conjunction with shorter TR. The second effect is that, with

shorter TR, there is better background suppression and superb delineation of the contrast-enhanced vessel.

Image contrast in fast GRE techniques

In multi-echo sequences such as those used for CE-MRA, the intensity of the signal generated is related to the amount of residual M_z available after the application of each RF pulse. The application of the initial RF pulses results in a gradual decrease in the amount of M_z until a state of equilibrium is reached, (when the available M_z remains constant) despite application of RF pulses (*signal saturation*). The higher the flip angle, the more intense the signal saturation. The relationship between TI and TR establishes the level of M_z at which the equilibrium is reached for a specific tissue (Figure 13.6). The use of RF pulses with partial flip angle applied in rapid succession does not allow recovery of M_z to any substantive degree for background tissue, resulting in signal suppression of the latter. In contrast, gadolinium, within the lumen of the vessel, by markedly shortening the speed of TI recovery for blood, allows a significantly higher 'equilibrium' M_z compared to the suppressed background tissue at the same TR.

k-Space filling schemes

One of the important goals of MR arteriography is the selective delineation of arteries without venous contamination. This is usually accomplished in CE-MRA by obtaining information during peak arterial opacification and limiting

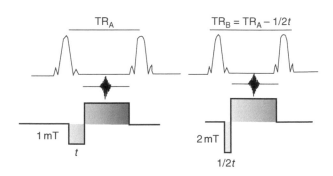

Figure 13.5 The effect of reducing duration of gradient lobes on TR. When the duration of the dephasing lobe (t) is reduced by 1/2, this reduces TR by that amount. 1mT refers to the gradient amplitude, TR$_A$ refers to the original TR, and TR$_B$ is the new TR after changing the gradient lobe duration.

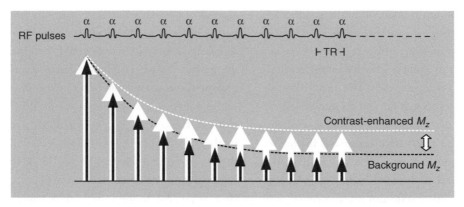

Figure 13.6 Generation of image contrast in GRE imaging with gadolinium-based contrast agent enhancement. The repeated application of multiple RF pulses with partial flip angle (α) results in the gradual reduction in longitudinal magnetization (M_z) available for the generation of MR signal (signal saturation). After a certain number of RF pulses, the M_z level reaches a state of equilibrium, which is dependent on the relation between the repetition time (TR) between successive RF pulses and the TI value for each tissue. As a consequence of the gadolinium-induced TI shortening, the M_z values at equilibrium are significantly higher in contrast-enhanced tissues (i.e., vessels) compared to the background tissues.

the acquisition time to the time that the contrast is in the arteries (arterial phase). As detailed in Chapter 12, information stored in the center of k-space is responsible for image contrast, while the periphery of k-space dictates image details. The ideal CE-MRA examination is timed so that the center of k-space is being filled at peak arterial contrast. The center of k-space can be filled by a variety of different schemes. In conventional MR imaging (non-contrast imaging) and in some CE-MRA applications, a linear sequential scheme is employed (Chapter 12, Figure 12.13). With this scheme, echo filling starts on one side of k-space and moves to the other side, passing through the center of k-space in a progressive linear fashion. Alternatively, a linear centric scheme can be used, in which the echoes stored in the center of k-space are collected at the beginning of image acquisition and are followed by the ones corresponding to the k-space periphery. Such a scheme can be utilized when the peak arrival of contrast can be predicted accurately and when the duration of arterial phase is short (brief arterio-venous transit times). Centric k-space filling is very sensitive to timing, and if the acquisition occurs prior to peak contrast opacification (early), or when the contrast concentration is changing rapidly, it can cause artifacts (Gibbs or truncation artifacts). Non-cartesian trajectories of k-space filling (e.g., radial, spiral, etc.) may be employed to obtain rapid and efficient filling of the center in comparison to the periphery of k-space (Chapter 12, Figure 12.14). Centric filling schemes are preferred in territories where venous contamination is more prevalent (i.e., CE-MRA of the carotids, pulmonary arteries, renal arteries, and distal leg arteries).

Imaging coverage and spatial resolution

To obtain a wide anatomic coverage while containing scan time, the 3D volume is placed with the largest dimension corresponding to the frequency-encoding direction. The remaining dimensions of the 3D volume are generally smaller and correspond to the two phase-encoding directions, which represent the time-consuming steps of image acquisition. The spatial resolution of a 3D CE-MRA image is usually higher in one dimension (frequency-encoding) than in the other, although isotropic voxel size may be obtained in many cases owing to the rectangular field-of-view (Chapter 12). Parallel imaging techniques are currently integrated in CE-MRA and this enables higher spatial resolution ($<1.0\,\text{mm}^3$ isotropic voxel size in some cases), with no increase in scan time duration.

Contrast injection

The goal of CE-MRA is good signal (contrast) separation between vessels and perivascular tissues (mostly fat) with adequate background suppression (reduced noise). Thus, a high enough concentration of contrast agent must be reached in the vessel lumen to lower the TI of blood below that of the surrounding fat (which is also characterized by a short TI). Another important consideration is that high contrast concentrations should be maintained throughout image acquisition. For most exams, matching contrast bolus duration to the scan time will ensure that an adequate concentration of gadolinium is obtained in the imaged vessel. Various gadolinium-based contrast agents are available for clinical MRA applications. By using an automatic power injector, a bolus of contrast agent is followed by a saline flash (20–30 ml) to maintain a compact bolus. The injected dose of contrast agent is usually between 0.1 and 0.2 mmol/kg body weight, with the lower dose employed to image short vascular beds (i.e., carotid and renal circulation) and the higher concentrations preferred for imaging of large vascular territories (i.e., thoracic and abdominal aorta). A value of 0.3 mmol/kg represents the maximum recommended dose for most of the commercially available contrast agents. The rate of contrast injection (2–3 ml/s) may be varied (in relation to patient characteristics, clinical indication, and acquisition time).

Timing of image acquisition

To obtain optimal arterial CE-MRA, image acquisition needs to be synchronized with the peak arterial contrast enhancement. CE-MRA protocols always include a time delay (*scan time delay*, T_{DELAY}) between the beginning of contrast injection and the start of image acquisition related to the time for the contrast bolus to travel from the site of injection to the artery of interest (*circulation time*, T_{CIRC}). There can be interindividual variability in T_{CIRC} related mainly to cardiac function and, to a lesser extent, to other demographic factors (Chapter 5). Different methods to estimate T_{DELAY} have been developed to account for these interindividual differences.

Guess method

With this method the T_{DELAY} is approximated, based on age and clinical history. Thus, a T_{DELAY} of 10–12 s may be reasonable in a young healthy subject, while a longer T_{DELAY} (25–30 s) is used in older subjects, or in the presence of diminished cardiac ejection fraction. The best guess method works in almost 90% of cases (note that the use of a longer contrast bolus may reduce the risk of wrong timing with the guess method).

Test bolus method

The test bolus method measures the actual time a small amount of contrast material (1–2 ml) takes to travel from the injection site to the vessel of interest (corresponding to T_{CIRC}). Images of the target vessel are sequentially acquired at a rate of 1 image/s during the test bolus injection for a total period of 40–60 s. The image frame with maximal intraluminal signal intensity is then used to determine the T_{CIRC} of the patient. To be reliable, the test bolus time needs to be measured at the same injection rate and the same amount of saline bolus as the actual injection. With the test bolus method, the correct T_{DELAY} for image acquisition can be mathematically derived, but the calculation will vary with the k-space filling scheme (Figure 13.7). In CE-MRA, the acquisition of the center of k-space (T_{CENTER}) has to be as close as possible to the time of peak contrast (T_{PEAK}). For practical purposes, T_{PEAK} may be considered as equal to the sum of T_{CIRC} and approximately half of the bolus time duration (T_{BOLUS}). Based on these assumptions, when a linear sequential k-space filling scheme is applied, a practical equation to calculate T_{DELAY} is:

$$T_{DELAY} = T_{CIRC} + T_{BOLUS}/2 - T_{SCAN}/2$$

On the other hand, when a linear centric filling scheme is employed, T_{DELAY} may be considered to be equivalent to T_{CIRC}.

Bolus detection method

With this method, CE-MRA acquisition is triggered by contrast arrival at the vessel of interest. This is accomplished through the repetitive acquisition of low resolution, background suppressed 2D images (inversion recovery prepared SSFP or fast low angle shot [FLASH] images) of the selected vessel during the actual contrast injection. When high intravascular signal due to contrast arrival is visualized, the CE-MRA acquisition is triggered either manually (by the operator) or automatically. The automatic triggering is based on continuous sampling of the signal intensity within a prescribed region of interest in the imaged vessel CE-MRA acquisition starts automatically when a prespecified increase in signal intensity is detected within the region of interest.

CE-MRA protocols

Setting up a CE-MRA examination

After preliminary scouts, rapid morphologic images (black-blood HASTE and bright-blood SSFP images) in three planes are usually obtained. These serve the dual purpose of defining the vascular territory and anatomy of interest and also provide a superior resolution 'road map' to plan the

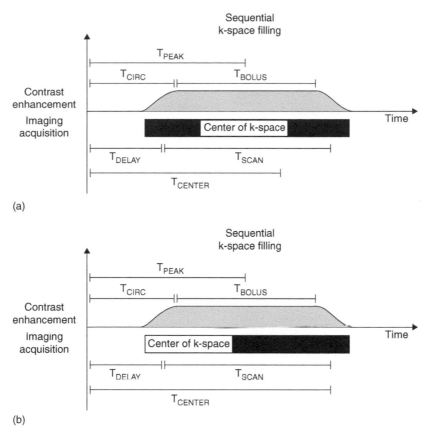

Figure 13.7 Scan time delay calculation from the measured circulation time in CE-MRA. The filling of the center of k-space is crucial in determining the final image contrast. To obtain optimal image contrast, T_{CENTER} has to be as close as possible to T_{PEAK} ($T_{CENTER} \approx T_{PEAK}$). As graphically represented in the figure, T_{PEAK} is equal to the sum of T_{CIRC} and approximately half of T_{BOLUS} ($T_{PEAK} = T_{CIRC} + T_{BOLUS}/2$). When a linear sequential filling scheme is applied, with the center of k-space acquired in the mid-portion of T_{SCAN}, T_{CENTER} is equal to the sum of T_{DELAY} and approximately half of T_{SCAN} ($T_{CENTER} = T_{DELAY} + T_{SCAN}/2$). Thus, a practical equation to calculate T_{DELAY} when linear sequential k-space filling is used may be derived ($T_{CENTER} \approx T_{PEAK} \Rightarrow T_{DELAY} + T_{SCAN}/2 = T_{CIRC} + T_{BOLUS}/2 \Rightarrow T_{DELAY} = T_{CIRC} + T_{BOLUS}/2 - T_{SCAN}/2$). In cases in which a linear centric filling scheme is employed, with the center of k-space acquired at the beginning of T_{SCAN}, T_{CENTER} may be considered to be approximately equal to the sum of T_{DELAY} and $T_{BOLUS}/2$ and a simplified equation to calculate T_{DELAY} for CE-MRA using linear centric k-space filling scheme may be obtained ($T_{CENTER} \approx T_{PEAK} \Rightarrow T_{DELAY} + T_{BOLUS}/2 = T_{CIRC} + T_{BOLUS}/2 \Rightarrow T_{DELAY} = T_{CIRC}$). T_{BOLUS} = bolus time duration; T_{CENTER} = time to the acquisition of the center of k-space; T_{CIRC} = circulation time; T_{DELAY} = scan time delay; T_{PEAK} = time to peak contrast; T_{SCAN} = acquisition scan time.

eventual CE-MRA exam. The 3D volume is prescribed and the plane may vary depending on the territory and the clinical question. Usually obliquely oriented planes are preferred for complete coverage of the aorta, while straight coronal planes are preferred for the pulmonary and carotid arteries. After optimizing scan parameters, including EKG gating (if this is required) and with breath-hold if indicated, an MRA acquisition is performed without contrast injection. This non-contrast acquisition serves the dual purpose of testing the sequence and procuring precontrast mask images for subsequent subtraction from the CE image acquisition. Once this is satisfactorily accomplished, the precontrast images are carefully examined for quality (signal) and artifacts. Once the mask images are satisfactorily procured, the actual CE-MRA is obtained by timing the image acquisition to peak arterial contrast, as detailed above. Finally, in most cases, the 3D sequence is repeated once or twice immediately after completion of the arterial phase CE acquisition. These delayed post-contrast acquisitions provide additional sets of images, which may be useful in case of inappropriate timing for the CE-MRA and may also provide venous phase images.

Single-station and multi-station MRA

CE-MRA protocols may involve a single vascular territory within the imaging field of view (*single-station MRA*) or may be engineered to image multiple contiguous vascular territories covering a large area (e.g., lower extremity vessels, thoraco-abdominal aorta, etc.) during the same imaging session (*multi-station MRA*). In one approach to multi-station MRA, contiguous stations are acquired during separate injection of contrast and after repositioning of the patient within the scanner (*multi-injection MRA*). However, multi-injection MRA is not preferred as it is limited by the total amount of contrast that can be administered (usually no more than 0.3 mmol/kg body weight) and by the lingering effects of residual contrast from the previous injection at the subsequent level. A more practical approach involves a moving-table technique in which the passage of a single contrast bolus from one station to the other is sequentially followed automatically, moving the scanner table through the center of the magnet, thereby covering the entire region of interest (*moving-table MRA*). For a multi-station moving-table CE-MRA, the scan time delay (T_{DELAY}) for the first station is measured by one of the methods described before. The T_{DELAY} for subsequent stations is derived by including the additional time the table takes to move from one position to the other (very short in modern scanners). With this approach, by keeping the acquisition scan time ($T_{IMAGING}$) for each station short (8–15 s), a total of 3–4 separate stations can be acquired in less than 1 minute.

Time-resolved MRA

MRA techniques based on repeated acquisition of 3D images at the same location over time have been recently introduced in clinical practice (time-resolved MRA). The rapidity of image acquisition obviates the need for precise arterial contrast timing with time-resolved MRA, besides providing arterial and venous phase information in a dynamic fashion. The ability to perform time-resolved imaging predicates rapid speed so that the temporal arrival of contrast in a vascular bed can be tracked over time. Image resolution also has to be satisfactory to enable clinical decision-making. Thus time-resolved imaging strives for compromise between adequate spatial and temporal resolution and this balance may be appropriately modified depending on the clinical question and application. Temporal resolution with most current time-resolved sequences relies on information sharing of k-space lines to circumvent time-consuming phase-encode steps. Time-resolved acquisition techniques such as the TRICKS (time-resolved intravascular contrast kinetics) and TREAT (time-resolved echo shared angiographic technique), when used in conjunction with parallel imaging, can effectively reduce temporal resolution to 200–300 ms/3D slab.

Echo sharing in time-resolved MRA

Time-resolved techniques are based on the use of shared echo lines, where data are shared from one 3D data set to other. The center of k-space is repeatedly sampled, while portions of peripheral k-space are sampled intermittently. This reduces the time to acquire the 3D volume and effectively improves temporal resolution. Figure 13.8 illustrates one particular approach whereby time for acquisition is reduced by two-thirds. The first acquisition is the only acquisition where the entire data set is obtained and all subsequent acquisitions share information.

Time-resolved MRA has tremendous applications in the evaluation of patients with peripheral arterial disease and is routinely incorporated for the assessment of atherosclerotic involvement of the distal leg vessels as part of hybrid imaging approaches (Chapter 22). It can also be used for the evaluation of suspected pulmonary vascular disease, for the evaluation of grafts, conduits, and collaterals.

Artifacts and pitfalls of CE-MRA

Multiple artifacts may compromise the diagnostic value of the images obtained with CE-MRA. Some of the most common pitfalls noted in CE-MRA are related to poor-quality images caused by failure to suspend breathing, poor timing of bolus injection, or inadequate setting for the image field of view (FOV).

Timing artifacts

Suboptimal timing of data acquisition relative to the peak arterial contrast arrival is a frequent source of image artifacts with CE-MRA. When image acquisition occurs too late with respect to the peak arterial enhancement, venous opacification may obscure the visualization of arterial vessels (*venous contamination*). Conversely, an early image acquisition may lead to incomplete arterial opacification. A characteristic artifact (Gibbs, truncation, or Maki artifact) is produced in cases where central k-space data sampling occurs during rapidly changing contrast concentrations.

Susceptibility artifacts

A variety of conditions can cause artifacts which may lead to *pseudostenosis* on CE-MRA images. Metallic clips and intravascular stents are common culprits and should always

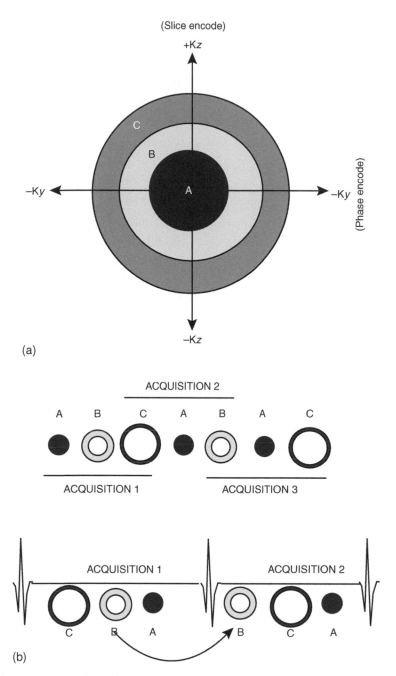

Figure 13.8 (a)　Graphical representation of k-space and its partition into 3 areas. The innermost area (A) corresponds to the center of k-space while regions B and C comprise outer k-space. **(b)** Echo (data) sharing schemes in time-resolved MRA. Each acquisition repeatedly samples A (center of k-space) but B and C are shared, with these areas being refreshed in every other acquisition. The second representation shows the sequence of acquisition with EKG gating. The center of k-space is sampled with every cardiac cycle, but is deliberately acquired during diastole to minimize artifact (reverse centric acquisition) while the periphery is shared.

be considered. The presence of highly concentrated gadolinium contrast agent in a contiguous vein can cause T2 shortening and may give the appearance of a vascular stenosis in the adjoining artery (*susceptibility artifact*). Furthermore, inappropriate positioning of the imaging volume with vessel exclusion may frequently produce pseudostenosis or vessel

occlusion, especially in tortuous arteries. Areas with signal drop-out on subtracted images may be due to a subtraction artifact and should be differentiated from masses by inspection of the raw, unsubtracted 3D data or complementary morphologic images. The reason for this artifactual signal drop-out on subtracted images is that unsaturated spins, especially at the edges of the FOV, may result in bright signal on the precontrast image, which if subtracted from corresponding areas on the post-contrast images may result in signal drop-out.

Aliasing artifacts

The use of small FOV in relation to the body size generates image aliasing that may preclude the adequate visualization of vessels close to the margin of the images (*wraparound artifacts*). Wraparound artifacts occur only in the phase-and-slice encoding direction and rarely in the frequency-encoding direction.

Resolution artifacts

Limited spatial resolution limits sensitivity to detect small lesions, such as intraluminal defects, small stenoses in vasculitis, and atherosclerotic disease. Partial voluming due to thick slices can give the appearance of stenosis or fail to detect intraluminal lesions partially obstructing flow. Imaging should, if possible, be performed on multiple planes to confirm findings.

CONCLUSIONS

Multiple different MR-based approaches have been developed for the imaging of the vasculature. In black-blood imaging, an SE sequence is modified to adequately null the signal produced by flowing blood. The resulting images allow visualization of the vessel wall and its pathologies. GRE imaging techniques are the basis for bright-blood techniques such as TOF-MRA, PC-MRA, and CE-MRA. TOF-MRA is frequently employed for assessment of intracranial vessels but has important limitations (e.g., long scan duration, flow-related artifacts, etc.) that restrict its widespread use. Vascular evaluation may also be obtained by PC imaging, where signal produced by moving protons is differentiated from stationary protons, through the application of flow-encoding gradients. PC imaging may also be applied to obtain velocity and flow information, with important applications in the assessment of stenosis severity. In CE-MRA, intravenous injection of a gadolinium-based contrast agent is used to produce high intravascular signal. High spatial resolution and fast acquisition are combined in a facile manner lending itself to use in a variety of clinical applications.

PRACTICAL PEARLS

- Multiple MR techniques have been developed to allow the study of vessel lumen and/or vessel wall with a combination of approaches being frequently used in the clinical setting.

- Vascular imaging may be broadly classified as 'black-blood' or 'bright-blood' modalities, based on the appearance of the vascular lumen following application of a pulse sequence.

- Black-blood imaging refers to spin-echo (SE) sequences modified with a double inversion recovery (IR) preparation pulse suppressing the signal produced by the flowing blood. Bright-blood MRA approaches are GRE-based (time-of-flight [TOF], phase-contrast [PC] MRA or contrast-enhanced [CE] MRA).

- Double IR prep of a SE sequence includes two sequential 180° RF inversion pulses prior to the 90° pulse (one non-slice-selective and a second slice-selective). Longitudinal magnetization of stationary protons (such as the protons in the vessel wall) is completely unaffected. These must be performed before contrast administration.

- To obtain images that are specific for arterial flow in TOF imaging, the saturation band must be applied distal to the slice, to suppress venous flow signal. In MR venography, the saturation band is applied proximally to suppress arterial inflow.

- 3D TOF-MRA is particularly helpful in vessels with rapid steady blood flow without respiratory motion (e.g., intracranial vessels).

- Accurate measurements using PC techniques are dependent on the selection of the appropriate velocity encoding (Venc) and a plane perpendicular to the imaged vessel.

- Centric k-space filling is sensitive to timing, and if the acquisition occurs prior to peak contrast opacification (early), or when the contrast concentration is changing rapidly, it may cause artifacts (Gibbs or truncation artifacts).

- Centric filling schemes are preferred in territories where venous contamination is more prevalent (i.e., CE-MRA of the carotids, pulmonary arteries, renal arteries, and distal leg arteries).

- A dose of 0.3 mmol/kg represents the maximum recommended dose for most of the commercially available contrast agents.

- To obtain optimal arterial CE-MRA images, image acquisition needs to be synchronized with the peak arterial contrast enhancement.

- To obtain optimal arterial CE-MRA images, image acquisition needs to be synchronized with the peak arterial contrast enhancement. When a linear sequential k-space filling scheme is applied, a practical equation to calculate time delay to start the scan is: $T_{DELAY} = T_{CIRC} + T_{BOLUS/2} - T_{SCAN/2}$, where T_{CIRC} is time for peak contrast opacification, T_{BOLUS} is the duration of bolus, and T_{SCAN} is scan time.

- Time-resolved techniques are based on the use of shared echo lines, where data are shared from one 3D data set to another. The center of k-space is repeatedly sampled, while portions of peripheral k-space are sampled intermittently.

FURTHER READING

Arena L, Morehouse HT, Safir J. MR imaging artifacts that simulate disease: how to recognize and eliminate them. Radiographics 1995; 15(6): 1373–94.

Bradley WG Jr, Waluch V, Lai KS, Fernandez EJ, Spalter C. The appearance of rapidly flowing blood on magnetic resonance images. AJR Am J Roentgenol 1984; 143: 1167–74.

Brown MA, Semelka RC. MR imaging abbreviations, definitions, and descriptions: a review. Radiology 1999; 213: 647–62.

Crawley AP, Wood ML, Henkelman RM. Elimination of transverse coherences in FLASH MRI. Magn Reson Med 1988; 8: 248–60.

Elster A, Burdette JH. Questions and Answers in Magnetic Resonance Imaging. St Louis, MO: Mosby, 2001.

Evans AJ, Hedlund LW, Herfkens RJ, Utz JA, Fram EK, Blinder RA. Evaluation of steady and pulsatile flow with dynamic MRI using limited flip angles and gradient refocused echoes. Magn Reson Imaging 1987; 5: 475–82.

Frahm J, Haase A, Matthaei D. Rapid three-dimensional MR imaging using the FLASH technique. J Comput Assist Tomogr 1986; 10: 363–8.

Hawkes RC, Patz S. Rapid Fourier imaging using steady-state free precession. Magn Reson Med 1987; 4: 9–23.

Higgins CB, de Roos A, eds. MRI and CT of the Cardiovascular System. Philadelphia, PA: Lippincott Williams and Wilkins, 2006.

Krause UJ, Pabst T, Kenn W, Wittenberg G, Hahn D. Time-resolved contrast-enhanced magnetic resonance angiography of the lower extremity. Angiology 2004; 55: 119–25.

Lee VS. Cardiovascular MRI: Physical Principles to Practical Protocols. Philadelphia, PA: Lippincott Williams and Wilkins, 2006.

Maki JH, Chenevert TL, Prince MR. Three-dimensional contrast-enhanced MR angiography. Top Magn Reson Imaging 1996; 8: 322–44.

Niendorf T, Sodickson DK. Parallel imaging in cardiovascular MRI: methods and applications. NMR Biomed 2006; 19(3): 325–41.

Nishimura DG. Time-of-flight angiography. Magn Reson Med 1990; 14: 194–201.

Prince MR. Contrast-enhanced MR angiography: theory and optimization. Magn Reson Imaging Clin N Am 1998; 6: 257–67.

Prince MR, Grist TM, Debatin JF, eds. 3D Contrast Angiography. Berlin: Springer, 1999.

Prince MR, Yucel EK, Kaufman JA, Harrison DC, Geller SC. Dynamic gadolinium-enhanced three-dimensional abdominal MR arteriography. J Magn Reson Imaging 1993; 3(6): 877–81.

Rofsky NM. MR angiography of the aortoiliac and femoropopliteal vessels. Magn Reson Imaging Clin N Am 1998; 6: 371–84.

Zhang H, Maki JH, Prince MR. 3D contrast-enhanced MR angiography. J Magn Reson Imaging 2007; 25(1): 13–25.

14

Contrast agents in MR angiography

Marc Sirol and Sanjay Rajagopalan

INTRODUCTION

Contrast agents are used in numerous imaging modalities to enhance tissue contrast or to provide an indication of organ function or flow. One of the major differences between magnetic resonance imaging (MRI) and other imaging modalities is that in MRI, the alterations in signal intensities of tissue depend on the effects of the contrast agents on the MR properties (i.e., water relaxation rates) rather than on the direct visualization of the contrast agent itself. Therefore, MRI contrast agents are imaged indirectly, by their effect on proton relaxation rates.

This chapter is intended to describe the basic principles of contrast agents used in MRI including their underlying chemistry, biophysics, and clinical safety. This chapter assumes that the reader has an understanding of basic principles in MRI including physics and image generation (see Chapter 12). While there are many kinds of contrast agents that have been used to change MR signal properties, including hyperpolarized gases, paramagnetic contrast agents, pH-indicating agents, and magnetization-transfer agents, we will focus primarily on agents that are used clinically to change water relaxation properties and provide an introduction to molecular contrast agents, which are likely to be important for vascular applications in the near future.

MAGNETIC PROPERTIES AND GENERAL PRINCIPLES

Clinical MRI methodologies rely on imaging protons located in the body tissues (mainly in water). In general, signal intensity at a given anatomic locus depends on the amount of water protons (proton density, PD) and on the relaxation times for longitudinal (T1) and transverse (T2) magnetization. The values of T1 and T2 for each tissue are influenced by a range of factors, some of which are intrinsic to the tissue and the external magnetic field B_0 that the body is being subjected to. The determinants of T1 and T2 relaxation and mechanisms of tissue contrast generation and manipulation are discussed in Chapter 12. The images are usually weighted to accentuate these specific aspects of tissue magnetic properties and may be broadly classified into T1-weighted, T2-weighted, or proton density (PD) weighted images.

Magnetism

Magnetic field strength is measured in units of gauss (G) or in Tesla (T, $1T = 10\,000\,G$). The earth's magnetic field is about $0.5\,G$. Magnetism or magnetic susceptibility represents the extent to which a substance becomes magnetized when placed in an external magnetic field. In quantum mechanics, nuclei containing an odd number of protons and/or neutrons (nucleons) have a characteristic motion or *precession* and are said to have a spin quantum number depending on the number of odd nucleons. *Precession* is a rotating motion or "wobble" of the nucleus about its own axis and results in the induction of a magnetic moment in the direction of the spin axis. The strength of the magnetic moment is a property of the type of nucleus. Hydrogen nuclei as well as possessing the strongest magnetic moment, is in great abundance in biological material. Consequently hydrogen imaging is the most widely used MRI procedure. When the direction of the induced magnetic moment M is in the same direction as B_0

then the effective field that the object is exposed to is enhanced. This magnetic field enhancement is referred to as paramagnetism (Figure 14.1). When the direction of the induced magnetic moment M is opposite to that of the external field, the effective field that the object is exposed to is diminished and the effect is known as diamagnetism. Magnetic susceptibility (χ) is typically defined as the magnitude of the induced magnetic moment M divided by the strength of the external field B_0. Most biologic materials have extremely small χ values ($<10^{-4}$) while paramagnetic materials have values many orders of magnitude above zero (see below).

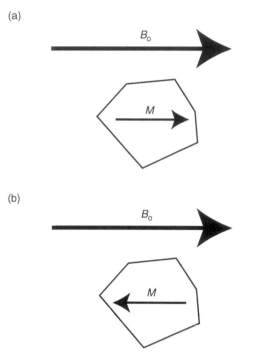

(a)

(b)

Figure 14.1 Effect of the exposure to an external magnetic field (B_0) for paramagnetic material (a) and diamagnetic material (b). M = induced magnetization.

Ferromagnetic agents

Ferromagnetic materials generally contain iron, nickel, or cobalt. Objects that are relevant to imaging that are ferromagnetic include aneurysm clips, pacemaker leads, metallic shrapnel, etc. These materials have a large positive magnetic susceptibility when placed in a magnetic field, i.e. χ is typically very large ($>10\,000$). Ferromagnetic materials are also characterized by being made up of clusters of 10^{17} to 10^{21} atoms called magnetic domains, that all have their magnetic moments pointing in the same direction. In contrast, in unmagnetized materials, the moments are randomly oriented. The ability to remain magnetized when an external magnetic field is removed is a distinguishing factor, when comparing paramagnetic, superparamagnetic, and diamagnetic materials. On MR images, ferromagnetic materials cause susceptibility artifacts, characterized by loss of signal and spatial distortion. Of note, susceptibility artifacts can occur even with fragments too small to be seen on plain X-rays.

Paramagnetic agents

Paramagnetic materials include ions of various metals like iron (Fe^{3+}), manganese (Mn^{2+}), copper (Cu^{2+}), chromium (Cr^{3+}), and gadolinium (Gd^{3+}). Paramagnetic materials consist of unpaired electrons in their outer orbitals, resulting in a positive magnetic susceptibility (Table 14.1). The magnitude of χ for paramagnetic materials is, however, several orders of magnitude lower than that in ferromagnetic materials. Paramagnetic substances can influence relaxation rates in two distinctly different but related ways: (1) through alterations in the local magnetic fields by changing the local magnetic susceptibility and (2) through an electron–nuclear dipolar interaction. The effect of application of an external magnetic field on a parmagnetic ion is an increase in T1 and T2 relaxation rates.

Table 14.1 The relationship between number of unpaired electrons in various metal ions and net magnetic moment

Atomic N	Ion	3d	4f	Magnetic moment (Bohr magneton)
24	Cr^{3+}	↑ ↑ ↑ _ _		3.8
25	Mn^{2+}	↑ ↑ ↑ ↑ ↑		5.9 (weak field)
26	Fe^{3+}	↑ ↑ ↑ ↑ ↑		5.9 (weak field)
29	Cu^{2+}	↑↓ ↑↓ ↑↓ ↑↓ ↑		1.7–2.2
63	Eu^{3+}		↑↓ ↑ ↑ ↑ ↑ ↑	(6.9)
64	Gd^{3+}		↑ ↑ ↑ ↑ ↑ ↑ ↑	7.9
66	Dy^{3+}		↑↓ ↑↓ ↑ ↑ ↑ ↑ ↑	(5.9)

Cr, chromium; Mn, manganese; Fe, Iron; Cu, copper; Eu, europium; Gd, gadolinium; Dy, dysprosium.

The paramagnetic metal ion used in most current cardiovascular applications is gadolinium (Gd^{3+} or Gd). Contrast agents containing Gd across a wide range of concentrations cause preferential T1 relaxation, resulting in an increase in signal on T1-weighted images. Figure 14.2 illustrates the exponential relationship between Gd concentration in blood and T1 relaxivity. Concentrations of at least 1 mM are required to get T1 of blood below that of fat (present around blood vessels in the form of peri-adventitial fat). It is important to note that Gd can also cause T2 relaxation and this effect may predominate at very high Gd concentrations, as is sometimes seen in the urinary bladder or in certain circumstances in the vasculature (high venous concentrations owing to slow flow). Enhanced T2 relaxation may cause a loss of signal (Figure 14.3).

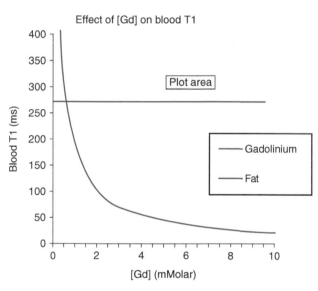

Figure 14.2 Effect of increasing gadolinium (Gd) concentration on T1 relaxivity of blood. A decline in T1 of blood below that of fat occurs at concentrations higher than 1 mM. Adapted from Rajagopalan and Prince.

Superparamagnetic agents

Superparamagnetic materials consist of individual domains of elements that have ferromagnetic properties in bulk. Their magnetic susceptibility χ is between that of ferromagnetic and paramagnetic materials. Examples of superparamagnetic materials include ferrites and magnetites (mixture of FeO and Fe_2O_3). Although ferrites shorten T1, their predominant effect is on T2 and T2*. The mechanism of their preferential effects on T2 is a consequence of the bulk effects of these particles on local field and resultant susceptibility effects. Thus, water protons in the vicinity of these particles become dephased, with consequent signal loss.

Diamagnetic agents

Diamagnetic materials have no intrinsic atomic magnetic moment, but when placed in an external magnetic field weakly repel the field (Figure 14.1), resulting in a small negative magnetic susceptibility ($\chi < 0$). Materials like water, copper, nitrogen, barium sulfate, and most tissues are diamagnetic.

Relaxivity

MRI contrast agents work through alteration of the relaxation rate of neighboring water molecules and consequent change of signal intensity. Since the contrast agent is typically present at several orders of magnitude lower concentration (0.1–1 mM) compared with water (55 M), the contrast agent must act catalytically to relax water protons in order to have a measurable effect. Although contrast agents can be visualized using a variety of pulse sequences (including spin-echo and gradient-echo techniques), optimization of imaging parameters

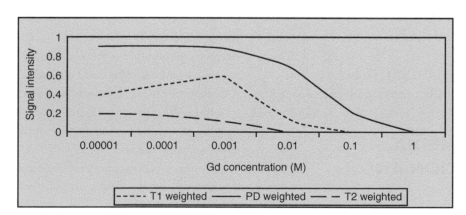

Figure 14.3 Non-linear relationship between gadolinium (Gd) concentration and signal intensity (SI) with different pulse sequence techniques. With T1 techniques, there is an initial increase in SI, resulting in positive contrast, followed by a significant decrease in SI at high Gd concentrations. With T2 and PD techniques no significant changes in SI are seen at Gd concentrations usually encountered in clinical conditions.

and an understanding of the effect of the contrast agent on signal intensity based on the pulse sequence is important.

The relaxivities values r1 and r2 respectively describe the catalytic efficiency of a contrast agent on T1 and T2 relaxation rates. Gd-containing contrast agents typically induce preferential shortening of T1, when used at concentrations indicated for clinical applications. The relaxivity values r1 and r2 respectively are very similar for Gd (4 and 5 mmol/ls respectively for Gd-DTPA as an example) one may incorrectly surmise that Gd has equal effects on T1 and T2 relaxation rates. This is, however, not true and Gd selectively shortens T1 more than T2. This is illustrated by the following example. Let us assume that after Gd injection, the T1 and T2 of tissue ($T1_{Tiss}$ and $T2_{Tiss}$) change to $T1_{TissGd}$ and $T2_{TissGd}$ respectively, where $T1_{Gd}$ and $T2_{Gd}$ are the relaxation times of the Gd agent alone and T1 TissGd or T2TissGd is the rate with the agent in the tissue. Since the resultant effect of the contrast agent on the T1 and T2 recovery rates of the tissue is a composite of the intrinsic properties of the tissue and that of the contrast agent, this may be expressed by the equations:

$$(1/T1_{TissGd}) = (1/T1_{Tiss}) + (1/T1_{Gd}) \qquad (1)$$

and

$$(1/T2_{TissGd}) = (1/T2_{Tiss}) + (1/T2_{Gd}) \qquad (2)$$

Now $1/T1_{Gd} = r1 * [Gd]$ while $1/T2_{Gd} = r2 * [Gd]$. Thus, it is apparent that there is a direct relationship between Gd concentrations and relaxation rates, with higher concentrations having a larger impact on relaxation rates (Figure 14.2). Let us assume that, for blood, $T1_{Tiss}$ is 1000 ms and $T2_{Tiss}$ is 100 ms. In addition, let us assume that, after injection of contrast, Gd achieves a concentration of 0.1 mmol/l. According to equation 1, $(1/T1_{TissGd}) = (1/1) + (1/T1_{Gd})$. Since $1/T1_{Gd} = r1 * [Gd]$ or $4 * 0.1$ mmol/l, $1/1/T1_{Gd} = 0.4$. Thus $1/T1_{TissGd} = 1.4$ or $T1_{TissGd} = 714$ ms (29% reduction in T1). On the other hand, $1/T2_{TissGd} = 1/0.1 + 5 * 0.1 = 10 + 0.5 = 10.5\,s^{-1}$. Thus $T2_{TissGd} = 95$ ms (5% decrease). Thus Gd at least at certain concentrations will produce a selective shortening of T1 over T2.

CONTRAST MEDIA CLASSIFICATION AND ATTRIBUTES

Table 14.2 lists current FDA approved contrast agents for human use while Table 14.3 includes agents in clinical development or preclinical testing. There are several ways in which MRI contrast agents may be classified. None of these schemas are all encompassing and all of the schemes show considerable overlap.

Classification of MR contrast agents can also be based on their specificity of uptake, mechanism of uptake, and requirement for activation. Based on this approach, contrast agents can be divided into three main groups: (1) non-specific agents, including both low molecular weight contrast agents, e.g. Gd-DTPA and high molecular weight blood pool agents; (2) targeted contrast agents, which are actively directed to a specific molecular target with an appropriate ligand; and (3) 'smart' contrast agents, also referred to as activated or responsive agents. An example of such an agent is EgadMe, a complex which contains a sugar moiety that prevents water from coordinating with Gd. In this water-inaccessible conformation, the contrast agent is 'inactive' and does not modulate T1. Galactosidase is an endogenously present enzyme able to enzymatically cleave the galactopyranose from the chelate, freeing a coordination site. The result is an irreversible transition of the contrast agent to an 'active' state by improving the accessibility of water to Gd.

An alternative scheme to classify contrast agents is as positive and negative contrast agents. Gd chelates, for instance, for the most part enhance T1 relaxivity and, therefore, result in enhanced signal intensity on T1-weighted sequences (positive contrast agents). Gd or other metals with unpaired electrons are typical positive contrast agents. Although the predominant effect is positive, these contrast agents can have negative effects on signal intensity at high concentrations of Gd (Figure 14.3). The effect of these agents on the SI of T2-weighted and PD-weighted images is minimal, except at very high concentrations.

Negative contrast agents are usually particulate aggregates that induce negative contrast and appear dark on MRI images. The predominant effect is on spin-spin relaxation through creation of local field inhomogeneities or T2* effects, which results in shorter T1 and T2 relaxation times. Examples of negative contrast agents include superparamagnetic iron oxide (SPIO) and ultra-small SPIO (USPIO). A special group of negative contrast agents are perfluorocarbons (perfluorochemicals) which, by their presence, exclude signal in protons responsible for the signal in MR imaging. These particles have been used in atherosclerosis imaging in order to detect and characterize specific sites or molecules of the atherothrombotic plaque in vivo, such as thrombus or platelet accumulation sites.

Finally, contrast agents may be classified by their effects on tissue contrast or by the predominant phase of distribution (e.g., extracellular, blood pool, protein bound, etc.).

Table 14.2 MRI contrast agents approved for clinical use

Generic name	Brand name and company	Chemical abbreviation	r_1, 0.5 T 37°C	r_2, 0.5 T 37°C	Osmolality[a] (osmol/kg)	Viscosity[a] (cP)	Normal enhancement pattern
Gadopentetate	Magnevist® Berlex, Schering	Gd-DTPA	3.8		1.96	2.9	Positive
Gadoterate	Dotarem® Guerbet	Gd-DOTA	3.6	4.8	1.35 (4.02)	2.0 (11.3)	Positive
Gadodiamide	Omniscan® GE Healthcare	Gd-DTPA-BMA	3.9		0.79 (1.90)	1.4 (3.9)	Positive
Gadoteridol	Prohance® Bracco	Gd-HPDO3A	3.7		0.63 (1.91)	1.3 (3.9)	Positive
Gadobutrol	Gadovist® Schering	Gd-DO3A-butrol	3.6		0.57 (1.39)	1.4 (3.7)	Positive
Gadoversetamide	Optimark® Mallinckrodt	Gd-DTPA-BMEA	4.7		1.11	2.0	Positive
Gadobenate	Multihance® Bracco	Gd-BOPTA	4.4	5.6	1.97	5.3	Positive
Mangafodipir	Teslascan® Amersham Health	Mn-DPDP	1.9	2.2	0.29	0.7	Positive
Ferumoxide	Feridex IV® Berlex; Endorem® Guerbet	AMI-25	24	107	0.2	0.34	Negative blood pool agent
Feurucarbotran	Resovist® Schering	SHU555a	20	190	0.33	1.0	Negative

[a] All values reported are for 0.5 M concentrations, except for values noted in parentheses, which represent 1 M; Mn-DPDP is 0.01 M while AMI-25 is 0.2 M. cP = centa-Poise where water has a viscosity of approximately 1cP.

Extracellular contrast agents

In general, three features are common to all the approved extracellular fluid agents: (1) they are Gd-based; (2) they contain a ligand (chelate) bound to Gd; and (3) they contain a single water molecule coordination site to Gd. Since free Gd^{+++} is highly toxic, the chelate is required to make the agent clinically tolerable. The safety of the complex therefore is dependent on the properties of the chelate, its binding to Gd, and the stability of the complex. The chelate must be non-toxic, demonstrate a very high affinity for Gd, and the resulting complex should be sufficiently soluble. The chelate must exhibit selective affinity for Gd^{+++}, as exchange with other metals in the body can result in non-specific chelation (transmetallation). Furthermore, the chelate

must exhibit slow dissociation, resulting in near complete excretion of the ion before the dissociation. Additional favorable attributes of Gd chelates include low viscosity and osmolality.

Most extracellular agents have very similar properties. They are all very hydrophilic, with similar relaxivities and excellent safety profiles. To date, two basic type of Gd chelates have been developed: linear and macrocyclic.

Linear non-ionic Gd chelates

Linear chelates include DTPA (diethylene-triamine pentaacetic acid) and DTPA-BMA (diethylene-triamine pentaacetic acid-bismethylamide). Figure 14.4 illustrates

Table 14.3 Experimental MRI contrast agents in various stages of development

Name of compound	Central moiety	Relaxivity	Distribution	Indication
Gadolinium-chelates				
MS 325				
Diphenylcyclohexyl phosphodiester-Gd-DTPA, Gadofosveset, EPIX Pharmaceuticals (Angiomark®)	Gd^{3+}		Intravascular, short elimination half life – blood pool agent	MR angiography, vascular capillary permeability
(Gd-DTPA)-17, 24 cascade polymer (gadomer 17,24)	Gd^{3+}	r1=11.9, B0 = 1.0 T, (r2 =16.5)	Intravascular – blood pool agent	MR angiography
Gadofluorine-8 (Gd-DO3A) derivative (gadofluorine)	Gd^{3+}	r1=17.4, B0 = 1.5 T, (r2=23.7)	Intravascular	Atherosclerosis
EP-2104R	Gd^{3+}	r1=72.0, B0 = 1.5 T	Intravascular	Fibrin (thrombus)
EPIX Pharmaceuticals Gd-DTPA-PEG polymers (polyethylene glycol)	Gd^{3+}	r1=6.0, B0 = 1.0 T	Intravascular	MR angiography, vascular capillary permeability
(Gd-DTPA)n-albumin, (Gd-DOTA)n-albumin	Gd^{3+}	r1=14.4, B0 = 0.23 T	Intravascular	MR angiography
(Gd-DTPA)n-polylysine	Gd^{3+}	r1=13.1, B0 = 0.23T	Intravascular	MR angiography
(Gd-DTPA)n-dextran	Gd^{3+}		Intravascular	MR angiography
MP 2269, 4-pentyl-bicyclo [2.2.2] octan-1-carboxyl-di-L-aspartyllysine-DTPA	Gd^{3+}	r1=6.2, B0 = 1.0 T	Intravascular	MR angiography
Gadoxetic acid, Gd-EOB-DTPA (Eovist®)	Gd^{3+}	Short T1 relaxation time	Hepatobiliary	Liver lesions
Liposomes, paramagnetic	Gd^{3+}		RES directed	Liver lesions
Polylysine-(Gd-DTPA)x-dextran	Gd^{3+}		Lymph nodes	Staging of lymph nodes
WIN 22181	Gd^{3+}	r1=9.5	Urinary tract	MR urography
Superparamagnetic iron oxides				
Ferrixan, carboxy-dextran coated iron oxide nanoparticles, SHU 555A (Resovist®)	Fe^{2+}	r1=25.4, r2=151	RES directed	Liver lesions – Blood pool agent
AMI-227 (Sinerem, Combidex®)		Fe^{3+}/Fe^{2+} r1=25, r2=160, B_0=0.47 T, Xm=0.34, r1=23.3, r2=48.9, B_0=0.47T	Vascular, lymph nodes, hepatobiliary agent	MR angiography, vascular staging of RES-directed liver diseases – blood pool agent
PION (polycrystalline iron oxide nanoparticles) PION-ASF or DDM 128 are larger particles	Fe^{2+}/Fe^{3+}	T2*enhanced, r2/r1=4.4, r2/r1=7	RES-directed lymph nodes, hepatobiliary system	Liver lesions, MR lymphography
MION, monocrystalline iron oxide nanoparticles	Fe^{3+}/Fe^{2+}	r1=3.7, r2=6.5, B_0=0.47 T, Xm=0.11	Vascular lymph v. (MION-46) tumors, FAB-MION, anti-myosin, FAB-MION	MR angiography, MR lymphography, tumor detection, infarction
Fe-HBED	Fe^{2+}		Hepatobiliary	Liver lesions
Fe-EHPD	Fe^{2+}		Hepatobiliary	Liver lesions
Fe O-BPA USPIO	Fe^{3+}/Fe^{2+}		Vascular	MR angiography, blood pool agent

Table 14.3 Continued

Name of compound	Central moiety	Relaxivity	Distribution	Indication
Manganese and dysprosium chelates				
MnCl$_2$ (Lumenhance®)	Mn^{2+}	Paramagnetic	Gastro-intestinal	Bowel marking
Manganese substituted hydroxylapatite PEG-APD (MnHA/PEG-APD)	Mn^{2+}	r1=21.7, r2=26.9, B$_0$=1.0 T	Intravascular	MR angiography
Mn-EDTA-PP (liposomes)	Mn^{2+}	r1=37.4, r2=53.2, B$_0$=0.5 T		
Magnetic starch microspheres	Mr^{2+}/Mr^{3+}	r1=27.6, r2=183.7, B$_0$=1.0 T	RES directed	Liver and spleen lesions
Sprodyamide, Dy-DTPA-BMA	Dy^{2+}	T2*enhanced, r1=3.4, r2=3.8, B$_0$=0.47 T, Xm=4.46 10^2	Intravascular	Blood flow, perfusion
Dy-DTPA	Dy^{2+}	T2*enhanced, Xm=4.8 10^2	Intravascular	Blood flow, perfusion
Albumin-(Dy-DTPA)x	Dy^{2+}	T2*enhanced	Intravascular	Blood flow, perfucion
Dy-tatraphenyl-porphyrin sulfonate, Dy-TPPS or Ho-TPPS	Dy^{2+}Ho^{2+}	High susceptibility	Tumor selective uptake	Tumor detection and control
Fatty emulsion	Fatty liquid	Short T1 relaxation time	Gastro-intestinal	Bowel marking
Vegetable oils	Fatty liquid	Short T1 relaxation time	Gastro-intestinal	Bowel marking
Sucrose polyesters	Fatty liquid	Short T1 relaxation time	Gastro-intestinal	Bowel marking
Barium suspensions and clay mineral particles OMP	Ba^{3+}, Al^{3+}, Si^{2+}	Diamagnetic, T2 short	Gastro-intestinal	Bowel marking

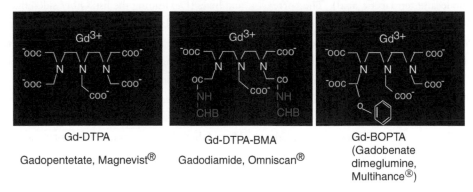

Gd-DTPA
Gadopentetate, Magnevist®

Gd-DTPA-BMA
Gadodiamide, Omniscan®

Gd-BOPTA
(Gadobenate dimeglumine, Multihance®)

Figure 14.4 Open-chain linear gadolinium (Gd) contrast agents approved for clinical use.

currently approved linear chelated Gd agents and includes Gd-DTPA [gadopentetate dimeglumine or Magnevist® (Berlex Laboratories)], Gd-DTPA-BMA [gadodiamide or Omniscan® (Amersham, GE Healthcare)], and Gd-BOPTA [gadobenate dimeglumine, or gadolinium benzyloxy-propionic tetraacetic acid, or Multihance®, Bracco Diagnostics]. Gd-DTPA (Magnevist®, Berlex Laboratories) was the first Gd agent to be developed. This agent is approved for use in pediatric and adult patients at a dose of 0.1 mmol/kg for non-angiographic indications. The dose for 3D contrast-enhanced angiography is higher (0.2–0.3 mmol/kg), but the FDA considers this an unapproved indication. There is little effect on signal intensity beyond doses of 0.2–0.3 mmol/kg. Thus, there is no need to exceed this threshold to obtain increased signal. A fixed volume based dose may also be used in angiography (30–40 ml), with modifications being made only in very large or very small patients. For time-resolved sequences, substantially smaller doses can be used (0.05 mmol/kg). Caution should be exercised in patients with renal impairment, although the agent is cleared by dialysis. Gd-DTPA-BMA or gadodiamide is derived by the substitution of two anionic donor groups ($^-CO_2$) with methylamide and is a neutral (non-ionic) linear chelate (Figure 14.4). This agent has a slightly lower thermodynamic stability than Gd-DTPA and some concerns have been raised about transmetallation. In particular, significant drops in serum zinc levels have been noted. This effect may indicate either chelation of zinc by the agent or substantial release of Gd^{+++}. The effect on contrast enhancement is the same as Gd-DTPA, at least in studies on imaging of head and spine. Gadodiamide is approved in the United States for administration at a dose of 0.1 mmol/kg of body weight for central nervous system imaging in adult and pediatric patients. In MRA, doses that are 2–3 fold higher than the dose used for non-angiographic applications may need to be used and specific guidelines by the manufacturer are not provided. Gadoversatamide (Gd-DTPA bis-methoxyethyl amide, Optimark®, Malinckrodt Medical, St Louis, MO) is a linear low osmolality non-ionic chelate that is FDA approved for use in non-MRA applications in the United States.

Cyclic Gd chelates

Cyclic chelates include HP-DO3A [1,4,7 tris(carboxymethyl)-10-2′hydroxypropyl-1,4,7,10-tetraazacyclododecane) and DOTA (1,4,7,10-tetraazacyclododecane tetraacetic acid). The corresponding Gd chelated agents include gadoteridol (Prohance®, Bracco Diagnostics, Wayne, NJ) and gadoterate dimeglumine (Dotarem®, Guerbet, France). Figure 14.5 provides the chemical structure of cyclic Gd chelates. In the United States only one macrocyclic chelate is available (gadoteridol). Partly owing to the macrocyclic ring, this preparation is more stable than the linear chelates. These agents are therefore less likely to cause release of Gd^{+++} leading to transmetallation and should be theoretically safer. The current approval for the agent is in the dose range of 0.1–0.3 mmol/kg for non-MRA uses. MRA evaluations typically require doses that are higher than non-MRA exams. Gadoterate dimeglumine is approved for use in Europe and is comparable to gadoteridol in terms of in vitro and in vivo stability. Gadobutrol (Gadovist®, Schering AG) is a non-ionic cyclical agent that is approved in Europe for use in MRA. The non-ionic (neutral) compounds (gadodiamide, gadoteridol, gadoversetamide, and gadobutrol) were designed to minimize the osmolality of the formulation. This was prompted by the distinct reduction in toxicity and side-effects brought on by the development of non-ionic X-ray contrast media. However, the injection volumes are much smaller for MRI than for X-ray and, thus, the overall increase in osmolality after injection of an MRI contrast agent is insignificant. One benefit of the non-ionic compounds is the ability to formulate them at high concentration (1 M) without drastically increasing the osmolality or viscosity (Table 14.2). These high-concentration formulations may be useful in fast dynamic studies such as perfusion and dynamic MRA.

Safety of Gd-containing extracellular agents

The safety records of the four longest approved Gd-based agents (gadopentetate dimeglumine, gadodiamide, gadoteridol, and gadoterate meglumine) were recently reviewed by Runge et al. These authors found that the four agents have approximately the same overall adverse event rates, with nausea (1–2%) and hives (1%) leading the list. Other side-effects include mild transitory headaches, vomiting, urticaria, and metal taste. Nearly all adverse events with these agents are transient, mild, and self-limiting. Nevertheless, there are reports of serious adverse reactions, including life-threatening anaphylactoid reactions and death for these agents. The best estimate puts the rate of these events at between 1/200 000 and 1/400 000 patients. Most of the Gd-based extracellular contrast agents are approved for pediatric use in pediatric patients above 2 years, although there are differences in their approval wording.

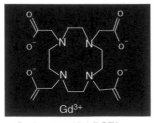
Gadoterate (Gd-DOTA, Dotarem®)

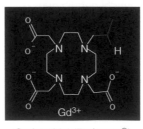
Gadoteridol (Prohance®)

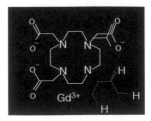
Gadobutrol (Gadovist®)

Figure 14.5   Macro-cyclic gadolinium (Gd) contrast agents approved for clinical use.

The package insert for these agents should always be consulted for the latest safety information. Precautions in the use of Gd-containing agents include use in patients with hemolytic anemia, sickle cell disease, pregnancy, lactation, renal failure, and severe allergies. Transient elevations in serum iron and bilirubin have been observed with higher doses of Gd agents, with a return to baseline levels within 24 hours. This effect is believed to arise due to release of Free Gd^{+++} with resultant hemolytic anemia. Thus, caution with their use has been recommended in hemolytic anemias. The use of Gd-containing agents in pregnancy is not recommended unless there are truly extenuating circumstances, as the agent crosses the placenta and is excreted in breast milk.

Gadodiamide and gadoversatamide have been reported to result in false or spurious hypocalcemia. The false lowering of calcium levels occurs only when the colorimetric assay to measure serum calcium is used. This artifact does not occur with gadopentetate dimeglumine (Magnevist®) or gadoteridol. Gadodiamide and gadoversetamide compete with calcium for the colorimetric reagent, but they do not affect other assays. This spurious hypocalcemia is likely caused by dissociation of Gd^{+++} from their ligands and complex formation with the chromophore used in the calcium assay. This interference is proportional to the Gd chelate concentration and is maximized by factors that lead to a high concentration of gadodiamide in the blood for extended periods of time, including high doses and use in patients with renal dysfunction. Recognition of this abnormality is important to avert inadvertent treatment of falsely low levels. Use of an alternate method for calcium measurement (non-colorimetric method or ionized calcium measurement) is recommended in these circumstances.

Blood pool agents

Extracellular agents have a major drawback in vascular imaging due to their rapid extravasation into the interstitial space and subsequent urinary excretion. This drawback has been partially overcome by the development of blood pool agents characterized by limited or totally absent diffusion across the vascular endothelium. The pharmacokinetic and physicochemical characteristics of blood pool agents have resulted in discrete subclasses of these agents. Rapid-clearance blood pool agents are characterized by a limited diffusion across normal endothelium (and consequently by a limited volume of distribution), with their clearance being equivalent to the glomerular filtration rate; this category includes macromolecular gadolinium chelates such as P792 (Vistarem®, Guerbet)

or Gadomer-17 (Schering AG). Slow-clearance blood pool agents, on the other hand, are confined to the blood compartment, with their body clearance further restricted. This category includes USPIO particles such as NC100150, large polymeric Gd chelates, or small Gd chelates that exhibit prolonged intravascular dwell time due to transient albumin binding. Blood pool agents provide the opportunity for alternative imaging strategies for three-dimensional MRA relative to methods used with extracellular contrast agents that rely on precise estimation of peak arterial contrast opacification. Blood pool agents make it possible to perform a steady-state imaging examination with contrast in both arteries and veins in addition to arterial phase imaging. Macromolecular Gd-labeled albumins include gadofosveset (MS 325, MS 32520, Vasovist®, ZK 236018, EPIX Pharmaceuticals), a gadolinium-based chelate that binds to serum albumin. This is the first agent for which an application has been filed at the FDA for primary use in MRA.

Protein-bound agents

MS-325 (EPIX Pharmaceuticals) and B22956 (Bracco Diagnostics) are Gd-based agents that bind reversibly to serum albumin. Albumin is the most abundant protein in plasma (concentration equal to 600–700 μM) and the binding to contrast agent induces significant effects on blood T1. Reversible albumin binding serves four purposes: (1) the albumin slows the leakage of the contrast agent out of the intravascular space; (2) the reversible binding still allows a path for excretion (the unbound fraction can be filtered through the kidneys or taken up by hepatocytes); (3) the bound fraction is 'hidden' from the liver and kidneys, leading to an extended plasma half-life; and (4) the relaxivity of the contrast agent is increased 4–10-fold upon binding to albumin. MS-325 is cleared mainly by the kidneys while B22956 has significant biliary clearance as well as renal excretion.

Gd-BOPTA (Multihance®) is composed of a weak protein-bound formulation that possesses 2-fold greater T1 relaxivity when measured in human plasma at 0.47 T ($9.7 \, l\,mmol^{-1}\,s^{-1}$, compared with $4.3–5.0 \, l\,mmol^{-1}\,s^{-1}$). This increased T1 relaxivity originates from a capacity to interact (in a weak and transitory fashion) with serum proteins, particularly albumin. The higher T1 relaxivity of this agent has been shown in numerous studies to induce a significantly greater enhancement of the intravascular signal intensity compared to that obtained with conventional gadolinium agents at equivalent dose. The optimal dose of Gd-BOPTA for acquisition of high-quality diagnostic MRA images is 0.1 mmol/kg body weight. Several studies in a variety of peripheral vascular beds have revealed significantly higher and longer-lasting signal intensity with Gd-BOPTA than with gadopentetate dimeglumine, when both contrast agents were administered at the same dose and injection rate. In renal MRA, Gd-BOPTA at a dose of 0.1 mmol/kg is comparable to gadopentetate dimeglumine at 0.2 mmol/kg.

Gadoxate disodium (Primovist®, Schering AG) is a water-soluble ethoxybenzyl derivative of Gd-DTPA and demonstrates weak affinity for albumin. This compound is taken up by the hepatocytes (approximately 30% of the dose goes to the hepatocytes) and is equally excreted renally and through bile in humans. Therefore, both dynamic and accumulation phase imaging can be performed after bolus injection.

SPIO and USPIO particles

The SPIO particles are superparamagnetic agents currently used for clinical liver imaging and other gastro-intestinal applications. SPIO particles consist of non-stoichiometric microcrystalline magnetite or ferrite cores, which are coated with dextrans [ferumoxide, (feridex®, Berlex Laboratories; Endorem®, Guerbet)], carboxydextran [Resovist® (Schering)] or siloxanes [Ferumoxsil (GastroMARK®, Advanced Magnetics); Lumirem®, Guerbet)] to form colloidal solutions. SPIO particles typically have cores containing more than one crystal of iron oxide and may have a range of particle sizes that determines eventual biodistribution and clinical application.

All particles must be <5 μm to avoid entrapment in lung, but large enough to be recognized by the reticuloendothelial system (RES) which removes them from the circulation. At low doses, circulating iron in SPIO particles decreases the T1 time of blood, but at higher doses the T2* effects predominate with signal loss in the targeted tissue (e.g., liver and spleen) with all standard pulse sequences.

USPIO particles usually consist of a crystalline iron oxide core containing thousands of iron atoms and a shell of polymer, dextran, or polyethyleneglycol, and they produce very high T2 relaxivities. The USPIO particles evade the RES but at the same time are too large to passively leak out of the vascular space and make very good blood pool agents. USPIO particles can be formulated as a stable suspension and can be administered intravenously. Besides having important differences in their biodistribution, USPIO particles also differ from SPIO in having a much greater effect on T2 than T1 (large r2/r1) and are used exclusively as T2 or T2* agents. USPIO particles have been evaluated in multi-center clinical

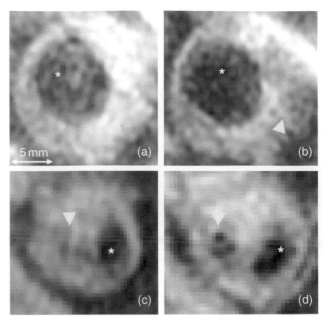

Figure 14.6 Pattern of USPIO-induced signal loss in atherosclerotic plaque imaging. T2* weighted (TE = 5.6 ms) axial MR images have been obtained through the common carotid artery. Compared to precontrast imaging (a and c), a diffuse (b) or focal (d) USPIO signal effect can be demonstrated on images obtained 36 hours after infusion. *: vascular lumen. Adapted with permission from Trivedi RA et al. Arterioscler Thromb Vasc Biol 2006; 26(7): 1601–6.

trials for lymph node MRI and MRA. Ferrumoxtran-10 (Combidex®, Advanced Magnetics) is an USPIO particle (20 nm) suspended as a colloid. It is currently being evaluated in clinical trials. USPIO particles, in view of their uptake by macrophages, have been used to image macrophage infiltration in atherosclerosis (Figure 14.6).

MOLECULAR IMAGING OF ATHEROSCLEROSIS

Contrast agents linked to antibodies or peptides targeting specific plaque components or molecules that localize to specific regions of atherosclerotic plaque are examples of strategies that have been employed to image atherosclerosis with MR. Macrophages have been imaged with iron oxide compounds (USPIO and SPIO particles), although these techniques have limitations relating to the difficulty of differentiating viable cells from resident iron deposits (i.e., hemorrhages).

Lipid emulsions to which paramagnetic chelates are bound allow a high pay load of the contrast agent to the surface of cells. Additional specificity to receptors may be conferred by combining this emulsion with a ligand such as an antibody. Examples of such refinements include agents that track angiogenesis through targeted peptidomimetics that allow binding to a specific peptidic motif (RGD) of the vitronectin receptor (αvβ3).

Additional targets of interest for imaging of atherosclerotic plaque with molecular specific MR contrast agents are oxidized low-density lipoprotein, tissue factor, endothelial integrins (e.g., E-selectin, P-selectin, intercellular adhesion molecule-1 [ICAM-1], vascular cell adhesion molecule-1 [VCAM-1], etc.), matrix metalloproteinases (MMPs), and extracellular matrix proteins such as tenascin-C.

Another recently developed imaging agent is a recombinant high-density lipoprotein (rHDL) molecule that incorporates Gd-DTPA phospholipids. Since the HDL particle is endogenous and does not trigger an immune reaction, and undergoes rapid transit in and out of the arterial wall, it could potentially serve as a contrast agent to image events dependent on HDL.

The ability to identify components of thrombus with molecular MRI may enable enhanced detection and characterization of both luminal thrombus and components of thrombus organized in an old atherothrombotic lesion. Therefore, selection of pivotal targets in the coagulation cascade, such as fibrin, tissue factor, platelet integrins, and factor XIIIa, may be necessary to identify areas of old or active thrombus formation. Thrombus imaging using either monoclonal antibodies or peptide ligands attached to Gd chelates has been performed in animal models and humans. Additionally, thrombi resulting from either plaque rupture or from blood stasis in an experimental model of carotid thrombosis have been identified using a fibrin-specific MR contrast agent. An example of enhancement in signal intensity of thrombus after contrast can be seen in Figure 14.7. Our group has also demonstrated thrombus enhancement in

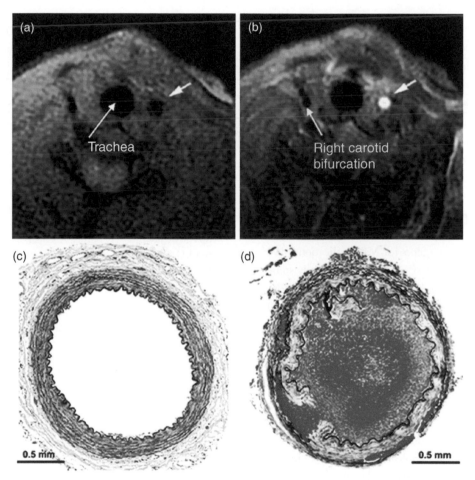

Figure 14.7 Transverse in vivo T1-weighted MR images of left (injured) and right (uninjured) carotid arteries in a guinea pig. MR imaging was performed before (a) and after (b) injection of a fibrin-targeted contrast agent (EP-1242). Thrombus in the left common carotid artery (white arrows) was not detectable on precontrast images as shown in (a). After EP-1242 injection, thrombus was readily detectable due to a dramatic contrast enhancement (b). Note that the contralateral right carotid artery does not display enhancement after EP-1242 injection. The lower row shows the corresponding histologic right patent carotid artery (c) and the left occluded common carotid artery (d) with an unorganized red blood cell-rich thrombus. (4 × magnification – sections stained with CME). From Sirol M, Aguinaldo JG, Graham PB, et al. Fibrin-targeted contrast agent for improvement of in vivo acute thrombus detection with magnetic resonance imaging. Atherosclerosis. 2005 Sep; 182(1): 79–85.

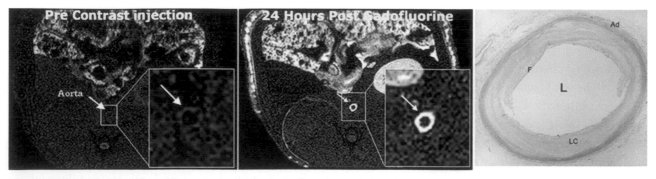

Figure 14.8 MR transverse image of a rabbit aortic plaque before and 24 hours after gadofluorine injection. Note how gadofluorine helps to improve atherosclerotic plaque detection in vivo. The corresponding histopathological section confirms presence of advanced atherosclerotic lesion. From Sirol M, Itskovich VV, Mani V, et al. Lipid-Rich Atherosclerotic Plaques Detected by Gadofluorine-Enhanced In Vivo Magnetic Resonance Imaging. Circulation 2004; 109(23): 2890–6.

chronic or organized thrombus using this fibrin targeted approach.

The utility of a new class of contrast agent, gadofluorine, has been recently demonstrated for plaque detection. Although gadofluorine is a non-targeted contrast agent, it dramatically improves plaque detection in experimental models of atherosclerosis (Figure 14.8). The marked ability of this contrast agent to enhance atherosclerotic plaque imaging when compared to conventional Gd chelates may be related to the inherent lipophilicity of gadofluorine.

CONCLUSIONS

A vast number of contrast agents for MR applications have been developed during the last years. However, only some Gd-based contrast agents and few iron-containing particles have been approved for clinical use. In particular, Gd chelates are characterized by an extremely favorable safety profile but, nevertheless, they have not been formally approved for MRA applications. The design objectives for the next generation of MR contrast agents will likely focus on prolonging intravascular retention, improving tissue targeting, and making use of additional contrast mechanisms. Chemical modifications of contrast agents and alterations in their affinity to macromolecules to confer higher intravascular retention have already led to the introduction of blood pool agents. In addition, a variety of vector and carrier molecules, including antibodies, peptides, proteins, polysaccharides, liposomes, and cells, have been developed to deliver magnetic labels to specific sites, thereby conferring tissue specificity. Technical advances in MR imaging will further increase the efficiency of current contrast mechanisms.

FURTHER READING

Balci NC, Semelka RC. Contrast agents for MR imaging of the liver. Radiol Clin North Am 2005; 43(5): 887–98.

Caravan P, Ellison JJ, McMurry TJ et al. Gadolinium(III) chelates as MRI contrast agents: structure, dynamics, and applications. Chem Rev (Washington, DC) 1999; 99(9): 2293–352.

Choudhury RP, Fusteeer V, Fayad ZA. Molecular, cellular and functional imaging of atherothrombosis. Nat Rev Drug Discov 2004; 3(11): 913–25.

Flacke S, Fischer S, Scott MJ et al. Novel MRI contrast agent for molecular imaging of fibrin: implications for detecting vulnerable plaques. Circulation 2001; 104(11): 1280–5.

Frias JC, Williams KJ, Fisher EA et al. Recombinant HDL-like nanoparticles: a specific contrast agent for MRI of atherosclerotic plaques. J Am Chem Soc 2004; 126(50): 16316–17.

Gries H. Extracellular MRI contrast agents based on gadolinium. Top Curr Chem 2002; (Contrast Agents I): 221: 1–24.

Johansson LO, Bjornerud A, Ahlstrom HK et al. A targeted contrast agent for magnetic resonance imaging of thrombus: implications of spatial resolution. J Magn Reson Imag 2001; 13(4): 615–18.

Kooi ME, Cappendijk VC, Cleutjens KB et al. Accumulation of ultrasmall superparamagnetic particles of iron oxide in human atherosclerotic plaques can be detected by in vivo magnetic resonance imaging. Circulation 2003; 107(19): 2453–8

Lauffer RB, Parmelee DJ, Dunham SU et al. MS-325: albumin-targeted contrast agent for MR angiography. Radiology 1998; 207(2): 529–38.

Louie AY, Huber MM, Ahrens ET et al. In vivo visualization of gene expression using magnetic resonance imaging. Nat Biotechnol 2000; 18(3): 321–5.

Perez JM, Josephson L, O'Loughlin T et al. Magnetic relaxation switches capable of sensing molecular interactions. Nat Biotechnol 2002; 20(8): 816–20.

Pirovano G, Kirchin MA, Spinazzi A. Contrast-enhanced MR angiography of the renal arteries: blinded multicenter crossover comparison of gadobenate dimeglumine and gadopentetate dimeglumine. Radiology 2005 Feb; 234(2): 399–408.

Ruehm SG, Corot C, Vogt P et al. Magnetic resonance imaging of atherosclerotic plaque with ultrasmall superparamagnetic particles of iron oxide in hyperlipidemic rabbits. Circulation 2001; 103(3): 415–22.

Runge VM. Safety of magnetic resonance contrast media. Top Magn Reson Imaging 2001; 12(4): 309–14.

Sirol M, Aguinaldo JGS, Graham PB et al. Fibrin-targeted contrast agent for improvement of in vivo acute thrombus detection with magnetic resonance imaging. Atherosclerosis 2005; 182: 79–85.

Sirol M, Fuster V, Badimon JJ et al. Chronic thrombus detection using in-vivo magnetic resonance imaging and fibrin-targeted contrast agent. Circulation 2005; 112: 1594–600.

Sirol M, Itskovich VV, Mani V et al. Lipid-rich atherosclerotic plaques detected by gadofluorine-enhanced in vivo magnetic resonance imaging. Circulation 2004; 109: 2890–6.

Tombach B, Heindel W. Value of 1.0-M gadolinium chelates: review of preclinical and clinical data on gadobutrol. Eur Radiol 2002; 12(6): 1550–6.

Trivedi RA, U-King-Im J-M, Graves MJ et al. In vivo detection of macrophages in human carotid atheroma: temporal dependence of ultrasmall superparamagnetic particles of iron oxide-enhanced MRI. Stroke 2004; 35(7): 1631–5.

Winter PM, Morawski AM, Caruthers SD et al. Molecular imaging of angiogenesis in early-stage atherosclerosis with {α}v{β}3-integrin-targeted nanoparticles. Circulation 2003; 108(18): 2270–4.

15

MR angiography of the extracranial and intracranial circulation with imaging protocols

Claudia Fellner and Franz A Fellner

INTRODUCTION

The intra- and extracranial vasculature are some of the most demanding vascular areas in the human body from an imaging perspective. Motion artifacts may compromise diagnostic reliability at the level of the aortic arch, intracranial vessels are small with multiple branches, and the time interval between the arterial and venous phase is very short, increasing the likelihood of venous contamination artifact. Magnetic resonance angiography (MRA) has revolutionized the non-invasive evaluation of the extracranial circulation and has firmly replaced intra-arterial angiography for the diagnosis of atherosclerotic disease in many institutions. However, for imaging of intracranial vessels, intra-arterial angiography may still be the 'gold standard' due to its selective visualization, and excellent spatial and temporal resolution. Nevertheless, intracranial MRA is increasingly used as a supplementary tool in diagnosis and follow-up examinations for many different vascular diseases, or as the sole diagnostic method. The advantages of MRA include absence of ionizing radiation and iodinated contrast agent and the ability to obtain additional soft tissue information in the same session, which can be extremely important in the diagnosis of disorders such as acute stroke. Additionally, it is possible to selectively obtain arterial or venous phase information.

Up to now, three different techniques have been used in the MRA evaluation of the extra- and intracranial circulation – time-of-flight (TOF), phase contrast (PC), and contrast-enhanced (CE-MRA. Different implementations of these basic techniques have found their way into routine clinical application. The preferred technique depends on the vascular territory, the clinical question, the technical equipment (including vendor-specific differences!), and, finally, on the experience of the performing physician. Application of two different MRA techniques might sometimes be advantageous, as this may yield complementary information. Table 15.1 lists common indications for MRA in the intra- and extracranial circulation. Concomitant MR imaging may often be required for a number of these indications. In acute stroke, MR imaging of the brain, including diffusion and perfusion imaging is increasingly used in combination with MRA to detect ischemic areas, tissue at risk, and vessel occlusion.

FUNDAMENTAL PRINCIPLES

Depending on the clinical question and the vascular territory, one or several MRA techniques may be used (CE-MRA, TOF, PC-MRA). In this section the main advantages and drawbacks of these common techniques as they pertain to the intra- and extracranial circulation will be discussed. Detailed information on the pulse sequence and other technical details of MRA can be found in Chapters 12 and 13.

Table 15.1 Indications for extracranial and intracranial MRA/MRI

Atherosclerosis
Fibromuscular dysplasia
Dissections and aneurysmal disease

Vascular malformations
- Arteriovenous malformations (AVM)
- Cavernous hemangioma
- Developmental venous anomalies (DVA)

Venous thrombosis
- Dural and cortical thrombosis
- Jugular vein thrombosis

Neoplasms
- Intracranial and extracranial tumors

TOF

Two-dimensional (2D) TOF

High sensitivity for slow flow and good background suppression are the most important advantages of 2D TOF. Therefore, this is an important method for imaging of intracranial veins. Determination of flow direction in larger vessels is done very easily with axial 2D TOF, selecting a cranial saturation slab in a first measurement and a caudal saturation in a second measurement. Spin dephasing effects, which may result in significant overestimation of stenoses, are the most important drawback of 2D TOF MRA. Furthermore, in-plane saturation effects and motion artifacts can significantly reduce diagnostic reliability. 2D TOF implementations typically incorporate gradient moment nulling (flow compensation) to decrease loss of phase coherence resulting from first order motion. Please refer to Chapter 13 for further details on the TOF technique.

Three-dimensional (3D) TOF

The most important application of 3D TOF is in the diagnosis of stenoses, occlusions, aneurysms, and vascular malformations of intracranial arteries. The advantage of 3D TOF over 2D TOF includes higher spatial resolution and intrinsically higher signal-to-noise ratio (SNR). Long acquisition time is an important shortcoming of 3D TOF, which is why this technique is most relevant in small arterial beds with high velocity of inflowing blood, such as the carotid and the vertebrobasilar circulation, that will allow superb depiction of TOF contrast

of unsaturated protons. Spin dephasing effects are diminished by selecting high spatial resolution. Furthermore, first-order flow compensation and an out-of-phase echo time as short as possible are advantageous. Spin saturation effects, a relevant disadvantage of 3D TOF, is reduced by application of a tilted, optimized, non-saturating excitation (TONE) or ramped RF pulse and/or by a multiple overlapping thin slab acquisition (MOTSA) technique. Adding a magnetization transfer (MT) prepulse will further decrease signal intensity of brain tissue and increase vessel contrast in intracranial MRA. Application of a water excitation technique to suppress subcutaneous and retro-orbital fat can also be done if necessary. Improved conspicuity of small intracranial vessels can be accomplished with a 3D TOF sequence after administration of paramagnetic contrast agents. This is because in 3D TOF, blood within the volume is partially saturated by the application of frequent radiofrequency pulses and the administration of a contrast agent allows faster recovery of longitudinal relaxation. Differentiation between arteries and veins, however, will no longer be possible in this case. Another general caveat of 3D TOF MRA in the assessment of intracranial vessels is that methemoglobin may produce high signal intensity and may prevent discrimination of flowing and stationary blood.

PC-MRA

Chapter 13 describes the basic principles of PC-MRA. Two-dimensional PC is well suited to give a quick overview of the vascular anatomy and additionally provide assistance with flow direction (especially in cases of flow reversal, such as in the subclavian steal syndrome). Flow direction can be determined within a single short measurement using phase maps (blood flowing in one direction is shown with high signal intensity, while flow in the opposite direction is displayed with low signal and stationary tissue is shown with intermediate signal intensity). Because of the inherent low spatial resolution of 2D PC it is not recommended for detailed anatomic diagnosis. Correct selection of velocity encoding (Venc) is a major problem of PC-MRA. Flow velocity in small arteries is similar to flow in large veins. Furthermore, flow velocity might vary in diseased vessels. The short acquisition time, however, allows for testing of different Vencs. The acquired data can then be used to optimize the Venc for a high-resolution 3D PC measurement.

Three-dimensional PC overcomes the drawback of reduced spatial resolution in 2D PC, but at the expense of significantly prolonged acquisition time (several minutes for

3D PC versus several seconds for a single 2D PC slab). MRA of intracranial veins is the most important application of 3D PC. Application of 3D PC may also help in the differentiation between flowing and thrombosed blood or for display of very small arterial vessels. Grading of stenoses will be suboptimal with 3D PC because of its high sensitivity to dephasing effects.

CE-MRA

CE-MRA is performed during the first pass of a paramagnetic contrast agent (gadolinium chelates). The rapid circulation times in the cerebral vasculature and the short arteriovenous delay mandate precise timing in the arterial phase of contrast while assessing arterial lesions. On the other hand, venous MRA may be performed either during the equilibrium phase or as part of a time-resolved acquisition (see the following section). CE-MRA of the cerebral arterial circulation mandates high resolution isotropic imaging (to visualize small intracranial vessels) with techniques to optimize acquisition of arterial phase data. This is typically performed during breath hold to prevent motion-related artefacts involving the aortic arch vessels (the arch moves with respiration). EKG gating is typically not required as cerebral vessels are not pulsatile vessels.

As the determination of the precise time of peak arterial contrast is critical, different methods can be used. Performance of a separate test bolus run, although more time-consuming and requiring a dedicated bolus of contrast (typically 2 ml), is reliable. The time to peak arterial contrast is then used to plan the actual CE-MRA run (for sequences centric with the time to peak ordering is exactly the same as the time delay prior to triggering the 3D CE-MRA acquisition, see also Chapter 13). Alternately, manual initiation of the 3D sequence with centeric ordering, while looking at real-time images of a slab generated by a low resolution scan preceding the actual CE-MRA, allows one to assess contrast arrival and trigger the CE-MRA acquisition ['fluoroscopically triggered' techniques such as Smartprep®, CareBolus®, BolusTrak®, contrast-enhanced timing-robust angiography (CENTRA), Chapter 13]. This generally needs more experience to precisely time maximal contrast opacification. If the sequence is started too early, reduced vessel contrast and line artifacts will be present (truncation or ringing artifact, Chapter 12). On the other hand, a delayed start will result in venous overlay artifact. Automated detection of the bolus arrival, although easier in this regard, does require some judgement in placement of the monitoring volume and definition of the triggering

threshold. A drawback of the bolus tracking protocols is that integration of a breath hold command is more difficult than in the bolus timing technique, as the exact time of sequence start is not known in advance and the breath hold command is difficult to hear for the patient during acquisition of the fluoroscopic sequence (with the coils around the neck it may be difficult to place the ear phones). The ordering of k-space is critical in cerebrovascular CE-MRA in view of rapid flow rates and easy venous contamination. Using an elliptic centric k-space ordering instead of a sequential linear technique allows one to maximize the chances of acquiring arterial phase data during peak arterial contrast and avoid venous overlap (Chapter 12, k-space schemes).

Time-resolved or multi-phase techniques

These do not need determination of circulation time and are therefore very easy to perform (Chapter 13). However, the acquisition time has to be short enough to separate the arterial from the venous phase. This generally means an acquisition time lower than 8 s for extracranial vessels and 4–6 s for intracranial vessels. In the simplest version of time-resolved MRA, this can be realized only at the expense of significantly reduced spatial resolution. Time-resolved MRA for the supra-aortic arteries is feasible to detect significant stenoses or occlusions of the carotid arteries. This technique needs only a minimum of patient cooperation (no breath hold required) and a minimum of contrast agent compared with other CE-MRA techniques. However, the origins of the supra-aortic arteries are often difficult to assess because of motion artifacts at the aortic arch. The use of dedicated neurovascular phased array coils for signal detection allows the implementation of parallel imaging techniques, while maintaining excellent spatial resolution. Parallel imaging is relevant, especially for time-resolved MRA of the intracranial arteries, as it allows marked reductions in acquisition times (by a factor of 2–4). Use of echo sharing techniques (TRICKS) additionally allows reductions in acquisition times (Chapter 13). Although this protocol is available for use through select vendors, detailed comparative data on its use in the clinical context and decision-making are not available. Imaging at higher magnetic field strength (3.0 T), in conjunction with the use of multi-channel phased array coils, provides sufficient SNR to support faster parallel acquisition protocols, leading to improved spatial resolution. This may allow superior depiction of smaller intracranial branches.

CLINICAL PROTOCOLS

The clinical protocols shown in this section can be implemented on clinical 1.5 T scanners with suitable gradient performance to allow cardiovascular applications. Most use a linear k-space ordering scheme and partial Fourier techniques in phase encoding and slice select direction, as well as a reduced slice resolution (typically the measured slice resolution is about 70% of the displayed slice resolution).

Extracranial circulation

CE-MRA is the MR modality of choice to image the extracranial circulation. Generally a bolus timing approach with linear k-space ordering is used for the reasons mentioned in the section on 3D CE-MRA. The time-resolved technique with reduced spatial resolution can be used as a screening technique for abnormalities in this territory.

Patient preparation

Adequate coil selection is the first important step to successful MRA of the supra-aortic arteries. A combination of head, neck, and spine coil or a dedicated head-neck coil covering the patient´s head and neck down to the aortic arch is optimal. Comfortable positioning of the patient with fixation of the head is recommended. Venous access (20 gauge) should be ideally placed in an antecubital vein in the right upper extremity (if possible) in order to avoid susceptibility artifacts of the contrast bolus in the left brachiocephalic vein onto the left subclavian or common carotid artery. The patient should be informed about the procedure and asked to pay attention to the breath hold command and not to swallow if possible. An automated dual injector is strongly recommended.

MRA acquisition

Anatomic localizers are obtained in the transverse and coronal orientation, followed by two sagittal 2D PC slabs positioned onto the right and left carotid arteries, as overall vessel survey (Table 15.2). This is followed by performance of a test bolus with a slice in the transverse orientation through the common carotid arteries serving as the locus of timing. Alternately, the coronal or sagittal orientation may be selected. Between 1 and 2 ml of contrast agent is injected at the same flow rate, followed by the same amount of saline flush (20–30 ml) as planned for the 3D CE-MRA sequence. For the latter, a coronal slab covering the extracranial arteries from the aortic arch to the circle of Willis is selected. Inclusion of the origins of all supra-aortic arteries and vessel loops is critical, in order that proximal stenosis at the level of the great vessel origins is not missed. A precontrast data set is separately acquired in order to improve vessel contrast by subtraction from the contrast-enhanced data set. Acquisition during breath hold is advantageous whenever

Table 15.2 Protocols for MRA of extracranial arteries

	Localizer	Vessel localizer	Test bolus measurement	CE-MRA with bolus timing	CE-MRA fluoroscopically triggered[a]	CE-MRA time-resolved
TR (ms)	20	21	1000	3.78	4.8	3.14
TE (ms)	5	5.3	1.65	1.54	1.48	1.28
Flip angle (degrees)	40	15	8	35	40	25
Number of slices	7	2	1	88	60	64
Slice thickness (mm)	10	40	10	0.8	1.0	1.1
Field-of-view (mm)	300×300	300×300	300×300	188×300	350×350	195×300
Matrix	128×256	192×192	158×256	160×512	432×432	104×320
Pixel size (mm)	2.3×1.2	1.6×1.6	1.9×1.2	1.2×0.6	0.8×0.8	1.9×0.9
Bandwidth (Hz/pixel)	180	260	380	410		490
Venc (cm/s)	—	40	—	—	—	—
Acquisition time (min:s)	0:19	0:26	60×0:01	0:22	0:58	6×0:08

a According to Willinek et al.

possible. For CE techniques with elliptic centric k-space ordering and long acquisition times breath hold during acquisition of central k-space lines (i.e. at the beginning of the measurement) is sufficient. For most patients, it is more comfortable to perform the breath hold during inspiration. Usually there is enough time for an adequate breath hold command, like 'breathe in, breathe out, breathe in, stop breathing' which takes about 9 seconds. It is important to note that the precontrast data set used for subtraction has to be acquired during the same breath hold phase.

Contrast regimen

Many different protocols for contrast administration can be found in the literature. In general, 0.1 mmol/kg body weight of a 0.5 molar gadolinium contrast agent (i.e. 16 ml for an 80 kg patient) with a flow rate of 2 ml/s can be used successfully; others have proposed using a fixed dose that can range from 20 to 30 ml independent of the patient's body weight as this is simple to implement. We prefer a dosage of 0.1 mmol/kg of Gd-BOPTA (MultiHance®, Chapter 14). This dosage can be reduced (to about one half) for data sets with lower spatial resolution. Another important aspect is the bolus length; as a rule of thumb this should be two-thirds of the acquisition time (Chapters 13 and 17).

Optional measurements and comments

If the time-resolved technique is applied, simultaneous start of the CE sequence and contrast injection is recommended as this will result in at least one precontrast data set. We employ this technique in patients with acute stroke for screening of severe stenoses or occlusions of the carotid arteries, as it is a very fast and robust method which requires only half the contrast dosage, compared to high-resolution techniques. The implementation of parallel imaging techniques further improves spatial and/or temporal resolution: Nevertheless, an acquisition time of 8.3 s, which can be realized without parallel imaging, is short enough in most patients to get an arterial phase without venous overlap. The protocols for 3D CE-MRA given in Table 15.2 use a rectangular field-of-view (FOV) to reduce the acquisition time without loss of spatial resolution. If array coils are employed, parallel imaging techniques can be chosen as an alternative to the rectangular FOV. A square FOV for the supra-aortic vessels yields improved display of subclavian arteries without wrap artefacts.

Intracranial circulation

TOF, CE-MRA, and PC-MRA are all used for the assessment of intracranial vessels. The choice of a specific MRA technique mainly depends on the clinical question, but also on the technical skills of the technologist performing the study, assuming that state of the art equipment is available. Three-dimensional TOF is by far the most commonly used technique for the assessment of intracranial arteries. CE-MRA is increasingly used for both, the arterial and venous circulation, and with the introduction of 3.0 T scanners and phased-array neurovascular coils, is likely to be increasingly used in this setting. Up to now, two-dimensional TOF or 3D PC is mainly used for the assessment of the venous circulation.

Patient preparation

A dedicated head array coil is employed for MRA of intracranial vessels as it provides for good SNR and allows application of parallel imaging techniques. Comfortable positioning and fixation of the patient's head are performed as usual. The venous access for contrast application is preferably in an antecubital vein.

MR examination

MRA of intracranial vessels is generally performed in combination with MR imaging. Therefore, dedicated vessel localizers are not necessary as preceding imaging sequences can be used to position the MR angiographic slab. Precise positioning of the transverse slab is of principal importance for 3D TOF because the slab is usually reduced to a minimum thickness to minimize acquisition time.

Three versions of 3D TOF for intracranial arteries are given in Table 15.3: a single slab for high-resolution measurement (for example for intracranial aneurysms), a MOTSA technique for display of a larger volume, and a fast screening sequence with reduced spatial resolution that is recommended in acute stroke to detect arterial occlusion. If parallel imaging is not available for this screening sequence, the acquisition time has to be shortened in another way, for example by increasing the slice thickness and/or reducing the number of slabs.

Intracranial veins are best visualized using 2D TOF or 3D PC (Table 15.3), the latter yielding superior spatial resolution (at the expense of prolonged acquisition time). If available, parallel imaging is recommended for both techniques. Two-dimensional TOF for display of intracranial veins can be applied either in the transverse or in the oblique sagittal

Table 15.3   Protocols for MRA of intracranial vessels

	3D TOF HR	3D MOTSA	3D TOF fast	2D TOF	3D PC	CE-MRA time - resolved
TR (ms)	39	39	36	27	16	3.29
TE (ms)	7.2	7.2	7.2	7.2	6.9	1.31
Flip angle (degrees)	25	25	25	60	10	20
Number of slices	64	3×32	4×24	100	150	40
Slice thickness (mm)	0.8	1.0	1.0	3.0	0.8	2.0
Field-of-view (mm)	163 × 200	163 × 200	179 × 220	179 × 220	161 × 230	167 x 250
Matrix	208 × 512	208 × 512	208 × 256	208 × 256	108 × 256	128 x 384
Pixel size (mm)	0.8 × 0.4	0.8 × 0.4	0.9 × 0.9	0.9 × 0.9	1.5 × 0.9	1.9 x 0.9
Bandwidth (Hz/pixel)	65	65	81	97	170	540
Venc (cm/s)	—	—	—	—	25	—
Acquisition time (min:s)	7:03	5:51	3:11[a]	5:26[a]	7:25	8 x 0:04[a]

[a] Using parallel imaging with an acceleration factor of 2. HR, high resolution.

orientation. If the sagittal orientation is selected, a tilt from sagittal to coronal orientation of about 10–20° is recommended to assure sufficient inflow of venous blood. In both cases the whole brain has to be covered from the superior sagittal sinus to the upper jugular veins. The 3D PC protocol given in Table 15.3 is optimized for the acquisition in the transverse orientation. Both sequences, 2D TOF and 3D PC, are designed for display of dural sinus. For smaller areas of interest, the slab thickness can be reduced or spatial resolution might be improved.

There are many different ways of applying CE-MRA for visualization of intracranial vessels, as a time-resolved technique for display of arteries and/or veins or as a single-phase technique with improved spatial resolution (fluoroscopically triggered or using a test bolus for correct timing). Table 15.3 shows an example of the time-resolved technique, a coronal slab with a temporal resolution of 4.4 s. This technique is well suited for arterial MRA. For intracranial veins a lower temporal resolution is sufficient, which means that improving the spatial resolution or increasing the slab thickness is possible.

Contrast regimen

For most applications 3D TOF is performed prior to application of contrast agent to avoid venous overlap. Nevertheless, application of contrast agent improves delineation of small arteries. According to our experience contrast application also increases reliability in follow-up examinations of coiled aneurysms. The contrast regimen for CE-MRA does not differ from that used for the extracranial

arteries. Simultaneous start of acquisition and contrast injection is recommended for a time-resolved technique. If a test bolus is used, positioning of the slice in the internal carotid artery is recommended.

CLINICAL APPLICATIONS

Extracranial circulation

Stenoses and occlusions

Stroke is one of the leading causes of death and disability in the Western world. The important benefit of carotid endarterectomy for symptomatic patients with severe carotid artery stenoses (70–99%) has been proven in two independent studies, the North American Symptomatic Carotid Endarterectomy Trial (NASCET) and the European Carotid Surgery Trial (ECST). The Asymptomatic Carotid Atherosclerosis Study (ACAS) has even shown some benefit for asymptomatic patients with stenoses greater than 60%. The grading of stenoses in these studies was based on intra-arterial catheter angiography, which has been regarded as the gold standard. For catheter angiography a risk of 1 to 4% for neurologic complications has been reported, with 0.4 up to 1% of these complications being severe. Therefore, non-invasive imaging techniques are essential in pre-operative imaging and screening.

Up to now, a large number of studies has been published comparing MRA to intra-arterial catheter angiography for grading of carotid stenoses. Most of them reached sensitivities between 90 and 100% and specificities between 80 and 100%

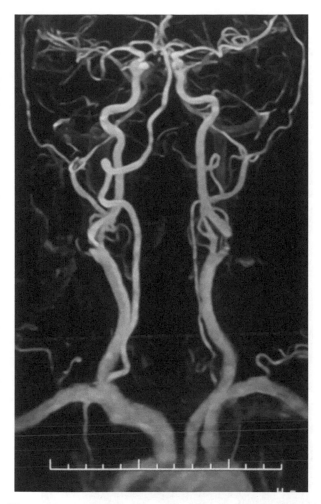

Figure 15.1 *Severe stenoses of both internal carotid arteries.* High-resolution CE-MRA with elliptic centric k-space ordering of the supra-aortic arteries reveals severe stenoses of both internal carotid arteries. The acquisition time for this high-resolution technique was 58 s. Courtesy of R. Schmitt, Department of Radiology, Herz- und Gefaessklinik, Bad Neustadt.

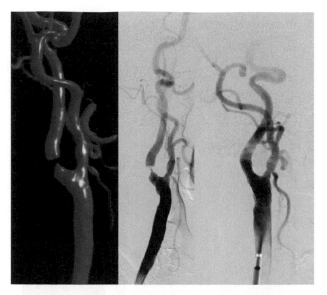

Figure 15.2 *Severe stenosis of the internal carotid artery.* High-resolution CE-MRA (volume rendering) (left) depicts severe stenosis of the internal carotid artery nearly identical to selective catheter angiography (middle). Catheter angiography was performed during the interventional session with stent implantation (right).

for detection of severe stenoses. Different MRA techniques with different measurement parameters were used in those studies, but there are only a few studies comparing different MR angiographic techniques with intra-arterial angiography. Another complicating aspect for comparison of MR and catheter angiography is the fact that catheter angiography uses only a very limited number of projections (usually 2–3 projections per side), whereas MRA allows multiple projections. This may result in underestimation of stenoses by catheter angiography in some cases. Especially in more recent applications, CE high-resolution techniques are applied with good to excellent accuracy compared to catheter angiography. Nevertheless, high-resolution 3D TOF focussing on the carotid bifurcation is still recommended by a few authors as an additional technique to improve accuracy.

Nowadays, CE-MRA has become the MRA method of choice because of its ability to cover extracranial arteries from the aortic arch to the circle of Willis (Figure 15.1). This is extremely important as recent re-evaluation of the NASCET data revealed that a significant number of strokes are caused by atherosclerotic disease outside the carotid bifurcation. Furthermore, significant tandem stenoses in the proximal or distal carotid circulation can represent a contra-indication for surgery and thus have to be detected prior to endarterectomy.

Besides MRA of the supra-aortic arteries, MR imaging of the brain can be performed during the same session to exclude ischemic lesions in a pre-operative examination.

Local signal loss has been regarded to be a relevant problem because exact grading of stenoses is impossible in this case. Occurrence of this effect depends on many factors. Nevertheless, the experience of several authors has shown that local signal loss with distal recovery of signal is a reliable indication of a severe carotid stenosis (Figure 15.2). Differentiation of total and near-total occlusion is another major concern in MRA of this territory as this distinction influences therapeutic decision-making. Application of high-resolution techniques is very helpful in both cases. Furthermore, inspection of source images or multi-planar reconstruction through the vessel lumen is mandatory in those cases.

Assessment of vertebral arteries is another issue to consider in MRA. Despite high-resolution CE-MRA and data

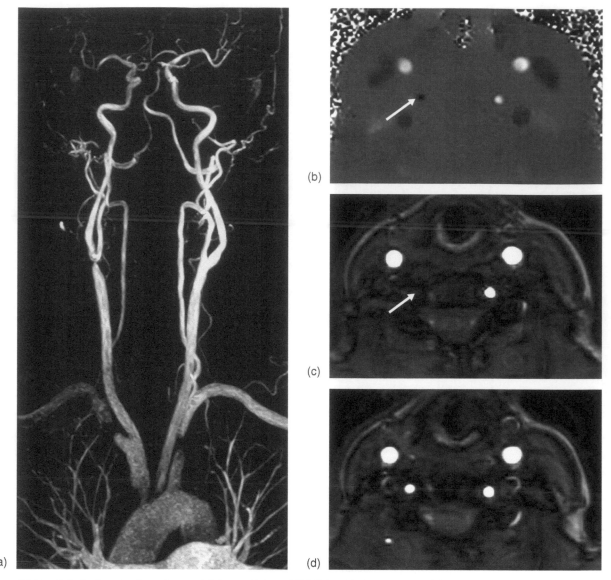

(a)   (b)   (c)   (d)

Figure 15.3 *Subclavian steal syndrome*. High-resolution CE-MRA with bolus timing (a) reveals severe stenoses of both subclavian arteries, the left common carotid artery (at the origin), the right common carotid artery (just below the bifurcation), and a stenosis of the brachiocephalic trunk. 2D PC (b) clearly depicts reverse flow in the right vertebral artery (arrow) consistent with subclavian steal. The reverse flow direction can also be demonstrated using 2D TOF with a cranial saturation pulse (c, low signal intensity, arrow) and another 2D TOF with caudal saturation pulse (high signal intensity, not shown); normalization of flow direction in the right vertebral artery (d) is seen after stent implantation in the right subclavian artery.

acquisition during breath holds, the origins of the vertebral arteries can still be difficult to assess in some patients because local signal loss due to spin dephasing effects may simulate severe stenoses at the origins. Furthermore, the distinction between hypoplastic and atherosclerotic vertebral arteries can be difficult.

Besides evaluation of stenoses of the supra-aortic arteries, additional information concerning the flow direction is of special interest in specific patients. In patients with *subclavian steal syndrome* the underlying cause of the disease, a severe stenosis or occlusion of the sublavian artery, can be

depicted with CE-MRA while 2D TOF or 2D PC-MRA has to be applied to show the reverse flow in the ipsilateral vertebral artery (Figure 15.3).

Fibromuscular dysplasia

Fibromuscular dysplasia mainly occurs in the young population, mostly young women. Renal arteries are more often affected than internal carotid and vertebral arteries, mono-as well as bilateral involvement may occur. High-resolution

CE-MRA is necessary to depict small variations in the vessel diameter.

Plaque characterization is another promising supplementary technique to MRA which can be performed in the same session. Multi-contrast imaging or even more advanced imaging techniques have been proposed to detect high-risk components within atherosclerotic plaques. Plaque imaging is not established in clinical practice yet, but might become a valuable tool for therapeutic planning in the future, based on vulnerability determinants, or in the assessment of moderate stenosis.

Duplex ultrasound (DUS) is currently the most important screening technique for patients who are suspected of having extracranial atherosclerotic disease as it is non-invasive, fast, economical, and relatively accurate. A major drawback, is that it is highly operator-dependent and intracranial vessels cannot be reliably assessed. Furthermore, extremely tortuous vessels or large calcifications may prevent correct grading of stenoses with DUS. In cases where DUS is not helpful, or in instances when the diagnosis is equivocal, DUS may be followed by MRA in lieu of catheter-based angiography prior to endarterectomy. CT angiography is another technique increasingly used for the delineation of extracranial arteries (Chapter 6). The spatial resolution is somewhat superior to MR and calcified plaques are easier to identify at the cost of ionizing radiation and iodinated contrast agent. One of the important limitations of CT angiography is the problem of overlapping bone and beam hardening artefacts related to vascular calcification which is not an issue with MRA.

Dissections

About 20% of ischemic infarction in young individuals (<30 years of age) is caused by dissection of cranio-cervical arteries. Dissections of the carotid or vertebral arteries may occur spontaneously or following trauma, for example caused by a motor vehicle accident, seemingly innocuous motion, or by chiropractic manipulations. The dissected vessels are located typically at the level of C1–C2. Predisposing factors for spontaneous dissection include hypertension, fibromuscular dysplasia, Marfan syndrome with cystic medial necrosis, Ehlers-Danlos syndrome, and alpha-1 anti-trypsin deficiency.

High-resolution CE-MRA is able to show the residual flow through the stenosed vessel similar to catheter angiography. Three-dimensional TOF including source images can be used to demonstrate the thickened vessel wall. In the subacute and early chronic stage methemoglobin within the intramural hematoma is depicted on transverse T1-weighted images with fat suppression; in the acute stage the hemorrhage is isointense to the surrounding tissue. According to our own experience, PD-weighted sequences with fat saturation are also well suited for imaging of the vessel wall. Furthermore, MRA and MR imaging are relevant tools for follow-up examinations to monitor regression of dissection and normalization of vessel lumen after therapy.

The combination of MRA and MR imaging has a very high sensitivity and specificity for detection of carotid dissections compared to catheter angiography. In contrast to catheter angiography, MR makes the display of the vessel wall and its pathologies possible. For the visualization of vertebral arteries, however, MR is inferior to intra-arterial selective angiography because of the smaller vessel dimensions.

Mass lesions and other pathologies

Vascular neoplasms

Neoplasms of the extracranial vessels are seen very rarely, with paraganglioma being the most common entity. Paragangliomas are benign tumors which are either derived from primitive neural crest ('glomus vagale paraganglioma') or arise from glomus bodies in the carotid body at the carotid bifurcation ('carotid body paraganglioma'); a third form of paragangliomas is located in the jugular fossa and tympanic cavity ('jugulotympanic paraganglioma'). Paragangliomas are well depicted on T2-weighted and T1-weighted post-contrast images with fat saturation; T1-weighted precontrast images show flow void effects due to fast flowing blood. 'Salt and pepper' appearance due to flow void in multiple small tumor vessels is typical for paraganglioma. Pre- and post-contrast 3D TOF has been reported to be the most effective technique for detection of paragangliomas, while time-resolved CE-MRA yields additional blood supply information. Nevertheless, intra-arterial angiography may still be required for detailed visualization of vascularity and for detection of very small paragangliomas.

In contrast to other vascular territories, *aneurysms* are rarely found in the extracranial circulation. CE-MRA is well suited for detection and exact localization of the aneurysm but has one major drawback: in the presence of a thrombus, the entire extent of the aneurysm cannot be delineated. Hence, T1- and T2-weighted images should be performed additionally.

Carotid artery false aneurysms are characterized by out pouching of the internal carotid artery with normal components of the arterial vessel wall. The vessel wall is partially or even completely disrupted. The out pouching of the internal carotid artery is seen on CE-MRA. MR imaging is recommended additionally for display of thrombosed parts of this lesion.

Venous thrombosis

Jugular vein thrombosis

This is an uncommon condition and may occur in conjunction with prothrombotic disorders or trauma. During the acute to subacute stage, thrombophlebitis with inflammation of the adjacent soft tissue is present which resolves in the chronic stage. Dynamic CE-MRA including arterial as well as venous phases will usually reveal the patency of the vessel. Transverse T1- and T2-weighted images (with and without fat saturation) are important to display the clot and to detect soft tissue inflammation.

Intracranial circulation

Aneurysms

Intracerebral aneurysms occur in 1 to 14% of the population, with an increased incidence in the case of a familial history. Aneurysms are subdivided into saccular, fusiform, and blister-like aneurysms. Saccular or berry aneurysms which generally arise from an arterial bifurcation are the most frequent subgroup. Ruptured aneurysms lead to subarachnoid hemorrhage, with a high risk for parenchymal intraventricular hemorrhage that sometimes may prove fatal. The risk for rupture of an intracranial aneurysm is assumed to be 1 or 2% per year. Besides surgical treatment (clipping of the aneurysm), endovascular treatment with Guglielmi detachable coils is increasingly employed today with low morbidity and mortality.

Selective intra-arterial catheter angiography is still the gold standard for detection and treatment planning of intracranial aneurysms; this is especially true for very small aneurysms. Important diagnostic information includes details about the size and the position of the aneurysm, the neck of the aneurysm, and the existence of concomitant lesions. Furthermore, differential diagnosis between an aneurysm and a simple vessel loop is essential. MR, however, has been reported to have a detection rate of 90–95% for aneurysms between 3 and 4 mm and is, therefore, increasingly used as a screening technique in patients with a familial history of aneurysms. Due to its high resolution, 3D TOF is the most important MRA method (Figure 15.4). Inspection of

the source images is essential for the detection of small aneurysms, which might be missed on maximum intensity projection (MIP) images. Further, advanced 3D post-processing techniques like shaded surface display (SSD) or preferably volume rendering (VR) (Figure 15.5) seem to be more sensitive for detection of aneurysms. CE-MRA or 3D PC-MRA is advantageous to separate flowing blood from thrombosed material within the aneurysm (Figure 15.4). Due to large thrombotic areas, the true size of giant aneurysms will be invisible for catheter angiography. In those cases MRA has to be supplemented by sectional MR (T1- and T2-weighted images) (Figure 15.4). If an aneurysm is found incidentally on MR imaging, 3D TOF has to be acquired additionally to search for further aneurysms.

Follow-up examinations of coiled aneurysms are currently performed using MR. Three-dimensional TOF and CE-MRA have been proposed to evaluate the patency of parent and branch vessels as well as the presence of aneurysm remnants or recurrences. Newer studies mostly favor CE-MRA over 3D TOF angiography. Nevertheless, the accuracy of 'conventional' 3D TOF might be improved using very high spatial resolution and/or very short echo times to reduce spin-dephasing effects; post-contrast 3D TOF can also be advantageous for this purpose. Three-dimensional TOF might regain some importance for intracranial aneurysms in the near future, because this technique is especially advantageous at 3 T. Increased spatial resolution and improved vessel contrast are expected to further improve diagnosis of intracranial aneurysms. Follow-up examinations of clipped aneurysms are not performed routinely with MR because of artifacts caused by the clip.

CT angiography is a promising, non-invasive technique for intracranial aneurysms (Chapter 6). Although spatial resolution of CT angiography is superior to MRA, CT has not been able to replace catheter angiography for intracranial aneurysms yet. One important disadvantage of CT angiography is the occurrence of bone artifacts near the skull base that makes post-processing and visualization of vascular structures challenging.

Vascular malformations

Arteriovenous malformations (AVM)

This is the most common form of vascular malformation. An AVM consists of feeding vessels, a nidus, and draining vessels. Hemorrhage of AVM is the most critical clinical manifestation and has a high mortality and morbidity. Treatment options

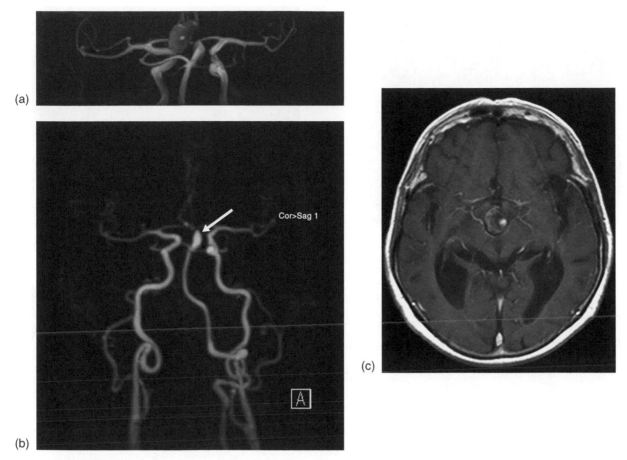

Figure 15.4 *Partially thrombosed aneurysm of the basilar artery.* High-resolution 3D TOF with water excitation (a) demonstrates a partially thrombosed aneurysm of the tip of the basilar artery. In contrast to 3D TOF, time-resolved CE-MRA (b) only shows the area of flowing blood within the aneurysm (arrow), whereas T1-weighted post-contrast imaging (c) visualizes all parts of the aneurysm.

include surgical, endovascular, radio-surgical, or a combination of these procedures. Selective catheter angiography is the method of choice, because display of afferent and efferent vessels is important in planning. Furthermore, the size of the nidus has to be determined exactly, as radiotherapy, for example, is especially successful in AVMs with a nidus below 3 cm. MRA and MR imaging, however, play an essential role in follow-up examinations after therapy. Three-dimensional TOF is valuable for this purpose (Figure 15.6), 3D PC or CE-MRA is preferable in the presence of subacute hemorrhage. Dynamic CE-MRA techniques have shown promising results for the display of AVMs, but the temporal and/or spatial resolution is still too low compared to catheter angiography.

Cavernomas

These are also called cavernous angiomas, and are considered to be benign vascular hamartomas, consisting of closely packed immature blood vessels without neural tissue between the vessels. Intralesional hemorrhage and/or calcification is frequently found. Although they are asymptomatic in most cases, cavernomas can cause neurologic symptoms like epilepsy; bleeding may lead to relevant complications. Cavernomas are characterized by a 'popcorn ball' appearance on T2-weighted images. Another typical sign is a low signal rim on T2-weighted images due to hemosiderin deposition and/or calcification, which causes prominent susceptibility effects on T2*-weighted images ('blooming effect'). T2*-weighted gradient echo techniques are most sensitive for detection of cavernomas; therefore, T2*-weighted imaging is mandatory in patients with cavernomas to detect or to exclude further cavernomas. MRA or catheter angiography is not indicated because cavernomas are 'cryptic angiomas' which are angiographically occult.

Developmental venous anomalies (DVAs)

In some cases, cavernomas are associated with DVAs. These are congenital cerebral vascular anomalies which

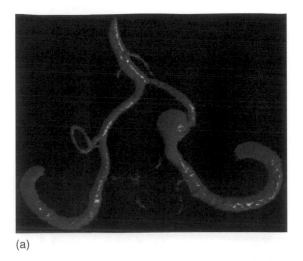

(a)

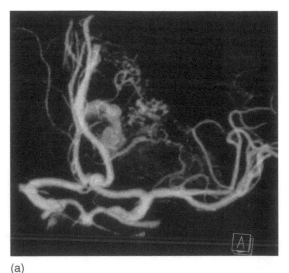

(a)

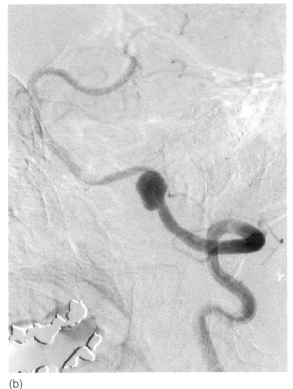

(b)

Figure 15.5 *Aneurysm of the vertebral artery.* 3D TOF (volume rendering) shows (a) an aneurysm in the V4 segment of the left vertebral artery; the findings in MRA are very similar to those yielded with catheter angiography (b).

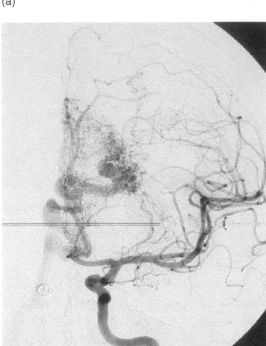

(b)

Figure 15.6 *Partially thrombosed AVM.* High-resolution 3D TOF acquired at 3.0 T (voxel size 0.4×0.4×0.4mm) clearly demonstrates (a) a partially thrombosed AVM with feeders originating from the A2 segment of the anterior cerebral artery, the pericallosal artery, and the M1 segment of the left middle cerebral artery. An ectatic draining vein is also seen. (b) Confirmation by catheter angiography. Courtesy of Ö Gürvit and H Lanfermann, Institute of Neuroradiology, University of Frankfurt.

consist of major mature veins. Typically, multiple medullary veins drain into a dilated transcortical collector vein. DVAs are mostly asymptomatic and are usually detected as incidental findings. The most reliable diagnostic sign is dilated medullary veins on post-contrast T1-weighted images (the so-called 'Medusa head' sign). MR imaging is superior to MRA for detection of DVA; if MRA is performed additionally, a technique optimized for slow venous flow (3D PC, 2D TOF, CE) has to be used.

Capillary telangiectasia

This is another venous malformation which is commonly asymptomatic. Capillary telangiectasias consist of a cluster of capillaries, often interdispersed within normal brain parenchyma, and are typically located in the pons. Faint brush-like enhancement on post-contrast T1-weighted images is characteristic for capillary telangiectasia. These appear iso- or hypointense on T2-weighted images. We have found that hypointense signal on diffusion-weighted images is helpful for differenting this from tumors. In some cases a draining vein can be detected on MR imaging.

Stenoses and occlusions

Stenoses of the intracranial arteries can be caused by atherosclerotic disease or arteritis (giant cell, Moyamoya, systemic lupus erythematosus, and primary arteritis of the CNS). Three-dimensional TOF may sometimes simulate stenoses and this should be kept in mind. Additional confirmation with a CE-MRA is recommended in equivocal cases. Catheter angiography may sometimes be required if the clinical situation warrants this. Three-dimensional TOF and/or high-resolution CE-MRA are valuable tools for planning and follow-up examinations of intra/extracranial anastomosis (Figure 15.7) or between the internal and the external carotid artery. Acute occlusion of intracranial arteries is the most common cause of stroke. Occlusions of larger vessels are reliably detected using a fast 3D TOF technique taking only 3–4 minutes (Figure 15.8). Besides diffusion and perfusion imaging, 3D TOF of intracranial arteries is a major component of an MR examination in acute stroke.

Tumors

For intracranial tumors, MRA is a valuable tool to supplement the information obtained from MRI. Displacement of larger vessels is reliably depicted with MRA. Depending on the vascular region of interest, TOF or CE-MRA may be used. Visualization of vascular anatomy as it relates to the tumor is invaluable for surgical planning: If the tumor is located near the sensorimotor cortex, the position of superficial veins as well as that of the tumor has to be known in order to avoid surgical complications. Before resection of extra-axial tumors, it may be very helpful for the neurosurgeon to visualize the displacement of the internal carotid, vertebral, and basilar arteries. Intracranial vessels above the skull base are usually well delineated on T1-weighted post-contrast 3D data sets. For this purpose a 3D data set with isotropic (or nearly isotropic) voxel size is used. Separating arteries from veins, however, is only possible taking into account anatomic information. A more dedicated visualization of arteries/veins in relation to the tumor position is possible through use of an MRA technique. Image fusion of the anatomic and the angiographic data set yields an optimal depiction of the vessel/tumor relationship, especially if color coding is used (Figure 15.9).

Neurovascular compression

Neurovascular compression may result in trigeminal neuralgia or hemifacial spasm if vessel loops are in tight contact with cranial nerves in the cerebellopontine angle. MRI/MRA may be performed in these patients to demonstrate the spatial relationship between vessels and cranial nerves. Cranial nerves as well as intracranial vessels are well depicted on a T2-weighted 3D data set with high spatial resolution. Distinguishing these two structures, however, can be difficult because both are hypointense on T2-weighted images. Therefore, an alternate strategy is preferred by most users. The combination of 3D TOF and a high-resolution T1-weighted 3D data set after application of contrast agent may be helpful. Intracranial vessels are well delineated on the T1-weighted data set as hyperintense structures, whereas cranial nerves have significantly lower signal intensity. Three-dimensional TOF source images are used to differentiate between arteries and veins.

Venous thrombosis

Intracranial venous thrombosis can affect dural sinus or cortical veins. Acute dural sinus thrombosis is an emergency indication for MRI/MRA. In this regard, 3D PC is superior to 2D TOF because thrombosed blood in the subacute stage appears hyperintense on TOF. Furthermore, saturation effects or insufficient inflow effects can simulate venous occlusion when using 2D TOF. When combined with sectional MR imaging (T2-weighted images as well as pre- and post-contrast T1-weighted images with a slice thickness of ≤3 mm) this is a reliable method for detection of sinus thrombosis. Time-resolved CE-MRA seems to be a promising technique for diagnosis of dural sinus thrombosis, but few data have been published on this topic.

Thrombosis of superficial cerebral veins can be associated with dural sinus thrombosis (Figure 15.10). The recommended method of diagnosis in the acute stage of cortical vein thrombosis is sectional MR imaging including a T2*-weighted gradient-echo sequence as this technique is very sensitive, even for small areas. In many cases, T2*-weighted images may be the only method that demonstrates cortical vein thrombosis. MRA has only a supplementary role in the case of cortical vein thrombosis.

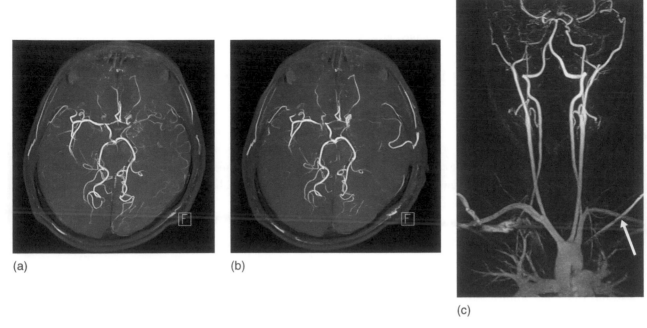

Figure 15.7 *Moyamoya disease before and after microanastomosis.* High-resolution 3D TOF with water excitation before (a) and after microanastomosis (b) between a branch of the external carotid artery and the middle cerebral artery on the left side as well as high-resolution CE-MRA with bolus timing after microanastomosis (c). Panel (a) also shows subtotal occlusion of the left middle cerebral artery and proximal stenosis of the right middle cerebral artery (M1 segment) due to Moyamoya vasculitis. Additionally, severe narrowing of the lumen of the right internal carotid artery is seen in (c). Significant foldover artifacts of both subclavian arteries (c) are caused by a rectangular FOV of 62% [crossing of the left subclavian artery and the right subclavian artery simulates a moderate stenosis (arrow)].

COMMON ARTIFACTS AND PITFALLS

Artifacts and pitfalls in MRA are mainly caused by specific drawbacks of individual MR techniques, post-processing techniques, or general problems related to the MR data acquisition. For the acquisition of reliable MR angiograms it is of great importance to know the disadvantages and pitfalls and to know how to avoid or reduce them. The most common artifacts will be discussed in this paragraph; typical drawbacks of individual techniques have already been presented in the section on fundamentals.

Artifacts and pitfalls related to a specific MR angiographic technique

Spin dephasing effects are a major problem inherent to all plain MRA methods and may result in overestimation or even simulation of stenoses in areas of turbulent flow. Thus, although 3D TOF MRA is the MR method of choice for diagnosis in intracranial vessels, due to its high resolution, stenoses in the carotid siphon can be simulated in rare cases (Figure 15.11). Additional application of a CE-MRA may be necessary to rule out the presence of a stenosis. Spin-dephasing effects in

3D TOF, which result in local signal loss, are a well-known problem in very large aneurysms. Due to the local signal loss, the true extension of the aneurysm is not seen with 3D TOF. Inspection of source images may be advantageous to detect small aneurysms, CE-MRA enables differentiation of flowing blood from thrombotic material (Figure 15.4). Another problem with 3D TOF occurs in the presence of hemorrhage (or thrombus) in the subacute state as methemoglobin is displayed as high signal intensity. CE or 3D PC MR angiographic techniques are recommended for those cases to differentiate between moving and stationary blood.

MOTSA is an important technique to reduce saturation effects in 3D TOF techniques; Venetian blind artifacts have been significantly diminished in most implementations. Nevertheless, the reliability of vessel delineation is sometimes reduced in the region of slab overlap and may simulate stenoses or dissected vessels.

Three-dimensional TOF with water excitation would be a desirable technique for delineation of superficial intracranial vessels and vessels near the orbit, but artifacts simulating stenoses or even occlusions have been reported for this technique. From our experience, those artifacts mainly occur in combination with MOTSA. Therefore, we apply water excitation only for single slab techniques. Furthermore, verification of stenoses found on

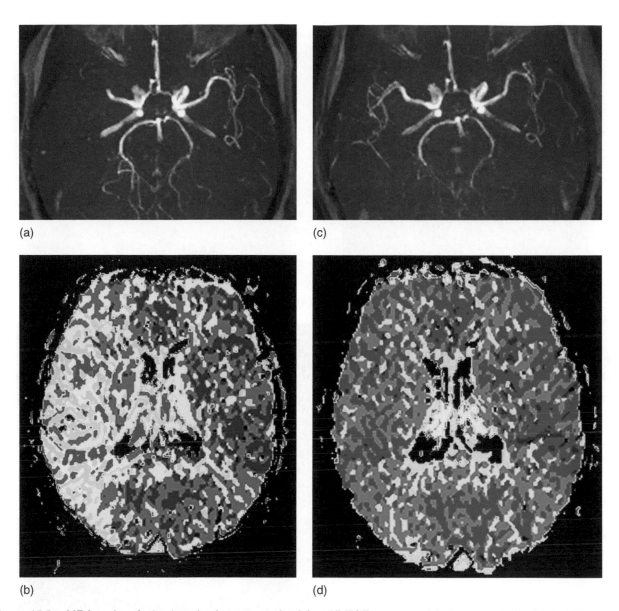

(a)

(c)

(b)

(d)

Figure 15.8 *MRA and perfusion imaging in acute stroke.* A fast 3D TOF sequence (a) shows occlusion in the M1 segment of the right middle cerebral artery in a patient with acute stroke; the mean transit time (MTT) map reveals significantly prolonged perfusion in the territory of the MCA (b). Follow-up examination one day after intravenous thrombolysis demonstrates complete recanalization of the middle cerebral artery (c) and consecutive normalization of the perfusion deficit (d) with complete resolution of the neurologic deficit.

water excitation images is recommended, using alternative MR angiographic techniques.

If 2D or 3D TOF is employed at the carotid bifurcation, two problems can arise: 2D TOF may simulate severe stenoses due to in-plane saturation effects and 3D TOF may simulate occlusion due to saturation effects within the slab.

Artifacts and pitfalls related to post-processing or display

Only the tissue with highest signal intensity is projected onto the MIP image (Chapter 4). If the vessel signal is too low, other tissues like subcutanous fat can mask the vessels. Targeted MIP or thin MIPs are techniques that use only a subvolume of the complete data set; in most cases these techniques are able to solve the problem. Inspection of source images and display of multiple projections can remedy this deficiency as well. Two vessels that seem to cross in the MIP image often simulate stenoses at the crossing point (Figure 15.7). Display of multiple projections is a very simple strategy to overcome this drawback. MIP is not the optimal post-processing method for complex vascular structures because of its projection basis, which does not allow the user to gain knowledge on the exact position of structure, three-dimensionally. Although multiple

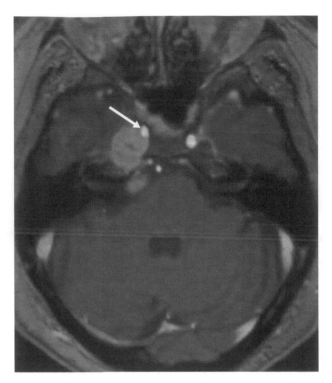

Figure 15.9 *Neurinoma of the trigeminal nerve.* Color-coded image fusion of a 3D TOF MR angiographic data set and a T1-weighted post-contrast 3D MP-RAGE data set reveals anterolateral displacement of the right internal carotid artery (arrow) by the neurinoma. Knowledge of the vascular topography may be essential for the neuro-surgeon to avoid complications, such as injury of the displaced artery, during the operation.

projections are helpful, 3D post-processing techniques like SSD, or preferably VR, are superior to MIP for 3D spatial relationships (Chapter 4).

General artifacts and pitfalls

Vessels out of the prescribed slab can appear falsely stenosed or occluded. This phenomenon can be observed especially at the origins of the supra-aortic vessels, carotid siphon, and for very elongated vertebral arteries. Careful positioning of the volume is recommended to solve this problem. Most applications of CE-MRA use a coronal 3D data set with a rectangular FOV to reduce acquisition time (Chapter 12). For supra-aortic arteries this procedure can result in significant foldover artifacts of the subclavian arteries (Figure 15.7). Application of parallel imaging techniques, if available, is recommended in combination with a square FOV to solve this drawback, mainly for visualization of subclavian arteries.

Artifacts caused by metallic implants appear as signal loss on MRA images (as these are gradient-echo images) and may simulate stenoses or occlusions. Intravascular stents and

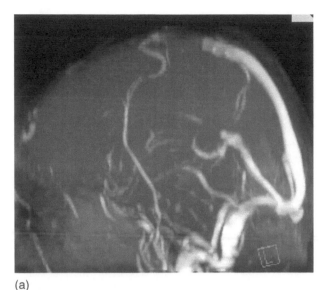

(a)

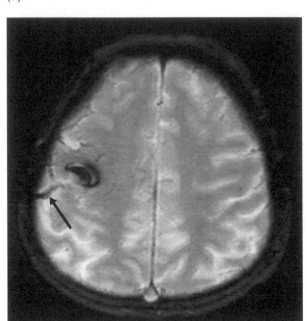

(b)

Figure 15.10 *Dural sinus thrombosis associated with cortical vein thrombosis.* 2D TOF (a) demonstrates acute thrombosis of the superior sagittal sinus. Associated corti-cal vein thrombosis (b, arrow) is only depicted on T2*-weighted sectional images.

aneurysm clips are the most common culprits. Some authors have recommended using a CE-MRA technique with very high flip angle (90° or more) after stent implantation to improve visualization of stents.

PRACTICAL PEARLS

- Use accurately timed high resolution for MRA (with sufficient signal-to-noise ratio) at short acquisition time to avoid venous overlap.

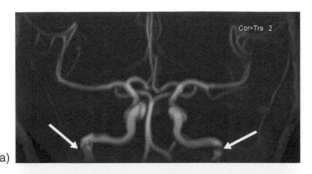

(a)

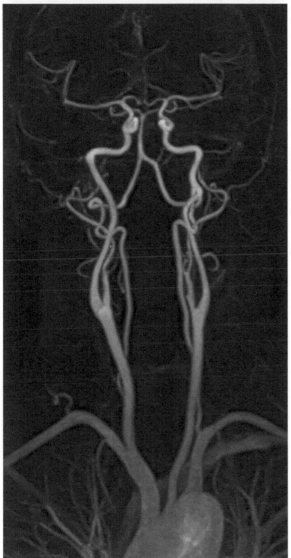

(b)

Figure 15.11 *Artifacts caused by spin dephasing in 3D TOF.* Spin-dephasing artifacts in the carotid siphon simulate stenoses on both internal carotid arteries in 3D TOF MRA (a, arrows), but these suspected stenoses were definitely excluded using CE-MRA (b).

- Venous access should be ideally placed in an antecubital vein in the right upper extremity (if possible) in order to avoid susceptibility artifacts in the left brachiocephalic vein.

- MIPs as well as source images and/or multiplanar reformations should be examined routinely while evaluating MR angiograms.

- In uncertain cases involving 3D TOF verify intracranial stenoses with CE-MRA, and vice versa.

- Apply additional MRA techniques and/or MR imaging in questionable findings.

CONCLUSIONS

MRA plays an important role in modern imaging of the extra- and intracranial vasculature as it is a fast and non-invasive method which offers exceptional soft tissue contrast without using iodinated contrast agents or ionizing radiation. While screening of the carotid arteries for atherosclerotic disease is usually performed with DUS, MRA has become the most relevant technique for the complete visualization of vessels from the aortic arch to the circle of Willis. Combining MRA and MR imaging is optimal to supplement DUS for diagnosis of carotid artery dissections. MRA and MR imaging are important techniques for delineation of tumors and other pathologies such as true and false aneurysms and venous thrombosis. While catheter angiography is still the gold standard for many intracranial applications, MRA is widely accepted in follow-up examinations of coiled aneurysms as well as for visualization of thrombosed aneurysms and for screening of patients with a familial history of intracranial aneurysms. In patients with acute stroke, MR is able to depict arterial occlusions and to yield rapidly, relevant information about the tissue at risk. Vascular malformations like cavernomas, DVAs, and capillary telangiectasias are best depicted on sectional MR imaging, whereas MRA is an important method for the follow-up examinations of treated AVMs.

Technical advances in hardware and contrast agents are likely to improve visualization of intracranial vascular structures in the future. Further initial results at 3 T have demonstrated that high-field imaging is likely to represent an additional and important step towards accomplishing this aim.

FURTHER READING

Arlart IP, Bongartz GM, Marchal G, eds. Magnetic Resonance Angiography, 2nd edn. Berlin, Germany: Springer, 2002, 2003.

Elgersma OE, Wust AF, Buijs PC et al. Multidirectional depiction of internal carotid arterial stenosis: three-dimensional time-of-flight MR angiography versus rotational and conventional digital subtraction angiography. Radiology 2000; 216: 511–16.

Fellner C, Lang W, Janka R et al. Magnetic resonance angiography of the carotid arteries using three different techniques: accuracy compared with intraarterial X-ray angiography and endarterectomy specimens. J Magn Reson Imag 2005; 21: 424–31.

Lombardi M, Bartolozzi C, eds. MRI of the Heart and Vessels. Milan: Springer, 2005.

Nederkoorn PJ, van der Graaf Y, Hunink MGM. Duplex ultrasound and magnetic resonance angiography compared with digital subtraction angiography in carotid artery stenosis. A systematic review. Stroke 2003; 34: 1324–32.

Osborn AG, Blaser SI, Salzman KL et al. Diagnostic Imaging. Brain. Salt Lake City: Amirsys, 2004.

Schneider G, Prince MR, Meaney JFM, Ho VB, eds. Magnetic Resonance Angiography. Techniques, Indications and Practical Applications. Milan, Springer 2005.

Tay KY, U-King-Im JM, Trivedi RA et al. Imaging the verebral artery. Eur Radiol 2005; 15: 1329–43.

Townsend TC, Saloner D, Pan XM, Rapp JH. Contrast material-enhanced MRA overestimates severity of carotid stenosis, compared with 3D time-of-flight MRA. J Vasc Surg 2003; 38: 36–40.

Westerlaan HE, van der Vliet AM, Hew JM et al. Time-of-flight magnetic resonance angiography in the follow-up of intracranial aneurysms treated with Guglielmi detachable coils. Neuroradiology 2005; 47: 622–9.

Willinek WA, von Falkenhausen M, Born M et al. Noninvasive detection of steno-occlusive disease of the supraaortic arteries with three-dimensional contrast-enhanced magnetic resonance angiography. A prospective, intra-individual comparative analysis with digital subtraction angiography. Stroke 2005, 36: 38–43.

Wutke R, Lang W, Fellner C et al. High-resolution, contrast-enhanced magnetic resonance angiography with elliptical centric k-space ordering of supra-aortic arteries compared with selective X-ray angiography. Stroke 2002, 33: 1522–9.

16

MR angiography of the pulmonary circulation

Hong Lei Zhang, Hale Ersoy, and Martin R Prince

INTRODUCTION

Although CT angiography (CTA) has become a primary technique for evaluating pulmonary arteries, it carries the risks of ionizing radiation and iodinated contrast. Accordingly, there is a need for a safer technique, particularly in young patients and patients with renal insufficiency or history of severe allergic reaction to iodinated contrast. Pulmonary MR angiography (MRA) is not as fast as CTA and thus must overcome respiratory motion and cardiac pulsation, as well as susceptibility artifact at air–tissue interfaces, while still being able to resolve small subsegmental pulmonary arteries. Early pulmonary MRA techniques focused on black-blood and time-of-flight approaches, which have been proved to be unreliable in evaluating the pulmonary circulation. However, three-dimensional (3D) contrast-enhanced (CE) MRA with EKG gating (Figure 16.1) can provide excellent visualization of the pulmonary arterial tree from the main pulmonary artery through the subsegmental branches. Additionally, when combined with post-contrast MR venographic evaluation of the abdomen, pelvis, and lower extremity, pulmonary MRA provides a comprehensive assessment for venous thromboembolic disease.

The general concepts regarding the execution of pulmonary MRA will be discussed in this chapter, followed by a description of the principal clinical applications of this imaging modality (Table 16.1).

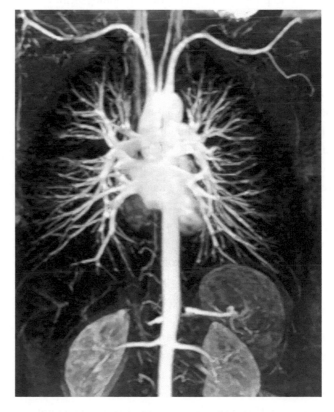

Figure 16.1 Coronal MIP of 3D EKG-gated contrast-enhanced MRA data set obtained during the injection of 30 ml Gd contrast. Note visualization of pulmonary arteries to the subsegmental level.

Table 16.1 Principal indications to pulmonary MRA

Pulmonary embolism
Pulmonary hypertension
Congenital abnormalities
Pre-ablation pulmonary vein mapping
Lung tumors

GENERAL PRINCIPLES OF PULMONARY MRA

There are a number of important technical principles that apply to pulmonary MRA. Pulmonary CE-MRA is obtained by applying a spoiled 3D gradient-echo sequence. The echo time (TE) should be less than 3 ms in order to minimize susceptibility artifact from air–tissue interfaces throughout the lungs and to minimize flow artifacts. This is generally not a problem on state-of-the-art, high-performance, 1.5 T scanners. However, 3 T imaging may be more challenging due to greater susceptibility, magnetic field inhomogeneities as well as dielectric effects.

In general, there are two approaches to performing 3D CE-MRA of the pulmonary arteries. The first approach is to acquire a single coronal 3D MRA with a large field-of-view (FOV) encompassing both lungs. This is performed with a single dose of paramagnetic contrast agent, typically 0.2–0.3 mmol/kg or 30 ml of gadolinium (Gd) chelate with parallel imaging which allows for a large number of slices. Since the coronal plane may have wrap-around artifact in the left–right direction, the FOV must be large enough to include both lungs as well as the arms and shoulders. Thus, a large FOV is often required. While wrap-around artifact can be somewhat reduced by elevating the arms over the head and using a narrow phased-array coil, it is virtually impossible to completely eliminate wrap-around from the shoulders. It may be possible to have a smaller FOV with acceptable wrap-around artifact if a phased-array coil with limited sensitivity in the left-to-right direction is employed. In this case, wrap-around from the distant edges of the arms and shoulders will be only a faint shadow superimposed on the brighter image of the lungs.

The second approach is to perform two separate sagittal acquisitions with smaller FOV and higher spatial resolution. This approach requires two separate Gd chelate injections. The wrap-around artifact is eliminated by frequency encoding in the S/I (superior-to-inferior) direction, phase encoding in the Anterior-to-posterior direction, and using the slice-encoding gradient to limit the

left–right dimension of the volume. The disadvantage of this method is that two separate data sets require two acquisitions and more complex data analysis. Another problem with this approach is that the sagittal volumes may not optimally cover the central pulmonary circulation, which can be an issue if the patient has an abnormality involving the main pulmonary artery. Since paramagnetic contrast is injected twice, it is necessary to reduce the volume of each injection down to 20 ml (or 0.15 mmol/kg). This smaller volume of the Gd chelate requires more precise timing of the bolus in order to assure that central k-space data is acquired during the pulmonary arterial phase of the bolus. The multicoil arrays used with parallel imaging, eg. a 32 channel coil, have higher SWR near the periphery of the lung where it is needed to resolve the smaller more distal branches.

Alternatively, data can be acquired with a time-resolved approach (Figure 16.2), which eliminates the need for bolus timing. However, time-resolved imaging requires a longer breath hold, which can be an issue in patients with pulmonary disease, such as pulmonary embolism or hypertension. Parallel imaging techniques in conjunction with echo sharing allow a shorter acquisition time for the same imaging volume with time-resolved MRA than is possible with conventional 3D CE-MRA. It is also possible to acquire more slices and phase-encoding steps on the sagittal plane, thereby improving spatial resolution.

After the acquisition of the pulmonary arterial phase images, an equilibrium phase imaging should also be acquired during another breath hold. It may be useful to acquire several sets of equilibrium phase data to ensure that at least one of them is obtained during complete suspension of respiration. The equilibrium phase is especially useful when the pulmonary arterial phase is not timed optimally or if it is degraded by motion artifacts. Equilibrium phase images are also useful for identifying other pathologies, such as enhancing lung cancers, metastases, and atelectasis. Equilibrium phase data may be the most valuable phase for assessing pulmonary veins and it is especially useful when using blood pool agents such as Vasovist (Gadofosveset trisodium injection, formerly known as MS325).

EKG gating and breath holding

EKG gating is useful to eliminate the pulsation artifact from the pulmonary arteries and motion artifact from the heart, which can smear over the adjacent vessels. EKG gating allows visualization of more distal branch vessels due to reduction in blurring.

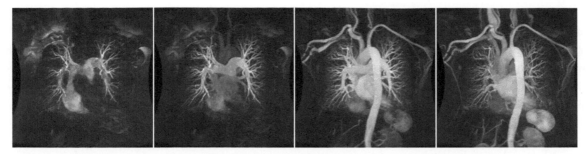

Figure 16.2 Time-resolved pulmonary MRA. Multiple phases show predominantly pulmonary arterial phase with minimal venous enhancement on the first two images, with later images showing enhancement of more vascular structures. The images were obtained in a normal subject using time-resolved MRA with 3D time-resolved imaging of contrast kinetics (TRICKS) at a 3.5 s temporal resolution and 40 ml Gd injected at 3 ml/s.

It is essential to acquire the data during breath holding. In patients with pulmonary disease, shortness of breath may limit the acquisition time to just 10 or 15 seconds. The breath hold duration can be lengthened by administering nasal oxygen. The rate of oxygen administration should not exceed 2 L/min in order to avoid suppression of respiratory drive in patients with severe obstructive lung disease. Prior to the actual scan, a test breath hold may be performed outside the gantry in order to determine the appropriate scan duration. In intubated patients, pharmacologic muscular relaxation may be useful to prevent spontaneous breathing during suspension of the ventilation. A respiratory therapist can help operate the ventilator for maximal effectiveness of the breath holding. Generally suspending respiration in maximum inspiration is less likely to induce spontaneous respiratory effort in the ventilated patient. In a patient unable to suspend breathing even for just a few seconds, it is best to acquire images over numerous respiratory cycles by using a longer acquisition (typically 40–60 seconds) and averaging multiple acquisitions. Because severely dyspneic patients generally tend to have minimal diaphragm movement during respiration, respiratory motion artifact can be largely eliminated with signal averaging. Navigator and respiratory bellows gating may also be helpful if available.

Post-processing

The 3D MRA data sets are best analyzed interactively on a computer workstation that is capable of performing subtractions, 3D reformations, and subvolume maximum intensity projection (MIP) images and volume rendering. Data should be reformatted for systematic identification of each pulmonary arterial vessel from the main pulmonary artery to the segmental branches in order to avoid overlooking small emboli. When a relatively high dose of Gd is used with thick slices, it may be possible to identify regions of greater suspicion for emboli by the presence of perfusion defects. It is also important to recognize that the MIP algorithm may not depict an embolus that is causing partial occlusion of a vessel. This potential pitfall can be overcome by scrolling through source images and thin multi-planar reformations.

Complementary sequences

Following 3D CE-MRA of the pulmonary vessels, it may be useful to acquire axial 2D steady-state free precession images. This may provide another chance to visualize the pulmonary arteries in case of insufficient breath holding for 3D CE-MRA. If there is pulmonary hypertension, 2D steady-state, free precession, double oblique views in the short axis, and 4-chamber and 2-chamber views of the ventricles can be helpful for the assessment of cardiac function, ventricular volumes and valvular insufficiency. Thrombus may appear bright on T1-weighted spin-echo images, although depending on the chronicity of the clot a variety of signal intensities are possible. In our experience this is not a reliable approach to identify pulmonary emboli. Post-Gd injection, inversion recovery prepared gradient-echo or steady state free precession SSFP imaging may be useful for identifying thrombi, especially in the proximal pulmonary arteries. Thrombus in this sequence typically appears dark at high inversion times and may take up a variable amount of contrast. Additional precontrast axial T1- and T2-weighted spin echo sequences may be helpful in patients with mediastinal masses. A potential future advantage of MRA is that blood pool contrast agents based on both Gd and iron oxides are under investigation for use in pregnancy. Blood pool agents are unlikely to cross into the fetal circulation iron oxides enter into the maternal iron stores which tend to be low in pregnancy.

Following pulmonary imaging, it may be useful to image the veins of the abdomen, pelvis, and thighs to evaluate for venous thromboembolic disease. This can be performed post-Gd using two large FOV coronal 2D or 3D gradient-echo volumes encompassing deep veins of the abdomen–pelvis and the thighs. Alternatively, if the Gd effect has begun to diminish, axial time-of-flight images can be acquired from the inferior vena cava down to just below the knee. These need not be contiguous slices if the time is limited. An axial gradient-echo acquisition with slice thickness of 3–5 mm and gap of 5–10 mm will not miss clot, because deep venous thrombus always occupies a segment that is longer than 1 cm. If the time-of-flight data are difficult to interpret, selective areas can be further evaluated with 2D phase contrast MRA using a Venc (velocity encoding) of about 30 cm/second in the S/I direction.

PRINCIPAL CLINCAL APPLICATIONS OF PULMONARY MRA

Pulmonary embolism

Pulmonary embolism is generally diagnosed by CTA or by ventilation/perfusion (V/Q) isotope lung scanning, with arteriographic validation in patients with indeterminate scan results or discordance between the V/Q scan results and clinical impression. V/Q scanning, however, provides only indirect evidence of pulmonary embolism since it is based upon unmatched ventilation–perfusion defects. For intermediate probability or indeterminate V/Q scans, further imaging is warranted. Because of the significant cost and potential morbidity physicians are reluctant to use pulmonary arteriography. As a result, treatment for pulmonary embolism may be undertaken without the benefit of a definitive diagnosis.

As cross-sectional imaging techniques, CTA and MRA can directly image arteries and provide a confident evaluation of patients suspected of a pulmonary embolism. Both CTA and MRA have developed into inexpensive, fast, accurate, and reliable tests for the assessment of pulmonary embolism. Data from multiple studies (Table 16.2) show credible evidence that 3D CE-MRA may supplant CTA for young patients and patients with renal insufficiency or a history of severe allergic reaction to iodinated contrast. Use of MRA may further accelerate with the availability of blood-pool contrast agents.

The disadvantages of MRA compared with CTA are the greater technical difficulty in performing and interpreting the exam and the greater difficulty in getting access to MR examinations due to the shortage of MR scanners. A major advantage of MRA is its ability to concomitantly examine the lower extremities for deep venous thrombosis as a single comprehensive exam lasting less than 45 minutes. Neither ultrasonic venography nor pulmonary angiography, if performed alone, can be comprehensive in identifying all patients with thromboembolic disease. The MRA/MR venography combination could even prove to be superior to CTA in conjunction with CT venography of the lower extremities owing to the higher diagnostic accuracy of MR venography when performed by experienced individuals.

Analysis of 3D CE-MRA data sets must include reformations in axial and several oblique planes in order to identify pulmonary arteries down to the segmental level. On older, slower scanners that require fewer slices to complete the study in a breath hold, the right middle lobe segmental artery is excluded because of its anterior course. Emboli are identified as intraluminal filling defects (Figures 16.3 and 16.4) just as on conventional catheter pulmonary arteriography or CTA. There may also be an associated wedge-shaped perfusion defect distal to the embolus. Data from numerous studies (Table 16.2) indicate the sensitivity and specificity of MRA for diagnosing pulmonary embolism are in the 75–100% range, which is superior to ventilation-perfusion imaging and comparable to CTA.

Table 16.2   Accuracy of 3D contrast MRA for pulmonary embolism

Author	Year	# of Patients	Sensitivity (%)	Specificity
Isoda	1995	18	80	95
Wolff et al	1996	34 (18[a])	68–76	93–95
Meaney et al	1997	30	75–100	95–100
Gupta et al	1999	36	85	96
Kreitner	2000	20	87	100
Kruger	2001	50 (15[a])	89	100
Goyen et al	2001	8	100	75
Oudkerk et al	2002	118	77	98
Ohno et al	2004	48	92	94

[a] Correlation with conventional arteriography available.

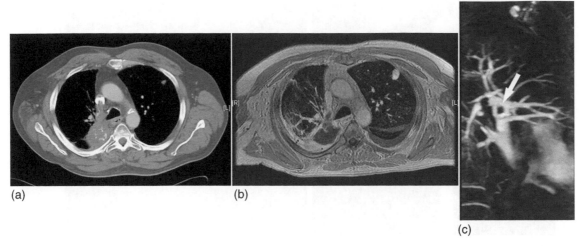

Figure 16.3 Pulmonary MRA for the detection of pulmonary embolism. Images refer to a 22-year-old male with known metastatic soft tissue sarcoma. (a) Chest CT demonstrates paravertebral soft tissue mass invading the hemiazygos vein and tumor extending into the lumen of the superior vena cava. At 15-day follow-up, a chest MRA is performed to re-evaluate the tumoral involvement of the superior vena cava. (b) The lumen of the superior vena cava is patent on axial 3D fast acquisition with multiphase efgre (FAME). (c) The 3D contrast-enhanced pulmonary MRA shows a filling defect in the right lower lobe artery (arrow), which is consistent with tumor embolus.

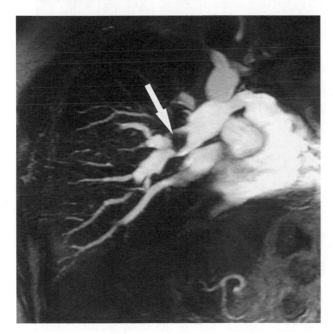

Figure 16.4 Oblique subvolume MIP of right pulmonary artery shows an intraluminal filling defect (arrow) indicating pulmonary embolus.

Pulmonary hypertension

In patients with pulmonary hypertension, pulmonary arteriography is employed to either exclude a diagnosis of chronic thromboembolic hypertension or, in the case of known thromboembolic hypertension, to prepare for surgical endarterectomy. Conventional arteriography is only performed as a last resort in these patients because of the 4-fold increased procedural mortality.

Cardiac MRI evaluation when performed in conjunction with pulmonary MRA can help in the assessment of left and right ventricular volume and function, and in the assessment of left to right shunts such as ostium secundum atrial septal defect as well as patent foramen ovale and tricuspid regurgitation. These findings may impact what kind of medical intervention these patients receive. Additional screening that may be performed as part of complete evaluation in the patient with pulmonary hypertension includes delayed enhancement imaging of the left ventricle to assess infiltrative disorders of the left and right ventricle (e.g. sarcoidosis) and phase contrast imaging of the aorta and pulmonary artery to calculate flow at these levels and derive Qp/Qs (flow in the pulmonary artery expressed as a ratio of the flow in the aorta). A ratio of greater than 1.1 may indicate a left to right shunt.

For pulmonary hypertension, 3D CE-MRA is performed in the coronal plane to demonstrate the central pulmonary arterial anatomy (Figure 16.5). The 3D nature of CE-MRA data actually provides a better delineation of the central pulmonary arteries than conventional angiography, where the catheter may be advanced into the pulmonary arteries beyond significant pathology. Pulmonary artery hypertension is diagnosed when the right pulmonary artery is greater than 28 mm in diameter and there is rapid proximal to distal tapering of the pulmonary arteries. One study found these criteria on 3D CE-MRA to be 89% sensitive and 100% specific for diagnosing pulmonary artery hypertension in 18 of 50 patients. In addition, 3D CE-MRA can accurately diagnose chronic pulmonary embolism, which is one of the

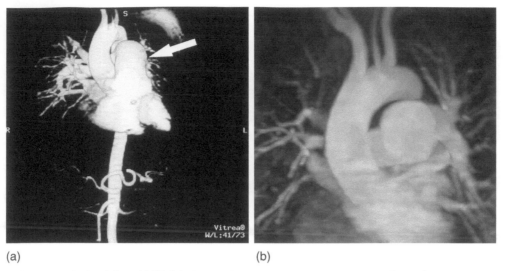

(a)   (b)

Figure 16.5   Volume rendering (a) and MIP (b) show enlarged main pulmonary artery (arrow) in pulmonary hypertension with rapid tapering of distal branches.

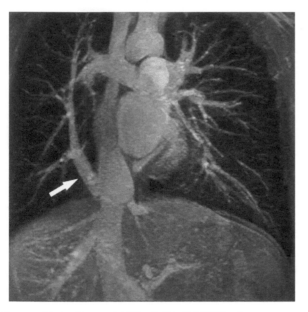

Figure 16.6   Coronal MIP of 3D Gd MRA shows anomalous drainage of right lower lobe pulmonary vein (arrow) into the supradiaphragmatic IVC.

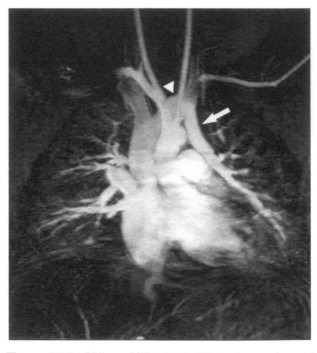

Figure 16.7   Oblique MIP of 3D MRA shows aberrant drainage of left pulmonary vein (arrow) to left brachiocephalic vein (arrowhead).

few correctable causes of pulmonary arterial hypertension. MRA can also diagnose pulmonary arterial involvement with Takayasu's arteritis or other vasculitis.

Pulmonary MRA of congenital abnormalities and anomalies

Three-dimensional CE-MRA is the technique of choice for evaluating the pulmonary circulation in young patients

with congenital heart disease. These patients are at higher risk of ionizing radiation and iodinated contrast because they will be having numerous pulmonary and cardiac imaging studies over their lifetime. CE-MRA is useful to diagnose congenital abnormalities of the pulmonary vasculature (Figures 16.6 and 16.7). Arterial anomalies tend to present early in life due to their effect on oxygenation and their common association with congenital heart disease.

Table 16.3 Pediatric pulmonary MRA for congenital abnormalities and anomalies

Author	Year	# of Patients	Sensitivity (%)	Specificity (%)
Pulmonary venous and other anomalies				
Berthezene	1998	1		
Masui	2000	23	96	100
Ferrari	2001	20 (19[a])	80	50
Godart et al	2001	6		96
Greil et al	2002	61 (25[a])	100	100
Congenital pulmonary artery or shunt stenosis				
Masui	2000	15 (31[a])	75	100
Kondo et al	2001	73	92.7	96.2
Geva	2002	32	100	100
Bernardes	2006	30	93.9	98.2
Sequestration				
Au	1999	1		
Kouchi	2000	1		
Gilkeson et al	2000	1		
Zhang	2001	1		
Deguchi	2005	1		

[a] Number of lesions.

In pediatric patients, 3D CE-MRA requires a higher weight-based dose because of the higher cardiac output of these patients relative to their size. Typically, up to 1 ml/kg is utilized to get adequate signal-to-noise ratio (SNR). Note that for a small baby this may only be 2 or 3 ml. CE-MRA is a particularly useful technique for sorting out pediatric vascular anomalies because there is no radiation exposure (Table 16.3). A study by Kondo et al showed high accuracy using breath-holding in patients greater than 10 years of age but allowing free breathing in younger, sedated patients. Even greater accuracy (100%) was achieved by Greil et al and Geva et al using general anesthesia and breath holding in all young patients. Greil et al found that 46% of 3D MRA examinations provided clinically important information not available from other sources. For example, in 8 patients MRA showed both the compression of pulmonary veins and the mechanism of compression (dilated atria post Fontan, scoliosis, or compression between the descending aorta and atria).

Fast multi-phase imaging is recommended in babies and toddlers to eliminate the complexities of bolus timing because of the fast transit time and small contrast volumes. To achieve short 3D acquisition time, slice thickness as large as 3–4 mm is acceptable, even in babies. With babies, it is also essential to use the smallest possible coil that they can fit into (e.g. a knee coil for neonates and a head coil or phased-array cardiac coil for larger babies). Although the dose is tiny in babies and infants, a dose per weight may be up to 1ml/kg to compensate for their proportionally higher cardiac output. Sequestration may also be diagnosed by 3D CE-MRA. The sequestered lobe is identified by T2 bright signal on single shot fast spin echo (SSFSE). The arterial supply and venous drainage are identified on 3D CE-MRA in order to assist with surgical resection and to discriminate intralobar from extralobar sequestration. Intralobar sequestrations commonly drain via pulmonary veins while the extralobar sequestrations have anomalous venous drainage.

CE-MRA can demonstrate vascular pathways in patients with pulmonary arterio-venous malformations because of the large size of the supplying arteries and draining veins. Small arterio-venous malformations, less than 5 mm, may be missed. Mapping out the anatomy prior to embolization helps to facilitate procedural planning, including coil sizing or embolization balloon sizing. It also reduces invasive procedural time and iodinated contrast requirements. Following coil embolization, however, the metal artifact may make it difficult to visualize the region of arterio-venous malformations by MRI unless the coils are platinum or titanium.

Pre-ablation pulmonary vein mapping

An effective treatment for atrial fibrillation is interrupting re-entry circuits by ablating myocardium where the pulmonary veins insert on the left atrium. This procedure is enormously simplified by first mapping the pulmonary vein anatomy with 3D CE-MRA. MRA is also useful for identifying pulmonary vein stenoses which may occur as a late complication of the ablation procedure and necessitate follow-up MR venograms. With increasing reliance on circumferential vein ablation rather than ostial approaches, this complication is, however, rare.

Lung tumors

The accuracy of 3D CE-MRA for staging lung tumors has not been extensively investigated, but our experience suggests that MRA may be useful for staging tumor patients who cannot tolerate iodinated contrast. MRA demonstrates the relationship of central tumors to the main pulmonary arteries and provides similar or superior information to CTA for preoperative surgical planning. A more comprehensive study by Ohno et al in 50 patients, 20 with surgical correlation, showed 3D CE-MRA to be superior to CTA in detecting vascular invasion. Obtaining delayed, equilibrium-phase images is important as mediastinal tumors and metastases may take a few minutes to enhance following Gd injection.

PITFALLS

There are several important potential pitfalls to be aware of when imaging the pulmonary arteries with 3D CE-MRA.

Susceptibility artifacts. These occur at air–tissue interfaces and can obscure image detail. Avoiding susceptibility requires keeping the (TE) short ($<$ 3 ms). Susceptibility artifact can also be caused by metal clips, coils and stents. Steel tends to cause much greater artifact than the relatively non-magnetic nitinol, tantalum and platinum devices.

Motion artifacts. Respiratory motion causes blurring, which can easily obscure subtle findings of a segmental or subsegmental embolus. When the data are corrupted by respiratory motion, it is better to make no effort to interpret the study rather than to provide false assurances that no embolus is identified.

Partial volume averaging. When emboli are only partially obstructing flow, they may be missed on thick MIP images.

Thus, it is important to interpret the source data interactively in multiple planes. Reconstructing with interpolation by zero filling also helps to maximize the chance of spotting emboli.

Misinterpretation of perfusion defects. Although perfusion defects are a marker of embolism, they can be seen with other pathologies, including bullae, emphysema, and tumor encasement of a vessel. They may also be positional due to the tendency for greater perfusion of the dependent portion of the lung.

Atelectasis. Atelectatic lung enhances dramatically. Although lung may be atelectatic as a result of pulmonary emboli, atelectasis is common in many clinical settings. It may also be rounded and simulate a mass.

CONCLUSIONS

Pulmonary MRA represents a valuable alternative approach to CTA for the evaluation of pulmonary circulation. CE-MRA provides the opportunity to obtain high-resolution 3D images depicting pulmonary vessels from the pulmonary trunk to the subsegmental branches. Major indications to pulmonary MRA are represented by patients with suspected pulmonary embolism, pulmonary hypertension (in conjunction with cardiac MRI), and congenital abnormalities. The main advantage with this modality is constituted by the absence of ionizing radiation and the good safety profile of Gd-based contrast agents. However, the execution of an adequate CE-MRA examination is particularly challenging and a high degree of expertise is required to avoid or promptly recognize any possible sources of artifact and to correctly interpret the images.

FURTHER READING

Au VW, Chan JK, Chan FL. Pulmonary sequestration diagnosed by contrast enhanced three-dimensional MR angiography. Br J Radiol 1999; 72: 709–11.

Bernardes RJ, Marchiori E, Bernardes PM, Monzo Gonzaga MB, Simoes LC. A comparison of magnetic resonance angiography with conventional angiography in the diagnosis of tetralogy of Fallot. Cardiol Young 2006; 16(3): 281–8.

Berthezene Y, Howarth NR, Revel D. Pulmonary arteriovenous fistula: detection with magnetic resonance angiography. Eur Radiol 1998; 8: 1403–4.

Deguchi E, Furukawa T, Ono S, Aoi S, Kimura O, Iwai N. Intralobar pulmonary sequestration diagnosed by MR angiography. Pediatr Surg Int 2005; 21(7): 576–7.

Ferrari VA, Scott CH, Holland GA, Axel L, Sutton MS. Ultrafast three-dimensional contrast-enhanced magnetic resonance angiography and imaging in the diagnosis of partial anomalous pulmonary venous drainage. J Am Coll Cardiol 2001; 37: 1120–8.

Geva T, Greil GF, Marshall AC, Landzberg M, Powell AJ. Gadolinium-enhanced 3-dimensional magnetic resonance angiography of pulmonary blood supply in patients with complex pulmonary stenosis or atresia: comparison with x-ray angiography. Circulation 2002; 106: 473–8

Gilkeson RC, Lee JH, Sachs PB, Clampitt M. Gadolinium-enhanced magnetic resonance angiography in scimitar syndrome: diagnosis and postoperative evaluation. Tex Heart Inst J 2000; 27: 309–11.

Godart F, Willoteaux S, Rey C, Cocheteux B, Francart C, Beregi JP. Contrast enhanced magnetic resonance angiography and pulmonary venous anomalies. Heart 2001; 86: 705.

Goyen M, Laub G, Ladd ME et al. Dynamic 3D MR angiography of the pulmonary arteries in under four seconds. J Magn Reson Imag 2001; 13: 372–7.

Greil GF, Powell AJ, Gildein HP, Geva T. Gadolinium-enhanced three-dimensional magnetic resonance angiography of pulmonary and systemic venous anomalies. J Am Coll Cardiol 2002; 39: 335–41.

Gupta A, Frazer CK, Ferguson JM et al. Acute pulmonary embolism: diagnosis with MR angiography. Radiology 1999; 210: 353–9.

Hoffmann U, Loewe C, Bernhard C et al. MRA of the lower extremities in patients with pulmonary embolism using a blood pool contrast agent: initial experience. J Magn Reson Imag 2002; 15: 429–37.

Isoda H, Ushimi T, Masui T et al. Clinical evaluation of pulmonary 3D time-of-flight MRA with breath holding using contrast media. J Comput Assist Tomogr 1995; 19: 911–19.

Kanne JP, Lalani TA. Role of computed tomography and magnetic resonance imaging for deep venous thrombosis and pulmonary embolism. Circulation 2004; 109: 115–21.

Kondo C, Takada K, Yokoyama U, Nakajima Y, Momma K, Sakai F. Comparison of three-dimensional contrast-enhanced magnetic resonance angiography and axial radiographic angiography for diagnosing congenital stenoses in small pulmonary arteries. Am J Cardiol 2001; 87: 420–4.

Kouchi K, Yoshida H, Matsunaga T et al. Intralobar bronchopulmonary sequestration evaluated by contrast-enhanced three-dimensional MR angiography. Pediatr Radiol 2000; 30(ll): 774–5.

Kreitner KF, Ley S, Kauczor HU et al. Contrast media enhanced three dimensional MR angiography of the pulmonary arteries in patients with chronic recurrent pulmonary embolism – comparison with selective intra-arterial DSA. Rofo 2000; 172: 122–8.

Kruger S, Haage P, Hoffmann R et al. Diagnosis of pulmonary arterial hypertension and pulmonary embolism with magnetic resonance angiography. Chest 2001; 120: 1556–61.

Maki DD, Siegelman ES, Roberts DA, Baum RA, Gefter WB. Pulmonary arteriovenous malformations: three-dimensional gadolinium-enhanced MR angiography – initial experience. Radiology 2001; 219: 243–6.

Masui T, Katayama M, Kobayashi S et al. Gadolinium-enhanced MR angiography in the evaluation of congenital cardiovascular disease pre- and postoperative states in infants and children. J Magn Reson Imaging 2000; 12: 1034–42.

Meaney JF, Prince MR. Pulmonary MR angiography. Magn Reson Imag Clin N Am 1999; 7: 393–409.

Meaney JF, Weg JG, Chenevert TL et al. Diagnosis of pulmonary embolism with magnetic resonance angiography. N Engl J Med 1997; 336:1422–7.

Ohno Y, Higashino T, Takenaka D et al. MR angiography with sensitivity encoding (SENSE) for suspected pulmonary embolism: comparison with MDCT and ventilation-perfusion scintigraphy. AJR 2004; 183: 91–8.

Oudkerk M, van Beek EJ, Wielopolski P et al. Comparison of contrast-enhanced magnetic resonance angiography and conventional pulmonary angiography for the diagnosis of pulmonary embolism: a prospective study. Lancet 2002; 359: 1643–7.

Prince MR, Grist TM, Debatin JF. 3D contrast MRA, 3rd edn. Springer Verlag, Heidelberg, 2003.

Schoepf UJ, Costello P. CT angiography for diagnosis of pulmonary embolism: state of the art. Radiology 2004; 230: 329–37.

Wolff K, Bergin CJ, King MA et al. Accuracy of contrast-enhanced magnetic resonance angiography in chronic thromboembolic disease. Acad Radiol 1996; 3: 10–17.

Woodard PK, Yusen RD. Diagnosis of pulmonary embolism with spiral computed tomography and magnetic resonance angiography. Curr Opin Cardiol 1999; 14: 442–7.

Zhang M, Zhu J, Wang Q, Shang D. Contrast enhanced MR angiography in pulmonary sequestration. Chin Med J (Engl). 2001; 114(12): 1326–8.

17

MR angiography of the thoracic aorta with protocols

Igor Klem, John D Grizzard, Dipan J Shah, Robert M Judd and Raymond J Kim

INTRODUCTION

Magnetic resonance imaging (MRI) plays a pivotal role in the diagnostic work-up of a broad spectrum of aortic diseases. In this chapter we will describe the MRI pulse sequences commonly used in the comprehensive assessment of the thoracic aorta, including assessment of the lumen and the wall, tissue characterization, and blood flow measurement. We will include a detailed description of clinical protocols aimed at providing 'hands-on' instructions for the image acquisition process as well as image data post-processing.

INDICATIONS

The common indications for thoracic MRA are listed in Table 17.1.

PULSE SEQUENCES

The fundamentals of pulse sequences used in MRA applications sequences are discussed in detail in Chapters 12 and 13.

Localizers

Steady-state free precession (SSFP) is the most commonly used sequence for localizer images.

Table 17.1   Indications for MRA of the thoracic aorta

- Imaging of aortic dissection
- Evaluation of thoracic aortic aneurysm
- Assessment of inflammatory aortic disease (immune, infectious)
- Evaluation of congenital anomalies of the thoracic aorta
- Evaluation of thoracic atherosclerosis
- Connective tissue diseases (Marfan's syndrome, Ehler–Danlos syndrome, and annulo-aortic ectasia)

Morphology and function

Half Fourier acquisition single-shot turbo spin-echo (HASTE). This double inversion recovery prepared turbo spin-echo sequence provides black-blood images with reduced image times, increased coverage per imaging time, improved lesion conspicuity, and reduced motion artifacts. This pulse-sequence is commonly used with fat suppression (Chapter 13).

Balanced steady state free precession (SSFP). This bright-blood technique has an exceptionally high signal-to-noise ratio with excellent contrast between blood and surrounding tissue. The *Cine*-SSFP sequence is used to depict functional changes of the structure imaged throughout the cardiac cycle. A single shot SSFP sequence with fast acquisition, designed to capture an entire image within one cardiac cycle can be performed rapidly to obtain an overview of the thoracic aorta analogous to HASTE-images (Chapter 13).

T1- and T2-weighted turbo spin-echo (TSE). T1 weighting is achieved by using a TR that is approximately 50 ms less than the patient's cardiac cycle (typically 500–1000 ms) and a short TE (5–20 ms). They are EKG-triggered and, due to long acquisition times, are sensitive to breathing and cardiac rhythm. Slow flow or stagnant blood may cause non-uniform vascular lumen signal intensity. T2-weighted TSE provide morphologic information comparable to T1-weighted images, and can also be useful to probe for tissues with long T2 characteristics (i.e. high water content).

Three-dimensional (3D) contrast-enhanced magnetic resonance angiography (MRA)

This has been reviewed in detail in Chapter 13. The correct timing of image acquisition relative to contrast injection is an important aspect of every MRA exam. Acquisition of the center of k-space data should correspond to peak concentrations of gadolinium contrast in the thoracic aorta with high and stable gadolinium concentrations lasting at least 1/2 to 2/3 of the scan duration. Hence an injection time 2/3 of the scan duration is recommended. In order to determine the correct sequence trigger time after the start of the contrast injection, equation (1) can be used for linearly ordered k-space acquisitions:

$$\text{Trigger time (s)} = \text{transit time} + (\text{contrast injection duration}/2)$$
$$- (\text{scan duration}/2) \qquad (1)$$

For pulse sequences with centric re-ordering, where the center of k-space is acquired at the beginning, the trigger time is equal to the transit time to maximal arterial opacification (Chapter 18). Transit time can be determined by the test bolus technique, using a 2D gradient-echo (GRE) sequence acquired at one image per second of the thoracic aorta in an axial or oblique sagittal view. A small bolus of contrast (1–2 ml) is injected, flushed with a saline bolus, and repeatedly imaged at the rate of 1 image/s. By visually inspecting the images or by using a signal intensity measurement tool in a region of interest within the aorta, the time to peak contrast in the thoracic aorta is determined: this is the transit time. Of note, the time to maximum signal intensity, not time to contrast arrival should be measured, and the region of interest should be placed in the center of the thoracic aorta, i.e. the arch, not in the ascending aorta close to the aortic root (this is especially important in patients with significant aortic insufficiency, as there may be a significant delay between the first arrival of contrast in the aortic root and the peak contrast concentration in the arch or descending aorta).

With some experience, a simpler and faster method can be used. The entire dose of contrast is injected and the same 2D GRE pulse sequence deployed for determining transit time is used to monitor contrast in real time (fluoroscopic triggering, 'care bolus'). The imaging plane usually should include the left ventricle and ascending aorta. When the scanner operator identifies the contrast appearing in the ascending aorta, imaging is switched manually to the 3D sequence. Some manufacturers provide an automated signal intensity measurement tool in a predefined region of interest in the aorta that automatically triggers the 3D sequence once a threshold is reached (automatic triggering).

Flow measurement

For flow measurements an EKG-gated flow-sensitive segmented k-space cine GRE technique is used (phase-contrast or velocity-encoded (Venc) MRI Chapter 13). This sequence is based on the principle that the phase of flowing spins relative to stationary spins along a magnetic gradient changes proportional to the flow velocity. The instantaneous velocities for each frame of the cine image during the cardiac cycle are integrated, thereby blood flow per cardiac cycle through the imaging plane is derived.

Tissue characterization

Both T1-weighted IR single shot SSFP and segmented k-space GRE sequences are used for delayed contrast-enhancement imaging. A tissue-specific inversion time can be used to null the signal from that tissue, thus providing evidence for the presence of thrombus. A thrombus can be identified, for example, in an aortic aneurysm, or in the false lumen of an aortic dissection by applying an inversion time of 600–800 ms; post-contrast this delay allows 'nulling' of signal from thrombotic material, making it appear black in the image.

CLINICAL PROTOCOL

The purpose of this section is to provide a comprehensive protocol for cardiovascular MRI evaluation of all portions of the thoracic aorta (Figure 17.1) and other relevant structures in the chest (aortic valve, heart, pericardium, and pleural space). This approach may need to be refined frequently based on the findings obtained during the scan. Thus additional evaluation using supplementary sequences may be warranted.

Preparation of the patient, scanner, and equipment

Breath holds of up to 20–30 s may sometimes be necessary for EKG-gated 3D MRA, and therefore education of the patient is important. Supplemental oxygen via nasal canula during the exam may increase breath holding capacity. A 20 gauge peripheral line is placed usually in the antecubital vein, and the power injector is prepared for intravenous injection of

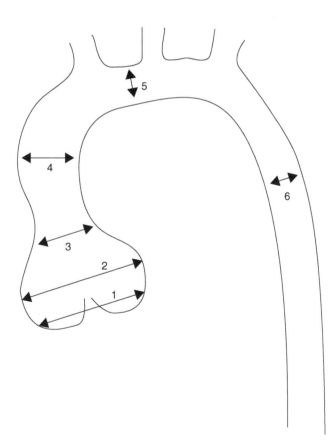

Figure 17.1   Schematic presentation of the thoracic aorta with the standard regions for aortic diameter measurements: 1=valve annulus, 2=aortic sinuses, 3=sinotubular junction, 4=tubular ascending aorta, 5=aortic arch, 6=descending thoracic aorta.

gadolinium contrast. The patient should be cautioned to avoid performing a Valsalva maneuver during breath holding, which may adversely impact the delivery of the contrast bolus. The patient is placed in the scanner bore headfirst and a phased-array coil is placed on the chest. If the patient is large and coverage of the lower part of the abdominal aorta is desired, an additional torso coil can be placed below the chest coil. The position of the patient in the scanner is chosen such that the heart is at the isocenter of the magnet.

Scan protocol

The scan protocol will be described in the order of the sequences employed during a typical thoracic aortic exam. Note, however, that some sequences and views are part of the standard 'core' protocol for the thoracic aorta (i.e. acquired in every exam) and some are supplementary, as shown in Table 17.2. All pulse sequences described here are EKG-gated, as the ascending aorta and arch are pulsatile structures. Our image acquisition protocol for the thoracic aorta consists of the following sequences. Table 17.3 outlines the specifications on these sequences.

SSFP – single shot localizers. Localizers are obtained in anatomic planes (axial, sagittal, coronal) during free breathing and in the standard cardiac axes (vertical and horizontal long axis, short axis) during breath hold. The cardiac localizers are useful if a standard cardiac exam is planned or if a cardiac exam is indicated based on the pathology identified.

T2-weighted single shot turbo spin-echo (HASTE). These images can be acquired rapidly, one entire image every cardiac cycle without breath holding, in the axial orientation starting from the level of the renal arteries up to the supra-aortic arch vessels, approximately 4–5 cm above the arch (Figure 17.2). Additional HASTE images are obtained in the sagittal and coronal planes covering the aorta as well as surrounding structures such as the pleural cavity (pleural effusion). In order to maximize spatial resolution, the field-of-view (FOV) in the read-out and phase-encode directions should be minimized as much as possible while still depicting the entire chest without causing 'wrap-around' artifacts. The coronal images usually require the largest FOV to avoid 'wrap-around' artifacts from the arms and shoulders. The SSFP single-shot sequence can be used in addition to HASTE images in the axial plane and are helpful in assessing luminal details. This set of images provides a general survey of the gross vascular anatomy and pathology (i.e. size of aorta, presence of dissection flap, or severe stenosis of arch vessels). They also form the basis for further image acquisition.

Table 17.2 Overview of the standard 'core' protocol and complementary protocols of thoracic MRI/MRA

Property of interest	Standard 'core' protocol		Complementary protocol		
	Pulse sequence	Orientation	Pulse sequence	Orientation	When applied
Localizers	bSSFP	Axial, coronal, sagittal			
Morphology/function	HASTE/bSSFP SS	Axial, coronal, sagittal			
	bSSFP cine	Axial, orthogonal[a], 'candy-cane'	bSSFP cine small field-of-view	Orthogonal[a]	• Exclude/confirm class 2–5 dissection[b]
			bSSFP cine (small field-of-view)	Aortic valve	• Type A dissection • Aneurysm of ascending aorta • Clinically suspected aortic regurgitation • Coarctation
			bSSFP cine	Standard cardiac exam	• Chronic dissection, first evaluation • Subacute dissection, stable patient • Concomitant cardiac disease
			T1 TSE	Axial	• Exclude/confirm class 2–5 dissection[b] • Inflammatory disease of aorta[c]
			T2 TSE	Axial	• Exclude/confirm class 2–5 dissection[b] • Inflammatory disease of aorta
Luminogram	3D GRE MRA	Oblique sagittal[d]			
Flow measurements			Venc	Aortic valve	• Aortic valve regurgitation
			Venc	Orthogonal to aortic wall	• Flow assessment of false/true lumen • Coarctation
Tissue characterization			IR SS bSSFP (IR GRE)	Axial	• Probing for thrombus in false lumen
			IR GRE	Standard cardiac exam	• Inflammatory disease of aorta[c] • Same as for cine standard cardiac exam

bSSFP, balanced steady-state free precession; HASTE, half Fourier acquisition single shot turbo spin-echo; SS, single shot; TSE, turbo spin-echo; MRA magnetic resonance angiography; IR, inversion recovery; GRE, gradient echo; Venc, phase-contrast MRI.
[a] Orthogonal to the aortic wall in 2 perpendicular views.
[b] See Figure 17.6.
[c] Pre- and post-contrast.
[d] If the course of the aorta is very tortuous or the subclavian arteries are of interest, a coronal/oblique coronal orientation is prescribed.

Table 17.3 Typical imaging parameters for pulse sequences used for MRI/MRA of the thoracic aorta

	2D SSFP SS (Localizer)	T2 w 2D HASTE	2D SSFP (Cine)	T1 w TSE	IR 2D GRE (care bolus)	3D GRE MRA	2 D GRE (Venc)	IR 2D SSFP SS
TR (ms)	3.4	800ᵃ	3.0	700	1000ᵃ	3.2	72	RR-50
TE (ms)	1.7	26	1.5	20	1	1.2	3	1
Flip angle (degrees)	60	160	50–80	180	8	30	20	50
Slice thickness (mm)	6	5	6	6	10	1.1–1.5	6	6
Gap (mm)	6	5	4	N/A	N/A	0	N/A	4
Number of slices/slab	N/A	N/A	N/A	N/A	N/A	52	N/A	N/A
Field-of-view (mm)	360	300–400	320–380	340	400	320–380ᵇ	320–340	360
Matrix (lines)ᶜ	83×128	160×256	192×256	146×256	240×256	240×448	115×256	104×192
Spatial resolution (mm)	3.5×2.8	1.1×1.1	1.4×1.5	1.9×1.3	1.6×1.6	1.0×1.0	2.1×1.6	2.8×1.8
Averages	1	1	1	1	1	1	1	1
Lines per segmentᵈ	1	1	12	1	1	1	3–5	1
Acquisition window (ms)	700	RR 50	RRᵉ	RR 50	N/A	RR50	RRᵉ	RR 50 ms
Gating	Prospective	Prospective	Retrospective	Prospective	Prospective	Prospective	Retrospective	Prospective
Acceleration factor	1	1	2	1	1	1	1	2
Bandwidth (Hz/pixel)	975	780	930	305	375	450	300	1130
Echo spacing (ms)	N/A	2.8	3.1	5.7	N/A	N/A	N/A	2.4
Breath hold	No/yesᶠ	No	Yes	Yes	No	Yes	Yes	No
Prepulse	No	Double IR	No	No	IR	No	No	IR
Readout order	N/A	N/A	N/A	N/A	N/A	Linear	N/A	N/A

SSFP, balanced steady-state free precession; SS, single shot; w, weighted; HASTE, half Fourier acquisition single shot turbo spin-echo; TSE, turbo spin-echo; GRE, gradient echo; MRA, magnetic resonance angiography; RR: RR interval; VENC, phase-contrast MRI; IR, inversion recovery.

ᵃ TR represents the time needed to acquire one image.
ᵇ For oblique sagittal orientation of 3D slab.
ᶜ Phase encoding×frequency encoding.
ᵈ Number of lines depends on heart rate and RR interval, 1 denotes maximum lines possible per RR interval.
ᵉ Retrospectively gated cine sequence with arrhythmia rejection algorithm.
ᶠ Multi-localizer with free breathing, standard cardiac localizer in breath hold.

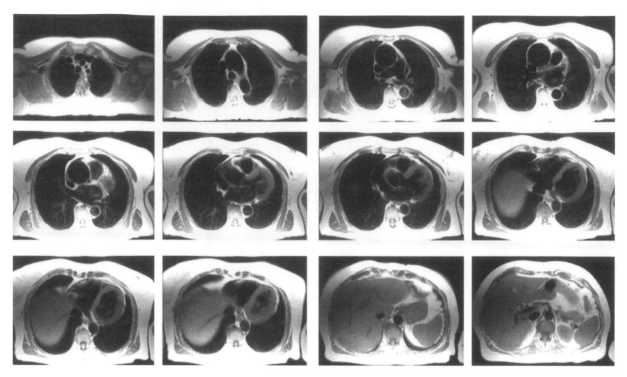

Figure 17.2 Stack of representative single-shot (one image per heart beat) dark-blood HASTE images in axial orientation, starting from the arch vessels and extending to the abdominal aortic branch vessels. The patient shown here has an ascending aortic aneurysm measuring 5.5 cm in diameter and a bicuspid aortic valve.

Segmented SSFP cine sequences. These are ideal to depict the anatomy as well as patho-physiologic events of the heart, the aortic valve, the aortic lumen, and wall during the cardiac cycle with excellent spatial resolution. Based on axial HASTE images we plan the acquisition of one or several SSFP cine angiographic images (approximately 6 s breath hold) of the thoracic aorta in a left anterior oblique sagittal view ('candy-cane'). This allows a quick representation of a large part of the aorta in one 2D image prior to the contrast-enhanced MRA (Figure 17.3). If the aorta has a very tortuous course, this technique may only capture portions of it in one 2D imaging plane. Cine images may also be obtained in representative axial views starting in the abdomen at the level of the renal arteries extending up to the supra-aortic arch vessels. The number of images we acquire is variable and depends on the findings from previous images and whether the scan is performed in an emergency situation. In a routine scan we would acquire 6 mm thick axial images at approximately 3 cm intervals, depicting landmark structures such as the ascending aorta at the root, level of pulmonary arteries, arch, and abdominal aorta at branch locations. In addition, images are acquired in orthogonal planes to the vessel wall to diagnose more subtle cases of dissection. For example, to correctly identify or exclude an intramural hematoma (based on the finding of wall thickening >0.5 cm), images must be

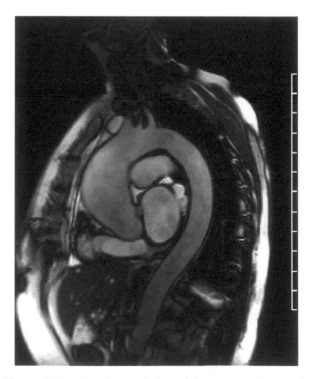

Figure 17.3 'Candy-cane' view of the same patient as in Figure 17.2, showing an ascending aortic aneurysm acquired with an SSFP cine sequence (one time frame from a cine image shown).

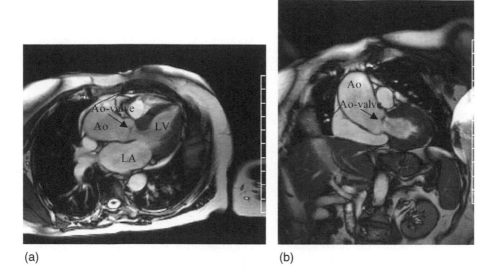

(a)   (b)

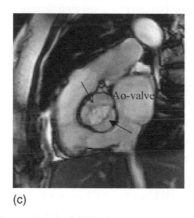

(c)

Figure 17.4 Planning of the aortic valve view using an SSFP cine sequence based on the 3-chamber view (3-CV) (a) and an orthogonal view to the 3-CV (b) showing the aortic valve plane. The imaging plane should be placed orthogonal to the valve, cutting through the valve leaflets. The through-plane motion of the valve during systole must be considered. To visualize the valve, scroll to a systolic frame which allows identification of the valve location during systole. Panel (c) shows a bicuspid aortic valve consisting of fused right coronary and non-coronary cusp (open arrow) and left coronary cusp (block arrow). Ao, aorta; LA, left atrium; LV, left ventricle.

acquired perpendicular to the aortic wall, as axial images may overestimate wall thickness if the vessel traverses the imaging plane obliquely, such as at the sinuses or sinotubular junction (where the vessel is oriented to the right and laterally). Additional small FOV cine images with phase oversampling to avoid 'wrap-around' artifact can be acquired to focus on specific regions of interest.

Given the frequent involvement of the ascending aorta in the pathologic processes, imaging of the aortic valve is often part of the imaging protocol. The slice orientation for the aortic valve is ideally planned based on two standard cardiac views: the 3-chamber view and an LVOT view (obtained in an orthogonal plane to the latter). The imaging plane for the dedicated small FOV acquisition of the aortic valve is placed perpendicular to the aorta on both images, cutting through the valve leaflets in a systolic time frame (Figure 17.4). Additional dedicated cardiac sequences may be obtained as indicated.

T1-weighted TSE was the traditional 'black-blood' technique used for imaging of the aorta, but it has been largely superseded by HASTE imaging. Occasionally, we perform a few complementary T1- or T2-weighted TSE axial images to support findings ascertained from previous techniques or to definitively exclude subtle forms of dissection such as intramural hematoma. The long image acquisition time, motion artifacts, and limited anatomic coverage reduce the usefulness of TSE for extended examination of the aorta. In suspected aortitis, black-blood prepared T1-weighted spin-echo images before (with/without fat saturation) and after contrast may provide evidence of aortic enhancement.

Three-dimensional contrast-enhanced GRE for aortic MRA. MRA is performed with an EKG-triggered GRE sequence in one breath hold. Based on the axial HASTE images a 3D slab in the oblique sagittal orientation is individually tailored to ensure that even an ectatic or tortuous aorta is contained within the imaging volume. Occasionally, if the course of the aorta is severely tortuous or the subclavian arteries need to be imaged as well. In this case, a coronal or oblique coronal slab is preferable; this, however, will require a larger FOV to avoid 'wrap-around' artifacts from the shoulders. The cranio-caudal extent of the 3D slab is visualized best on the sagittal and coronal HASTE images, and coverage from the proximal portion of the arch vessels cranially to the abdominal aorta below the renal arteries should be accomplished. A rectangular FOV with an anteroposterior phase-encoding direction allows minimization of phase-encoding steps. A trigger delay of typically 200–250 ms is used to eliminate any data acquisition during early systole. The typical imaging time is 20–25 s, but this may be reduced further by: (1) decreasing slices per volume; however, this comes at the expense of reduced spatial coverage or reduced spatial resolution (i.e. increasing the slice thickness). (2) Eliminating EKG gating and performing a non-gated acquisition, although this is suboptimal as aortic motion will degrade the image quality slightly (especially in the ascending aorta); it is acceptable if the alternative is significant artifact from insufficient breath holding. (3) Use of parallel imaging (Chapter 12).

A preliminary non-contrast scan is obtained to act as a mask image for later subtractions, and to ensure adequate scan coverage. Then a contrast-enhanced scan is performed using linear encoding of k-space. This type of data acquisition scheme is less sensitive to small triggering variations than sequences with centric ordering of k-space. A fluoroscopic triggering technique is convenient where the gadolinium-enhanced 3D MRA is triggered in real-time, typically in a location that allows visualization of the left ventricle and proximal aorta. Once the contrast is injected, the scanner operator monitors these images in real time. When the contrast enhances the left ventricle and enters the ascending aorta, the patient is instructed to breathe out and hold his/her breath and at the same time the 3D GRE sequence is started. After the first set of angiographic images is acquired the patient is allowed to take two breaths, then a second venous or equilibrium-phase image is acquired. This second data set is acquired to visualize slowly filling structures such as the false lumen in an aortic dissection, and to have a back-up image if the first image was suboptimal either due to early triggering or inadequate breath holding.

A gadolinium dose of 0.2 mmol/kg bodyweight delivered by an MRI-compatible power injector is ideal. The injection rate is calculated so as to result in contrast injection duration equal to 2/3 of the imaging time. The following simple equations are used to calculate the contrast dose for commercially available 0.5 mmolar contrast agents and the injection rate:

Body weight (kg)×0.2＝X mmol Gd (2)
X mmol Gd×2＝Y ml contrast (assuming 0.5M contrast) (3)
Injection time (s)＝2/3 imaging time (s) (4)
Injection rate (ml/s)＝Y ml contrast ÷ injection time (s) (5)

For example, if a patient weighs 80 kg, the contrast dose is 16 mmol (equation 1); with a usual 0.5 mmolar concentration we would inject 32 ml of contrast (equation 2). If the imaging time of the tailored pulse sequence is 24 s, the injection time would be 2/3 of that, which is 16 s. The injection rate is 32 ml contrast in 16 s or 2 ml/s (equation 4). A saline flush of 20 ml is injected at a rate of 1.5 ml/s to ensure that the entire contrast bolus has entered the circulation. Injection in the right arm is generally preferred because injection in the left arm may result in artifacts in the aortic arch from undiluted contrast in the left brachiocephalic vein (T2 shortening effects of Gd, Chapter 14).

Phase-contrast velocity MRI images may be acquired for: (1) assessment of severity of aortic valve regurgitation; (2) discrimination of the true from the false lumen in aortic dissection; (3) identification of the presence and direction of blood flow in the false lumen; and (4) the evaluation of aortic coarctation severity. For the assessment of aortic regurgitation, phase-contrast images in an orthogonal view to the ascending aorta approximately 1 cm above the aortic valve are obtained to measure through-plane blood flow. Phase-contrast images in orthogonal planes to the long axis of the aorta may be required depending on the site of aortic dissection. For assessment of coarctation, one image at the narrowest site of the coarctation, one just below the coarctation, and a third image at the level of the diaphragm are obtained. The image location is determined on the 3D angiographic data by scrolling along the long axis of the aorta, the imaging plane being perpendicular to the aorta in two orthogonal views. The operator on the scanner performs this procedure.

T1-weighted delayed contrast enhancement images for tissue characterization. These images are acquired only: (1) if a dissection is present to rapidly assess thrombus formation in the false lumen, (2) for assessment of the aortic wall in cases of suspected aortitis (in addition to post-contrast T1-weighted spin-echo images), and (3) if a cardiac exam is performed. For assessment of thrombus formation, we acquire T1-weighted images using a single-shot SSFP sequence with an inversion prepulse in the axial orientation covering the entire thoracic and abdominal aorta, starting from above the arch vessels extending down to the edge of the FOV. An inversion time of 600–800 ms is used to null the signal from thrombus and thus differentiate thrombus from blood, and image acquisition is started approximately 10 minutes after contrast injection.

For the assessment of inflammation of the aortic wall we acquire, in addition to T1- and T2-weighted TSE images, standard segmented IR GRE images in planes orthogonal to the vessel. Images are acquired pre- and post-contrast (approximately 10 minutes after contrast injection) and the inversion time is chosen to null signal from the vessel wall on the precontrast images, using the identical inversion time for the post-contrast images.

For tissue characterization of the myocardium standard cardiac views identical to the cine images are acquired using a segmented 2D IR GRE pulse sequence during breath hold.

Image post-processing and analysis

For morphologic images (bright-blood and black-blood images) no specific image post-processing is required. Three-dimensional contrast-enhanced MRA requires image post-processing for image interpretation and display of findings. The 3D data are best post-processed and analyzed on a separate workstation with 3D reconstruction capabilities.

Image post-processing. There are usually three 3D data sets: one baseline precontrast data set, the arterial, and a late phase data set. First, a digital image subtraction (arterial phase minus baseline) is performed. The resulting 3D data set is then reduced in size to limit the data-containing volume to the structures of interest. This is important because an MRA can result in a large amount of data (>1 gigabyte) which may impose a considerable storage burden on the image archiving and retrieving system. We create a range of very thin, parallel MIPs (thickness corresponding to the image acquisition thickness and a double thickness gap between images) usually in the axial orientation over the entire volume. This results in 40–80 images depending on the vascular structure that was imaged, which are saved in a cine format.

Next we create a rotating MIP image of the entire volume. Overlying enhanced structures, such as the cardiac chambers, pulmonary vasculature, and lung fields, obscure the view of the thoracic aorta. These structures can be cropped manually to reduce the image content to the aorta and branches.

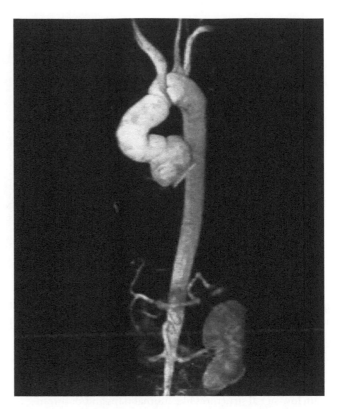

Figure 17.5 Volume-rendered image of the thoracic aorta in a patient after surgery for dissected ascending aortic aneurysm and bicuspid aortic valve showing the ascending aortic tube graft and residual dissection of the aortic arch. One representative frame of a cine image consisting of 36 images with 10° increments is shown.

Volume rendering techique (VRT) reconstructions can provide a better 3D appreciation of the aortic anatomy, although they are prone to artifacts and should not be used for primary image interpretation (Chapter 4). The appreciation of the aorta contour from all angles can be improved by creating VRT images, which rotate 360° around the long (cranio-caudal) axis. This is created by displaying VRT frames in 10° steps (36 images) in a cine format (Figure 17.5).

Image analysis and interpretation should always be performed by careful investigation of the source images by creating double-oblique MPRs or thin MIPs of the 3D data set in multiple planes to depict the vessels of interest. Subvolume MIPs can be created to highlight specific regions. By visual inspection of the MRA images, information regarding the size of the aorta (presence of aneurysm or stenosis/coarctation), the 3D course (aortic elongation and kinking), presence of a dissection flap (Figure 17.6) or other disease of the aortic wall (rough surface in atherosclerotic disease, penetrating ulcers), as well as aortic branch vessel pathology can be obtained. For the detection of dissection flaps, source images and MPRs must be carefully analyzed because the algorithms

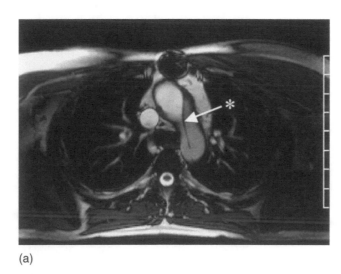

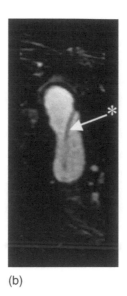

(a)   (b)

Figure 17.6   Intimal flap (marked with *) is seen as a linear structure separating two lumens of the aortic arch in a SSFP cine image (a) and a thin MIP 3D contrast enhanced image (b). Same patient as in Figure 17.5.

used for MIP and VRT (Chapter 4) may obscure voxels that contain low signal structures like intimal flaps and/or thrombus. By comparing the early arterial phase data with the late phase 3D images, contrast uptake in the false lumen and degree of communication can be assessed.

We have standard locations to measure the aortic diameter that are performed on cross-sectional images (Figure 17.1). Of note, the luminal diameters on contrast images do not represent the outside vessel diameters, which can be measured on the bright-blood or dark-blood morphologic images. The aortic valve annulus is another important location of measurement (to size prosthetic valve size), and is best measured on a cine image depicting the aortic valve.

Phase-contrast MRI

Aortic regurgitation. Visual inspection of the regurgitant jet on cine images across the aortic valve provides information on whether regurgitation is present and may be used to qualitatively evaluate severity of regurgitation. Aortic regurgitation can be quantified by measuring through-plane blood flow in the ascending aorta traveling in the antegrade and retrograde direction by phase-contrast MRI. The regurgitant volume is the retrograde or negative flow portion of the flow curve, and the regurgitant fraction is calculated by dividing the regurgitant volume by the stroke volume or antegrade flow.

Aortic coarctation. The peak velocity across the narrowest portion is estimated based on the through-plane images at the level of the coarctation, and the pressure gradient is calculated based on the modified Bernoulli equation ($\Delta P = 4 \cdot V_{max}^2$). For quantification of collateral blood flow, we measure blood flow just below the coarctation and at the level of the diaphragm (see subsequent section on congenital anomalies of the thoracic aorta).

Aortic dissection. This is done by evaluating for the presence of blood flow in true and false lumen. Flow measurements together with morphologic assessment are useful to identify the true and false lumen and to assess whether the lumens are communicating. (Also refer to the section on MRA for diagnosis of aortic dissection and Chapter 8.)

T1-weighted delayed contrast enhancement images are interpreted visually for the presence of thrombus (black) in the false lumen of aortic dissection, where all other structures appear brighter (i.e. various intensities of gray). In the cardiac exam hyperenhanced (bright) areas in the myocardium represent myocardial infarction and/or scar.

CLINICAL APPLICATIONS

MRA for diagnosis of aortic dissection

Classic dissection of the aortic wall results in an intimal flap separating two lumina, the true and false lumen. The Stanford and De Bakey classifications are commonly used in clinical practice to help in management (Chapter 8). With advances in imaging modalities it has become possible to image more subtle pathologies of the aortic wall, such as intramural hematomas and penetrating atherosclerotic ulcers, and this in turn has led to an alternate classification scheme to allow inclusion of these variants of aortic dissection (Chapter 8). The choice of the initial imaging study depends on the availability of the modality and the experience of the emergency room and imaging staff. The wider availability and ease of performance of computed tomography (CT) represents a major advantage versus MRI for the assessment of acute dissection (Chapter 8). It is also argued, sometimes correctly, that in the acutely unstable patient who is sedated and on multiple intravenous drips, MRI offers logistical challenges compared to CT. However, despite these disadvantages, MRI protocols tailored to the emergency situation may allow MRI to rival CT and transesophageal echocardiography as the first-choice imaging technique. In chronic dissection, MRI appears to be the ideal modality, providing comprehensive information, reproducible measurements, and relative patient comfort without ionizing radiation and nephrotoxic contrast agents.

The image acquisition protocol for the evaluation of dissection may need to be adapted based on the acuity of presentation. In acute dissection, in order to minimize scan duration, only the standard core protocol is acquired (Table 17.2), which can be done in <20 minutes. If the diagnosis of type A aortic dissection is made, the scan is concluded after additional assessment of aortic valve.

The following details are required in patients referred to MRI for clinically suspected aortic dissection:

- *Confirmation of diagnosis* is accomplished by demonstration of an intimal flap separating two lumina (Figure 17.6), or identification of more subtle forms of dissection.

- *Class and extent of dissection* are best assessed by manipulating MPRs or thin MIPs on the 3D workstation. A wall thickness greater than 0.5 cm is considered a diagnostic criterion for intramural hematoma, and is best assessed on cine images taken perpendicular to the vessel wall. Identification of the *entry site*, which is the site of the proximal intimal tear, is important because surgery or some forms of interventional therapy are aimed at occluding the tear site. Sometimes a *re-entry site* can be identified; occasionally several tears are present. The exact location of the intimal tear can be determined on the cine images, where the presence of a jet from the true into the false lumen may be seen.

- *The true and false lumens* need to be identified and their relative orientation has to be described. Characteristically, the cross-sectional area is smaller in the true lumen than in the false lumen. There is systolic antegrade flow, and the mean and peak velocities are significantly higher in the true lumen. In the true lumen unidirectional flow is found,

whereas bidirectional flow is often present in the false lumen with a broad range of retrograde blood flow. There is systolic expansion of the true lumen, which is more often localized in the inner aortic aspect. Thrombus may be encountered in the false lumen and blood flow and velocities decrease in the false lumen if thrombosis occurs.

- *Communicating dissections* are present if forward, reverse, or delayed flow is detected in the false lumen on the phase-contrast MRI images or on contrast-enhanced MRA.

- The presence of *fluid extravasation* into the pericardium, the left pleural cavity and/or mediastinum, and fluid around the aorta are signs of imminent rupture.

- The presence and severity of *aortic regurgitation* has to be assessed, and the surgeon requires a measurement of aortic valve annulus diameter.

- The origin and involvement of *branches* need to be carefully assessed. The dissection may extend into the coronary and carotid arteries, celiac trunk, mesenteric arteries, and renal arteries. The dissection may either directly extend into the branch vessel, causing static obstruction, or the dissection flap may extend into the lumen at the site of the branch vessel and cover the origin like a curtain (dynamic obstruction).

An example of a short scan protocol (approximately 20 minutes) in a patient admitted to the intensive care unit with aortic intramural hematoma is shown in Figures 17.7–17.10. Apart from aortic wall thickening, the findings on 3D MRA (smooth inner aortic wall lumen, not shown), absence of flow on phase-contrast MRI images (not shown), and thrombus by IR single-shot SSFP images (Figure 17.9) helped differentiate intramural hematoma from classic dissection.

MRI is the method of choice for serial imaging in chronic dissection and aneurysm and aids in the assessment of aneurysm expansion, progression of residual dissection, malperfusion syndromes through side branch occlusion, new in situ dissection or aneurysms adjoining the surgical anastomosis site in the event of prior repair, and endoleak in the event of previous endovascular stenting.

MRA for thoracic aneurysmal disease

Circumferential dilatation of the ascending aorta >4 cm or of the descending aorta >3 cm is classified as a fusiform aneurysm, whereas an eccentric out pouching that results in a focal increase in aortic diameter >1 cm compared to immediately adjacent normal aortic diameter is a saccular aneurysm. The risk for rupture rises abruptly as a thoracic aneurysm

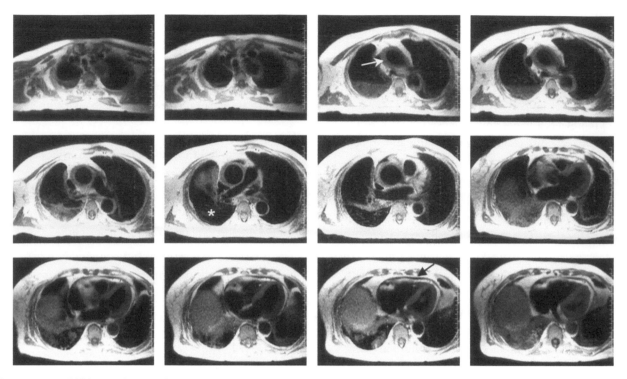

Figure 17.7 MRI scan in a patient with acute chest pain suggestive of acute aortic syndrome. Representative HASTE images show a structure with high signal intensity surrounding the ascending aorta (intramural hematoma, white arrow), beginning just above the aortic valve and extending approximately 9 cm distal to the origin of the left subclavian artery. Pericardial effusion (black arrow) and pleural effusion (marked with *) are present.

reaches a size of 6 cm (20% at 5 years). Serial imaging may allow detection of patients with expanding aneurysms (the average annual growth rate for all thoracic aneurysms is ≤0.1 cm/year). An ascending thoracic aortic aneurysm with a diameter of ≥5.5 cm is considered an indication for surgery, except for high-risk groups such as Marfan's syndrome or those with significant aortic regurgitation with left ventricular dilation where surgery is recommended at diameters ≤5.0 cm. Ascending aortic aneurysms commonly involve the aortic valve and MRI is the modality of choice to assess for related problems such as aortic regurgitation and stenosis.

For descending thoracic aortic aneurysms surgery is performed later (diameter >6 cm). MRI is particularly well suited for serial follow-up and provides accurate and reproducible measurements. The following details should be provided by an MRA evaluation in suspected thoracic aneurysmal disease: confirmation of diagnosis, location and extent, maximal aortic diameter and diameter in standard locations (see Figure 17.1), involvement of arch vessels and concomitant stenosis/pathology, aortic valve morphology and function, and left ventricular function. Measurements must be made on reconstructed MPR images, perpendicular

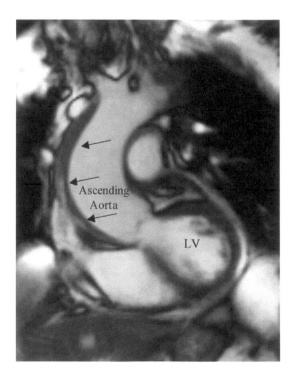

Figure 17.8 Cine image in a truncated candy-cane view of the same patient as in Figure 17.7, showing the intramural hematoma in the ascending aorta (black arrows). LV, left ventricle.

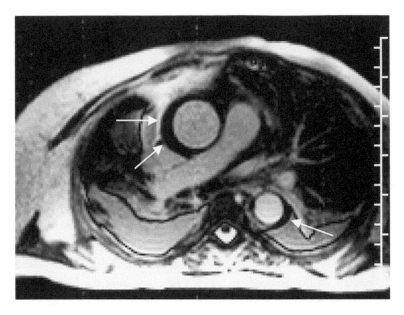

Figure 17.9 IR single-shot SSFP image with an inversion time of 800 ms showing thrombus formation in the aortic wall (white arrows).

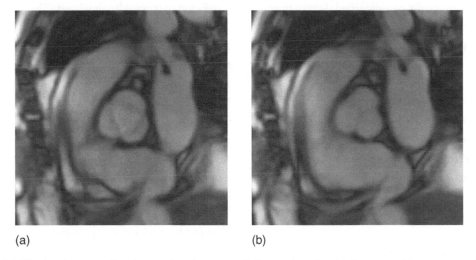

(a)   (b)

Figure 17.10 SSFP cine images showing no involvement of the aortic valve by intramural hematoma. (a) Systolic time frame of the cine image with open tricuspid aortic valve; (b) closed valve.

to the long axis of the vessel as axial images may be misleading. Special attention to perform serial diameter measurements in patients with known aneurysms in exactly the same location is important.

MRA for inflammatory disease of the thoracic aorta

The majority of the literature on MRI assessment of aortitis is based on T1- and T2-weighted spin-echo images. Currently, the wall thickness (>2 mm) and contrast enhancement on T1-weighted TSE images may be used as markers of inflammatory activity for serial assessment. A maximum wall thickness >2 mm (on pre-contrast T1-weighted images or SSFP cine images) has been found to be consistently indicative of aortitis compared to normal individuals who had a wall thickness of <2 mm. Wall thickening, however, can be non-specific and must be considered within the appropriate clinical context and differentiated from other causes such as intramural hematoma or atherosclerotic plaque. In addition to wall thickness, contrast enhancement on post-contrast T1-weighted images has been used as a marker of acute inflammation. Post-contrast enhancement of the aortic wall on T1-weighted images has been suggested as being indicative of aortitis, however this may occur in atherosclerotic involvement of the vessel wall as well and thus clinical context may be important. T1-weighted IR GRE sequences have also been used to evaluate aortitis, with a short inversion time (50–125 ms) to null signal from the blood pool on post-contrast images. If the inversion time is set to null signal from precontrast aortic wall, a marked increase in signal intensity after contrast (using the same inversion time) may be indicative of inflammation in that area. However, further research is necessary to confirm the mechanisms of increased signal intensity of aortic wall on post-contrast images (ongoing inflammation vs angiogenesis, or both). Further research to define what 'normal' contrast uptake is in the aortic wall is also needed. Earlier studies suggesting that T2- or 'edema'-weighted images may serve as a surrogate for inflammation have not been confirmed in subsequent studies. In cases of infectious aortitis, saccular 'mycotic' aneurysms may develop. This feature and inflammation can be identified by contrast uptake on T1-weighted images in conjunction with signs of fluid extravasation into surrounding tissue. The specific aspects to report in an MRA for assessment of aortitis include location and spatial extent of involvement as evidenced by wall thickening in the aorta and its branches, contrast enhancement of the vessel wall and periaortic tissue, on T1-weighted images, presence of aneurysms, stenosis, or dissection, and other complications that include involvement of contiguous structures (e.g aortic valve, coronary and branch vessels, etc.).

MRA for congenital anomalies of the thoracic aorta

The only anomaly of relevance to an adult MR angiographer is coarctation of the aorta and will be briefly discussed. Coarctation is a congenital anomaly affecting the thoracic aorta, with frequent association with other anomalies such as the bicuspid aortic valve. The following aspects should be considered while evaluating coarctation: morphology of the entire thoracic aorta to exclude concomitant dissection, visualization of the coarctation segment, the pressure gradient across the coarctation, evaluation of collateral blood flow (if coarctation is present), and information on the aortic valve (cine images of the valve and phase-contrast MRI to quantify stenosis/regurgitation). Once the morphology and location of the coarctation are characterized the severity of stenosis must be assessed. Three different methods have

been described: (1) Determination of percent luminal diameter stenosis at the site of the coarctation relative to distal segments [e.g diameter at coarctation/(diameter of ascending aorta+diameter of descending aorta midway between coarctation and diaphragm/2)], (2) peak coarctation jet velocity and estimated pressure differential by the modified Bernoulli equation, and (3) quantification of collateral blood flow.

The luminal diameter stenosis, although a useful morphologic parameter, does not provide hemodynamic information. Further, there is no specific cut-off value that can possibly determine a threshold for intervention. The peak coarctation jet velocity similarly may not reflect severity, since with increasing degree of stenosis, collateral blood flow increases, diverting the blood away from the coarctation and effectively reducing peak and mean velocity at the coarctation site. This parameter will thus not reflect the true degree of aortic narrowing and peak velocity as measured by phase-contrast MRI and coarctation diameter are inversely but only weakly correlated. The amount of collateral blood flow, on the other hand, does depend on the degree of narrowing at the coarctation site. Blood flow measurements in the proximal descending aorta and at the level of the diaphragm in the healthy subject usually reveal a slight (approximately 7%) decrease in total blood flow. In patients with significant coarctation, there is a reversal of this normal decrease to an increase (by around 80% in total flow from proximal to distal). The amount of collateral blood flow has been shown to correlate well with the luminal diameter stenosis at the coarctation and clinical parameters of severity. Thus, if there is reversal of the normal pattern of blood flow decrease in the descending aorta, the narrowing may be considered significant. The presence of left–right shunts, as in persistent ductus arteriosus, must be ruled out. Further, in a few patients no increase in collateral support may be seen, even in the presence of a significant stenosis.

MRI for the evaluation of thoracic atherosclerosis

MRI is indicated to detect atherosclerotic involvement of the arch, the great vessels, and the descending thoracic aorta, particularly in patients with embolic cerebrovascular accidents of uncertain source. Large and/or mobile atheromatous lesions, particularly common in the arch, are associated with cryptogenic stroke. Atheroma is best visualized using black-blood sequences (Chapters 12 and 13).

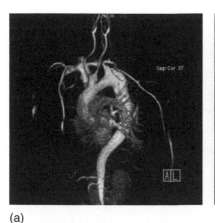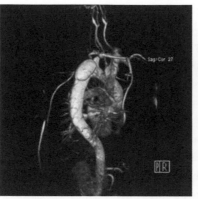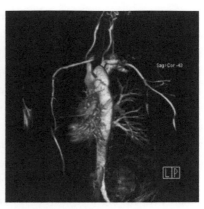

(a)

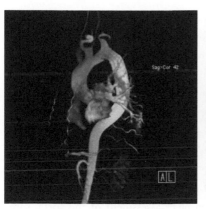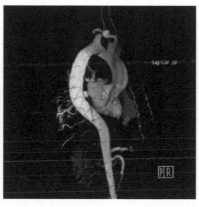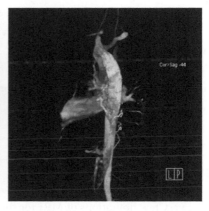

(b)

Figure 17.11 Patient with Ehler–Danlos syndrome IV presenting with a localized type B aortic dissection. Shown are three representative views of a rotating VRT image of the aorta (a). The same patient after treatment of dissection by stent placement shown in the same views as in (a). (b) Note that complete assessment of the intrastent lumen is possible.

MRI for the evaluation of connective tissue diseases

Marfan's syndrome, Ehler–Danlos syndrome (Figure 17.11), and annuloaortic ectasia are diseases affecting the thoracic aorta and are typified by cystic medial degeneration that results in a weakened aortic wall that can lead to dilatation, aneurysm formation, and eventually dissection and/or rupture. The approach to these diseases mirrors that detailed in prior sections on dissection and aneurysm formation.

DIAGNOSTIC ACCURACY OF MRA IN COMPARISON WITH OTHER TECHNIQUES

The MRI assessment of aortic luminal diameter is highly accurate and reproducible using both morphologic sequences as well as 3D angiography, and is considered an optimal modality for initial evaluation and serial imaging follow-up. MRI has been shown to have excellent accuracy for detection of aortic dissection, with sensitivity and specificity both reaching 100%. High accuracy has been shown for detection of intimal flaps in both types A and B dissection, identification of entry and re-entry, and detection of thrombus, aortic regurgitation, and complications. The vast majority of studies were performed in the early 1990s using sagittal spin-echo and GRE cine images. These techniques not only require long imaging times but do not fully exploit the diagnostic potential of contemporary pulse sequences and techniques. Contrast-enhanced MRA alone, for example, was shown to be useful in the diagnosis of aortic dissections, with a sensitivity and specificity of 100%. The use of SSFP sequences alone may provide excellent results for the detection of aortic dissection. Three-dimensional MRA appears to be more accurate in the detection of classical intimal flaps and evaluation of supra-aortic branch vessel disease than morphologic black-blood and SSFP images, but the latter are still necessary to identify intramural hematomas and pathology of surrounding structures. The value of an integrated approach using all of the currently used sequences in dissection remains unproven, but is likely to be very sensitive and specific for this condition.

Studies evaluating patients with suspected or known dissection with MRI and TEE (transesophageal echo) have shown comparable results for the two techniques, with monoplanar TEE having a somewhat lower specificity in the ascending aorta and arch which is improved by multi-planar TEE. Evaluation of the arch vessels with multi-planar TEE is comparable to MRI, however, the abdominal aorta and its branch vessels are outside the field-of-view of the TEE probe. MRI has equivalent sensitivity and specificity when compared with CT. However, CT does not provide hemodynamic information or information on flap dynamics, nor does it provide information on concomitant aortic valve involvement.

LIMITATIONS

There are very few limitations of MRI for the evaluation of the thoracic aorta. Metallic implants such as older stents or coils, although MRI safe, can cause severe image artifacts. Modern stent materials (e.g. nitinol) allow direct visualization of intrastent lumen (Figure 17.11). Compared to current multi-slice CT scanners, MRI requires longer scan times and the spatial resolution is still inferior; however, MRI provides a wide range of complementary information in addition to morphology. In estimating velocities and pressure gradients across very small orifices such as coarctation, the spatial resolution of phase-contrast MRI might preclude accurate measurements. In addition, in areas with highly turbulent blood flow, dephasing of protons and partial volume effects may render phase-contrast images inaccurate. Therefore, in these situations indirect methods such as described for evaluation of coarctation are preferable to direct measurements.

COMMON ARTIFACTS AND PITFALLS

Artifacts noted in the evaluation of the thoracic aorta are broadly applicable to the evaluation of arterial territories in

general. Of importance are artifacts mimicking aortic dissection, which can occur frequently (in up to 64% in one study evaluating traditional techniques such as T1-weighted spin-echo images and GRE cine images). With experience, differentiation can usually be made between artifacts and true pathologic findings. Artifacts may be characteristic to each specific pulse sequence used and their recognition and prevention require prior knowledge and training in MRI techniques.

Anatomic structures mimicking dissection

Anatomic structures around the aorta, which can be mistaken as dissection on axial morphologic images, are the superior pericardial recess (Figure 17.12) or, rarely, the left brachiocephalic vein.

Aortic ulcer mimicking a dissection

Although use of 3D gadolinium-enhanced angiography is mandatory in the complete assessment of the aorta, some MRI laboratories still rely on conventional spin-echo morphologic imaging for assessment of the thoracic aorta in order to obviate the need for contrast. Figure 17.13a is an example of a patient who appears to have an aortic dissection on a conventional axial spin-echo image. However, on reviewing the 3D gadolinium-enhanced angiogram, one can ascertain that this in fact is a penetrating aortic ulcer. This patient actually was referred with a diagnosis of a localized aortic dissection by an outside laboratory that performed only spin-echo imaging as part of their thoracic aortic protocol (Figure 17.13b).

Incomplete coverage of anatomy

The imaging volume of the 3D data set must cover the entire aorta and proximal portion of the branch vessels as well as the major part of the abdominal aorta, ideally down to the bifurcation/iliac arteries. The reason is that pathologies of the thoracic aorta are frequently associated with involvement of more distal vessels. For example, in a series of patients with intramural hematoma in the ascending thoracic aorta, some patients had isolated intimal flaps in the abdominal aorta.

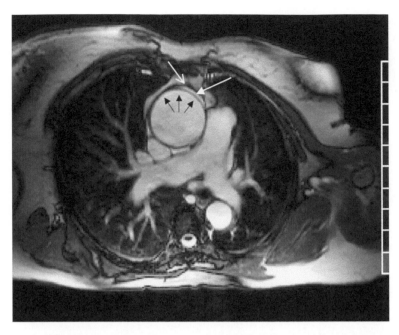

Figure 17.12 Superior pericardial recess (closed white arrow) must not be mistaken for dissection flap. Common SSFP artifacts: phase cancellation at pericardial fat–fluid (within pericardial recess) interfaces causing dark stripe artifacts (white open arrow). Faint pulsatile flow artifacts within aortic lumen (black arrows).

'Bright-blood' or SSFP-specific artifacts

SSFP sequences are susceptible to magnetic field inhomogeneities and pulsatile flow. Metallic structures such as clips and sternal wires in the vicinity of the aorta create local field inhomogeneities which cause local susceptibility artifacts. Highly pulsatile flow can cause subtle asymmetric rings in the aortic lumen. Phase cancellation dark stripe artifacts occur predictably at fat/water interfaces. Because all SSFP-specific artifacts occur very predictably, they seldom pose a relevant limitation in clinical practice (Figure 17.12).

'Black-blood' artifacts (turbo spin-echo imaging artifacts)

Black-blood images require inflowing blood into the imaged slice that was exposed to a non-selective inversion prepulse (Chapters 12 and 13). In areas of stagnant or reversed blood flow, signal from blood is incompletely nulled, causing image artifacts which may obscure a dissection flap. Similarly if the patient is very tachycardic, and image acquisition occurs before the signal from blood is nulled, the signal from blood may have similar intensity to the dissection flap, posing problems in differentiating the intimal flap from surrounding blood. HASTE images must be acquired prior to contrast administration, otherwise T1

relaxation is shortened to the point where nulling blood signal becomes impossible.

Artifacts in 3D contrast MRA

Optimal triggering is essential for acquisition of image data during the arterial phase. If the acquisition of center of k-space data coincides with a phase of rapid changes in T1 relaxation (early triggering), one or more dark longitudinal stripes within the aortic lumen may occur (ringing artifact). In contrast, late triggering may cause venous opacification to obscure the aorta, which itself may already be poorly opacified. Areas with signal drop-out on subtracted images may be due to a subtraction artifact and should be differentiated from masses by inspection of the raw unsubtracted 3D data or complementary morphologic images. The reason for this artifactual signal drop-out on subtracted images is that unsaturated spins, especially at the edges of the FOV, may result in bright signal on the pre-contrast image, which, if subtracted from corresponding areas on the post-contrast images, may result in signal drop-out.

CONCLUSION

MRI evaluation of the thoracic aorta is a comprehensive tool for the evaluation of a wide array of disease processes. While the standard acquisition protocol can be applied to any

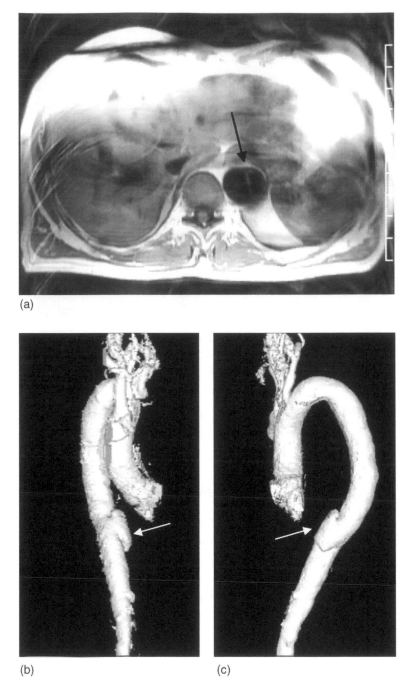

(a)

(b)   (c)

Figure 17.13   Clinical case example of an aortic ulcer which mimicks as an aortic dissection on conventional spin-echo images. (a) Conventional axial spin-echo image at the level of the diaphragm. Notice arrow pointing to what appears to be an anteriorly-posteriorly directed aortic dissection flap. (b, c) Different orientations of a surface-shaded display of the thoracic aortic 3D gadolinium angiogram. Arrow points to a penetrating aortic ulcer.

patient, specific clinical situations demand patient-specific modification of protocols to address specific clinical questions. MRI evaluation provides specific information in the evaluation of dissection, inflammatory disorders, and congenital anomalies that are currently not feasible with other modalities. These advantages include the ability to derive hemodynamic and physiologic information that may be critical in the patient with thoracic aortic disease.

PRACTICAL PEARLS

- Pronounced motion of the ascending thoracic aorta during the cardiac cycle can cause a fine dissection membrane, especially in more subtle forms of aortic dissection, to be obscured on 3D contrast MRA images. Therefore, a comprehensive imaging protocol for suspected aortic dissection in the ascending aorta should include pulse sequences detailing aortic wall morphology, such as SSFP images in the axial orientation and in planes orthogonal to the aortic wall, as well as HASTE and TSE (T1- or T2-weighted).

- Indirect signs of dissection found on the standard exam, such as presence of aneurysm, aortic regurgitation, and pericardial, mediastinal, or pleural effusion, should alert one to thoroughly investigate the aorta with multiple techniques.

- HASTE images in all three anatomic orientations acquired rapidly without breath hold at the beginning of the study provide a decent amount of information to produce a limited report, even if the study has to be terminated early due to patient intolerance.

- If breath holding is a problem, free-breathing images with multiple averages (cine, phase-contrast MRI) or real-time sequences (cine) provide an alternative.

FURTHER READING

Chatzimavroudis GP, Oshinski JN, Franch RH et al. Quantification of the aortic regurgitant volume with magnetic resonance phase velocity mapping: a clinical investigation of the importance of imaging slice location. J Heart Valve Dis 1998; 7(1): 94–101.

Choe YH, Kim DK, Koh EM et al. Takayasu arteritis: diagnosis with MR imaging and MR angiography in acute and chronic active stages. J Magn Reson Image 1999; 10(5): 751–7.

Erbel R, Alfonso F, Boileau C et al. Diagnosis and management of aortic dissection. Eur Heart J 2001; 22(18): 1642–81.

Isselbacher EM. Thoracic and abdominal aortic aneurysms. Circulation 2005; 111(6): 816–28.

Kim RJ, Shah DJ, Judd RM. How we perform delayed enhancement imaging. J Cardiovasc Magn Reson 2003; 5(3): 505–14.

Krinsky GA, Rofsky NM, DeCorato DR et al. Thoracic aorta: comparison of gadolinium enhanced three-dimensional MR angiography with conventional MR imaging. Radiology 1997; 202(1): 183–93.

Kunz RP, Oberholzer K, Kuroczynski W et al. Assessment of chronic aortic dissection: contribution of different EKG-gated breath-hold MRI techniques. AJR 2004; 182(5): 1319–26.

Murray JG, Manisali M, Flamm SD et al. Intramural hematoma of the thoracic aorta: MR image findings and their prognostic implications. Radiology 1997; 204(2): 349–55.

Nielsen JC, Powell AJ, Gauvreau K et al. Magnetic resonance imaging predictors of coarctation severity. Circulation 2005; 111(5): 622–8.

Nienaber CA, Spielmann RP, von Kodolitsch Y et al. Diagnosis of thoracic aortic dissection. Magnetic resonance imaging versus transesophageal echocardiography. Circulation 1992; 85(2): 434–47.

Nienaber CA, von Kodolitsch Y, Nicolas V et al. The diagnosis of thoracic aortic dissection by noninvasive imaging procedures N Engl J Med 1993; 328(1): 1–9.

Pereles FS, McCarthy RM, Baskaran V et al. Thoracic aortic dissection and aneurysm: evaluation with nonenhanced true FISP MR angiography in less than 4 minutes. Radiology 2002; 223(1): 270–4.

Prince MR, Narasimham DL, Jacoby WT et al. Three-dimensional gadolinium-enhanced MR angiography of the thoracic aorta. AJR 1996; 166(6): 1387–97.

Solomon SL, Brown JJ, Glazer HS et al. Thoracic aortic dissection: pitfalls and artifacts in MR imaging. Radiology 1990; 177(1): 223–8.

Steffens JC, Bourne MW, Sakuma H et al. Quantification of collateral blood flow in coarctation of the aorta by velocity encoded cine magnetic resonance imaging. Circulation 1994; 90(2): 937–43.

Svensson LG, Labib SB, Eisenhauer AC et al. Intimal tear without hematoma: an important variant of aortic dissection that can elude current imaging techniques. Circulation 1999; 99(10): 1331–6.

Wolff KA, Herold CJ, Tempany CM et al. Aortic dissection: atypical patterns seen at MR imaging. Radiology Nov 1991; 181(2): 489–95.

18

MR angiography of the abdominal aorta with protocols

Javier Sanz and Sanjay Rajagopalan

INTRODUCTION

The abdominal aorta is a common site for the development of arterial disease in humans. The infrarenal abdominal aorta is the most frequent site of involvement in atherosclerosis and aneurysmsal disease. Extension of a thoracic aortic dissection into the abdomen is not uncommon. In addition, the abdominal aorta may be involved in other pathologic processes, such as arteritis or infection.

Magnetic resonance imaging (MRI) in general, and contrast-enhanced magnetic resonance angiography (MRA) in particular, are widely employed for the non-invasive evaluation of pathology in the abdominal aorta and its branches. MRI may serve as an initial diagnostic modality, although ultrasound is more commonly used due to its lower cost and widespread availability. More often, MRI is employed as a confirmatory diagnostic modality, when detailed anatomic information is needed before an intervention, or as a follow-up tool in subjects requiring surveillance of known disease. Its outstanding image quality, its non-invasiveness the absence of ionizing radiation, and the lack of significant nephrotoxicity of currently employed gadolinium-based contrast agents make MRA an excellent alternative to computed tomography (CT) angiography, and the preferred imaging modality for the evaluation of abdominal aortic pathology in many centers.

In this chapter a review of the practical aspects of MRI techniques applied to the abdominal aorta will be presented. In addition, the most common clinical indications for abdominal MRA will be discussed (Table 18.1). The evaluation of the

Table 18.1 Principal indications to MR angiography of abdominal aorta
• Aneurysm of the abdominal aorta
• Dissection of the abdominal aorta
• Atherosclerosis of the abdominal aorta
• Inflammatory disease of the abdominal aorta

arterial branches arising from this vascular segment, such as the renal or visceral arteries, is addressed in detail in other chapters of this book. Similarly, the use of MRI for abdominal venography or visceral assessment is beyond the scope of this review.

IMAGING SEQUENCES

A complete evaluation of abdominal aortic pathology should include not only visualization of the luminal patency and caliber, but also of the vessel wall, where initial involvement may occur. Therefore it is important to combine MRI techniques that provide superb luminal delineation with sequences that are suited for depiction of anatomy and characteristics of the arterial wall.

Anatomic vascular imaging

For a quick initial evaluation of vessel and perivessel anatomy, single-shot black-blood imaging [i.e., half-acquisition Fourier-transformed single-shot turbo spin echo

(HASTE) or single-shot fast spin echo (SSFSE)] is typically performed. These images can also be used to determine the anatomic landmarks subsequently employed for planning the contrast-enhanced MRA. In addition, image quality is generally sufficient to rule out the presence of significant wall thickening, such as in cases of complex aortic plaque or mural thrombosis. If a more detailed assessment is desired (for example in atherosclerotic plaque characterization, evaluation of inflammatory thickening, 'edema' and clot) high-resolution double inversion-recovery (IR) fast spin-echo sequences with different weightings (T1, T2, proton density) may be employed. The use of fat saturation in black-blood imaging, by suppressing signal deriving from the perivascular fat, can facilitate the visualization of the outer border of the arterial wall. In some circumstances, adequate blood nulling may not be possible depending on the image orientation and/or the presence of slow flow, common in aneurysms or dissections. Especially in these cases, bright-blood techniques based on the use of spoiled gradient-echo (SPGR) or steady-state free precession imaging (SSFP) sequences can be useful to delineate the vessel lumen as well as anatomic vascular relations. Cine images with gated SSFP are useful in subjects with aortic dissection, where the evaluation of the dynamic behavior of the intimal flap or the pulsatility of the true or false lumens may be of interest. They can also be used as an alternative to contrast-enhanced MRA when the latter is not possible or is hindered by imaging artifacts. Although at the expense of longer examination times, cine SSFP sequences provide high-quality images of aortic pathology, accurate depiction of disease extent, and good differentiation of the vascular lumen and wall.

Luminal depiction of the abdominal aorta and branches

For MRA, three-dimensional (3D) contrast-enhanced techniques with SPGR sequences are by far the most widely used approach. Alternative non-contrast methods are infrequently used at the present time. Two-dimensional (2D) and 3D time-of-flight techniques are usually not employed in the abdomen because of long acquisition times as well as sensitivity to slow flow, breathing artifacts, or imaging plane orientation. Two-dimensional phase contrast (PC) angiography is occasionally useful to determine the presence and direction of flow (for example, in a communication between the true and false lumen through an intimal tear in cases of dissection). In addition, it may provide quantitative measures of flow rates

if needed. In some cases, time-resolved contrast-enhanced MRA, which enables evaluation of the dynamic behavior of the contrast agent during its transit through the abdominal aorta and thus the characteristics of flow, may also be employed.

Electrocardiographic gating is needed for most of the sequences mentioned before, including black-blood imaging, cine SSFP, PC imaging, and contrast-enhanced MRA. For this purpose, peripheral gating is sufficient most of the time and the placement of precordial EKG leads is rarely necessary.

IMAGING PROTOCOL

Patient preparation

Before starting the examination, the patients are instructed about the procedure and provided with breathing instructions. Especially with contrast-enhanced MRA, it is essential to avoid respiratory motion artifacts for optimal image quality. For the rest of the sequences, breath holding generally improves image quality and also reduces variability in the position of anatomic structures within images that will be employed to prescribe the 3D MRA volume. End-expiratory breath holds usually assure a more consistent position of the diaphragm. However, some patients may find it easier to maintain apnea in end inspiration. For subjects with difficulties in performing prolonged breath holds, single-shot techniques offer good image quality even during free breathing. If this is the case, it is important to remember that anatomic position may vary slightly in these images, and to increase the slab dimensions when prescribing the 3D MRA. The latter should anyhow be performed during apnea. Apart from technical considerations on imaging parameters that may decrease scanning time (reviewed later), brief hyperventilation preceding the breath hold or oxygen supplementation may increase the subjects' ability to hold their breath. A peripheral intravenous access ($\leq$22 gauge) is placed in a large vein in the arm (usually in the antecubital fossa or the forearm). The arms are placed on the chest or, alternatively, raised above the head, to avoid *wrap-around* artifacts in coronal acquisitions.

Contrast considerations

Gadopentate dimeglumine (Gd-DTPA) is the most commonly employed contrast agent in clinical practice. Therefore, the doses and protocols in this chapter will refer to Gd-DTPA. Other contrast agents may offer advantages in specific situations, and are discussed in Chapter 14 of this book. For adequate signal enhancement and image contrast, the T1 of blood must be shortened below that of the background tissue, especially fat (270 ms). This requires a minimum dose of 0.1 mmol/kg, but better results are achieved with a double dose (0.2 mmol/kg). In cases with severe aneurysmal dilatation, or in the event of low cardiac output (due to decreased systolic function), a dose of 0.3 mmol/kg may be preferable. The contrast is administered with an automatic power injector and is followed by a flush of saline (20 ml). The injection rate usually ranges between 1.5 and 2 ml/s. The total duration of the injection (and therefore the rate of administration) should be adjusted to the length of the acquisition (scanning time). Although injections shorter than the scanning time (about 2/3) provide good results, an attempt to match the injection time and the scanning time should be made.

As with any contrast-enhanced MRA technique, it is essential to precisely time the acquisition of the central k-space lines to the maximal blood concentration of the contrast agent (peak luminal signal intensity). The 'best guess' approach is rarely used for abdominal MRA, because the time for the contrast to arrive at the abdominal aorta (20–25 s on average) is highly variable amongst patients and depends on multiple factors such as injection site, age, hemodynamic status, etc. In our laboratory the test bolus technique is usually preferred. This is based on the injection of a small dose (2–3 ml) of contrast at the same rate as expected during the MRA. The arrival of the contrast to the area of interest (generally at the level of the renal arteries take-off) is monitored with a low frame rate 2D imaging sequence (1 frame/second). The time point of maximal signal intensity at that level is determined visually, or alternatively it can be precisely measured by plotting signal intensity versus time using specialized software. The advantage of the test bolus technique is the knowledge of the contrast transit time in each patient, which assures maximal signal enhancement at a precise time point in a consistent fashion. The disadvantage includes the fact that this requires a small additional contrast dose that may increase the signal of background tissue and slightly prolong examination time. In addition, the bolus travel time and kinetics (because of the different volumes) may vary between the bolus test and the actual MRA acquisition. Alternative methods that overcome these limitations include automated bolus detection or 'fluoroscopic' triggering. In the former, the signal intensity within a region of interest at the level of the abdominal aorta is measured repeatedly to detect the arrival of the contrast. When the signal surpasses a user-defined threshold, the acquisition is automatically or manually started. Contrast arrival is monitored in real time with a fast 2D sequence, usually in the sagittal or coronal planes, while the patient is told to breathe in and out repeatedly. When the contrast arrives at the lower thoracic aorta, the patient is instructed to stop breathing and the 3D MRA acquisition is started manually by the operator. The main limitation of these real-time techniques is that they are more susceptible to technical or human errors.

In centric or elliptical centric k-space filling MRA techniques, image acquisition is started at the time of maximal signal intensity. Using the test bolus technique, this corresponds to the delay between the beginning of the injection and peak contrast enhancement (contrast travel time). We usually add 1–2 s as a precaution to avoid early initiation of the scan, because fast changes in gadolinium concentration during central k-space filling may lead to severe ringing artifacts. If a sequential phase-ordering scheme is employed, the acquisition should start before maximal enhancement, and this is calculated with the formula:

$$\text{Imaging delay} = \text{contrast travel time} + (\text{injection time}/2) - (\text{scanning time}/2)$$

where contrast travel time is considered equal to the time to peak contrast.

Scan protocol

In our laboratory, we employ a 1.5 Tesla magnet (Magnetom Sonata©, Siemens, Erlangen, Germany) with a high gradient performance (40 mT/m maximum amplitude, slew rate 200 mT/m/ms). Although adequate image quality can be sufficient when the body coil is used, a phased-array surface coil should be always preferred as signal receiver because it results in improved signal-to-noise (SNR) ratios. The coil is placed so that the largest number of coils is oriented across the abdomen (in alignment with what will be the phase-encoding direction of the MRA scan) for maximal exploitation of parallel imaging techniques.

In the next paragraphs we will describe our routine protocol for abdominal MRA. The scanning parameters for the different sequences are detailed in Table 18.2. This protocol can generally be performed in less than 30 minutes. Modifications in the sequences employed and/or anatomic coverage may be required depending on the particular indication or study findings. In general, the image volume

Table 18.2 Imaging parameters

	Single-shot black-blood	Single-shot SSFP	Test bolus	Contrast-enhanced MRA	Post-contrast SPGR
Acquisition	2D	2D	2D	3D	3D
TR (ms)	N/A	4.3	1000	3.1	3.2
TE (ms)	25	2.1	1	1.2	1.4
TI (ms)	N/A	N/A	300	N/A	N/A
Flip angle (degrees)	160	79	50	25	15
Band width (Hz/pixel)	781	488	980	500	590
Fat saturation	No	Yes	No	No	Yes
Slice thickness (mm)	6	6	20	1.3	2.5
Gap (%)	30	30	N/A	N/A	N/A
Partitions/slices	20–30	20–30	1	72	120
Orientation	Axial/sagittal/coronal	Axial/sagittal/coronal	Axial	Coronal	Axial
Saturation bands	a-p	No	No	No	c-c
Field-of-view (mm)	360×270–360	360×270–360	360×360	360×360	360×270
Phase direction	a-p/r-l	a-p/r-l	a-p, r-l	r-l	a-p
Matrix (lines)	256×125–166	256×144–192	128×100	320×275	256×146
Pixel size (mm)	2.2×1.4	1.9×1.4	2.8×2.8	1.3×1.1	1.8×1.4
Averages	1	1	1	1	1
Partial Fourier	4/8	Off	Off	Slice direction (6/8)	6/8
Parallel imaging	No	Yes	No	Yes	Yes
Acceleration factor	N/A	2	N/A	2	2
Reference lines	N/A	24	N/A	24	24
Duration (s)	22–33	11–13	1	19	17
Other	Interleaved	Interleaved		Slice interpolation 69%	

SSFP: steady state free precession; MRA: magnetic resonance angiography; SPGR: spoiled gradient echo; TR: repetition time; TE: echo time; TI: inversion time; a-p: antero-posterior; c-c: cranio-caudal; r-l: right-left; N/A: not applicable. The values for field-of-view, matrix, pixel size and number of slices, as well as duration of acquisition, are based on average-sized patients and may vary for different individuals.

extends from the diaphragm past the aortic bifurcation. If the initial sequences reveal pathology extending proximally or distally to the abdominal aorta (i.e. a thoraco-abdominal aneurysm) the imaging protocol is modified accordingly. Except for initial low-resolution single-shot SSFP localizers, all acquisitions are performed during apnea.

Precontrast imaging

We usually start with axial, sagittal, and coronal stacks of intermediate-weighted HASTE images (Figure 18.1). Subsequently, we perform single-shot SSFP acquisitions in the same orientations. Together, these images display the intra-abdominal course and dimensions of the aorta, and differentiate the lumen and wall of the artery (Figure 18.2). Each of these acquisitions may be performed in one or more breath holds depending on the patient's respiratory capacity.

Contrast-enhanced MRA

The next step is setting the scanning parameters for the contrast-enhanced MRA (Figure 18.1). The imaged volume is prescribed from the previous acquisitions ensuring complete coverage of the area of interest. A sagittal plane offers the advantage of a smaller phase field-of-view (FOV) and shorter imaging times if only the abdominal aorta is to be assessed. However, this is infrequently the case as evaluation of the visceral, renal, and common iliac arteries is also desirable. Therefore, a coronal orientation with various degrees of obliquity is most often employed.

Imaging time must be kept within reasonable limits for patients to be able to maintain the breath hold during the acquisition. A scanning duration of 15 to 20 seconds works well in most instances. A major improvement during recent years was represented by the advent of parallel imaging techniques, which result in significantly shorter scan times.

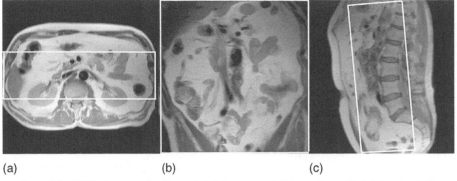

Figure 18.1 Examples of HASTE images in the axial (a), coronal (b), and sagittal (c) orientations. The white boxes demonstrate the typical image volume for contrast-enhanced abdominal angiography. The 3D slab is set in an oblique coronal orientation, usually including the visceral branches and the renal arteries.

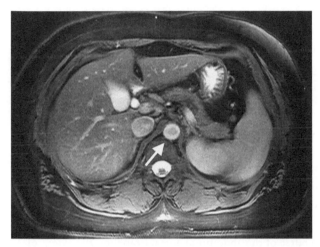

Figure 18.2 Axial image of a normal abdominal aorta (arrow) obtained with a fat-suppressed single-shot SSFP sequence. The vessel lumen is clearly visualized as hyperintense (arrow).

Although this comes at the cost of lower SNR, the large increases in T1 relaxivity associated with the contrast agent usually compensate for this loss and enable excellent image quality. Therefore, we generally apply parallel imaging techniques and use the saved time to increase anatomic coverage and/or spatial resolution. We usually employ the generalized autocalibrating partially parallel acquisition (GRAPPA) algorithm, with an acceleration factor of 2. If the subjects can perform prolonged breath holds (i.e. ≈25–30 s) or if there are concerns on the available SNR (for example in obese subjects where the coil may be far from the aorta) parallel imaging may not be applied. The FOV is reduced as much as possible, but always ensuring avoidance of *wraparound* artifacts. When possible, we employ a rectangular FOV with the phase-encoding direction in the shortest anatomic axis, usually antero-posterior for sagittal and axial views, or right-to-left for coronal acquisitions. The repetition time (TR) and echo time (TE), typically in the order of 3–4 ms and 1–1.5 ms, respectively, are set at the minimum possible. Other approaches can decrease imaging time, although with associated penalties in SNR. These include increasing the bandwidth (which will allow for further decreases in TE and TR), acquiring fractional echoes and/or a fraction of phase-encoding steps (partial Fourier schemes).

For abdominal imaging we usually employ a centric phase-encoding ordering approach, which offers the advantages of simpler timing calculations and fewer chances of breathing artifacts during the acquisition of central k-space lines. This enables one to 'risk' an excessively long period of apnea without resulting in significant breathing artifacts if the patient cannot maintain the breath hold in the last portion of the scan. In addition, if the bolus duration is shorter than the scanning time, it is less likely to cause 'ringing' artifacts. Additional advantages include avoidance of venous contamination artifact as the central portions of k-space correspond to peak arterial enhancement rather than venous.

Ideally, spatial resolution should be as high as possible, within the time constraints imposed by the required anatomic coverage and the patient's ability to perform prolonged breath holds. Isotropic or near-isotropic voxels are preferable because they allow for smoother 3D image reconstructions that facilitate diagnostic evaluation, although this is more important in the evaluation of aortic branches. Therefore, we try to reach a spatial resolution in the order of 1–1.5 mm in all three spatial directions. Further increases in displayed spatial resolution can be achieved by using zero-filling interpolation without additional increments in scanning time.

After all the parameters for the contrast-enhanced MRA scan have been defined, a precontrast acquisition is performed to confirm adequate anatomic coverage, to rule out significant artifacts related to inadequate FOV or secondary to parallel imaging, and to test the patient's ability to maintain the breath hold during the scanning time. In addition, this acquisition will serve as a mask for subsequent subtraction of background signal (particularly fat tissue) from post-contrast images. This requires that the scanning parameters of both acquisitions match exactly, so if artifacts are noted in the precontrast scan that result in protocol modification, the acquisition needs to be repeated. Because a successful subtraction depends on identical position of structures during pre- and post-contrast acquisitions, these images should be acquired within a short interval.

After the precontrast scan, the test bolus is administered and its arrival to the abdominal aorta monitored with an inversion-recovery prepared SSFP sequence repeated every second. This occasionally may already reveal important information about blood flow dynamics, such as differential flow through the false versus the true lumen in a dissection. After determining the contrast travel time, gadolinium is injected and the actual MRA obtained during maximal arterial enhancement, as described above. After the end of the first MRA, the patient is allowed to breathe again and a second acquisition is immediately repeated. This 'venous phase' can be useful, for example, to depict late filling of the false lumen in a communicating aortic dissection or parenchymal perfusion through branches involved by the disease. Additional phases are acquired if appropriate.

Post-contrast imaging

The last portion of the examination includes a post-contrast T1-weighted fat-saturated axial 3D SPGR sequence. In this acquisition the lumen of the aorta is clearly differentiated from the wall after the administration of contrast, the extent of plaque or thrombus is well visualized, and abnormalities in organ perfusion may be more evident than during the arterial or venous phases of the contrast transit. Additionally, these images may display peri-aortic inflammatory changes or contrast leaks. In the evaluation of patients with stents or prosthetic grafts, where the presence of endoleaks is a particular concern, it is useful to perform the same sequence both before and after the administration of gadolinium, to enable an easier interpretation of post-contrast images.

Time-resolved MRA

Time-resolved MRA techniques allow obtaining a similar 3D volume within a few (5–9) seconds to display multiple phases of contrast transit. There are several approaches for time-resolved MRA, described previously in this book. We occasionally employ the technique known as time-resolved imaging of contrast kinetics (TRICKS), in which the central lines of k-space are sampled more often than peripheral lines. Final images are reconstructed by combining the acquired central k-space lines and interpolated peripheral lines from different time points. With time-resolved techniques, the dynamics of blood flow can be studied, and adequate timing of image acquisition is no longer an issue as there will be precontrast, arterial, and venous phases throughout the scan. This ultrafast acquisition comes at the expense of decreased spatial resolution, usually in the partition thickness, resulting in anisotropic voxels. TRICKS imaging can be useful in the evaluation of endoleaks in aortic stent grafts.

Image analysis

It is important to first review the unsubtracted MRA source images to avoid potential artifacts or errors associated with the process of subtraction. Volume-rendered reconstructions may be useful to provide 3D images of the course of the abdominal aorta, branches, the extent of potential abnormalities, and relationships with surrounding structures. Maximum intensity projection (MIP) reconstructions are usually preferable for diagnostic purposes (Figure 18.3). MIPs can depict limited or extensive vascular segments in any desired plane orientation, which is particularly useful to obtain accurate measurements of the cross-sectional arterial diameter. In addition, MIP images provide high contrast between the vessel and background tissue. However, these post-processed images may result in artifacts and pitfalls. A thick MIP may overlook an eccentric plaque, an intimal flap, a focal stenosis, or the presence of arteries with a small caliber (such as accessory renal arteries). Thus, it is mandatory to additionally review multi-planar reformats (MPRs) or the source images. Furthermore, it must always be remembered that, in contrast-enhanced MRA, only the lumen displays high signal intensity (Figure 18.4). Therefore, it is important to assess MRA findings in conjunction with precontrast spin-echo or SSFP sequences. As an example, a large mural thrombus may be overlooked in the contrast-enhanced MRA and the degree of

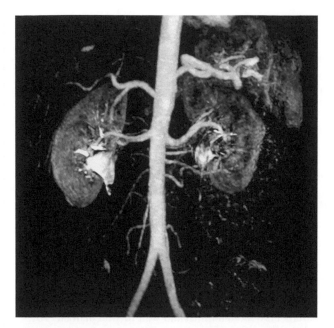

Figure 18.3 Coronal maximum intensity projection (MIP) reconstruction of a normal abdominal aorta. Note the smooth appearance of the lumen and the absence of significant narrowing in the aorta or any of its branches.

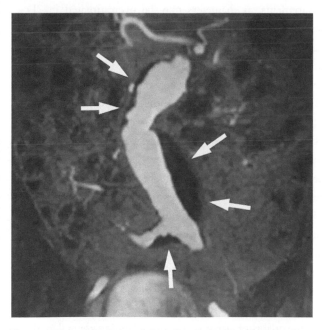

Figure 18.4 Maximum intensity projection (MIP) reconstruction of an unsubtracted contrast-enhanced abdominal angiogram. There is extensive mural thrombosis (arrows) that appears dark in spoiled gradient-echo images, facilitating the diagnosis. Note that measurement of the luminal diameter alone would clearly underestimate the severity of the disease process.

aortic dilatation largely underestimated, if only the lumen is measured. In this regard, wall-to-wall rather than luminal diameters are more meaningful as markers of the severity of disease.

CLINICAL INDICATIONS

Abdominal aortic aneurysms

An abdominal aortic aneurysm (AAA) is usually diagnosed when the aortic dimension dilatation exceeds 1.5 times the normal abdominal aortic diameter (obtained from an unaffected suprarenal segment or from available normograms) or, more generally, if the aortic diameter is ≥3 cm. The abdominal aorta is the most common location of aortic aneurysms, with an estimated prevalence close to 5% in necropsy or screening studies. In approximately 90% of the cases, the aneurysm occurs in the infrarenal segment, and extension into the iliac arteries is seen in approximately one-third of these subjects. Concomitant aneurysms involving other vascular territories, such as the thoracic aorta or the femoropopliteal arteries, are not uncommon. Increasing age, male gender, smoking, arterial hypertension, hyperlipidemia, atherosclerosis, chronic obstructive pulmonary disease, and positive family history for aortic aneurysms are all associated with the development of AAAs of degenerative etiology. Other causes include connective tissue disorders (Marfan's or Ehlers–Danlos syndromes), inflammatory processes (i.e. vasculitis), infection (micotic aneurysms), trauma, or prior dissection. Most degenerative AAAs are fusiform, although many saccular aneurysms are also related to atherosclerosis (Figure 18.5).

General diagnostic evaluation

The majority of patients with AAA are asymptomatic, and the abnormality is discovered incidentally during physical examination or an imaging test. When symptoms occur, they consist of lower abdominal or back pain. Because of the high prevalence of AAA in the population, the US Preventive Task Force recommends screening all males 65–75 years old with a history of smoking. The recommendations of the Society of Vascular Surgery and the Society for Vascular Medicine and Biology include all men 60–85 years old, women in the same age range with cardiovascular risk factors, or both men and women >50 years old with a family history of AAA. Ultrasound is the preferred test for screening or initial evaluation, because it is safe, widely available, and relatively inexpensive. CT is generally considered the diagnostic method of choice for a complete characterization of the aneurysm and in the planning of interventions. Although traditionally reserved for subjects with renal insufficiency or an allergy to iodinated contrast media, current contrast-enhanced breath-hold MRA techniques represent a robust

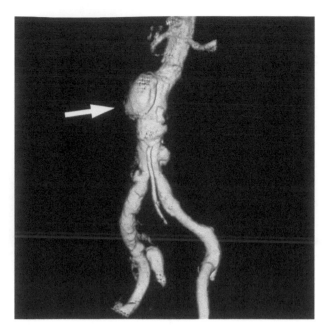

Figure 18.5 Volume-rendered reconstruction of a contrast-enhanced angiogram showing a saccular aneurysm (arrow) in the anterior wall of the infrarenal aorta. Additional luminal irregularities suggest atherosclerotic etiology.

alternative to CT and are increasingly replacing its use in many centers. MRI offers accurate determinations of aneurysm dimensions and extent when compared with intra-operative findings, and can detect associated stenoses in abdominal branches with sensitivity and specificity surpassing 90%.

Patient management

Serial imaging is recommended yearly for aneurysms measuring >4 cm and every 6 months if they exceed 4.5 cm. The annual rate of maximum diameter progression of an AAA is in the order of 10% per year, although there is substantial individual variability. Rapid expansion of the aneurysm (>0.6–1 cm/year) is generally a marker of increased risk for rupture. Other risk factors include female gender, smoking, chronic obstructive pulmonary disease, arterial hypertension, family history, or an eccentric morphology. However, the maximum diameter is the most important predictor of rupture, and the risk increases sharply above 6 cm. Therefore, repair of an asymptomatic AAA is usually indicated when the maximum diameter reaches 5.5 cm in men and 4.5–5 cm in women. Rapid growth, development of symptoms, young age, or other high-risk features may prompt an earlier intervention. Elective surgical repair with a prosthetic graft is the stan-

dard therapy, with an average operative mortality of 2–4%. Alternatively, endovascular repair with stent grafts in patients with an adequate anatomy offers reduced early postoperative morbidity at the expense of increased cost and higher rate of re-interventions, with no overall mid-term survival benefit.

Role of MRI

MRI is useful in the initial evaluation, as a serial follow-up modality, and in characterizing features that define the indication and suitability for either open or endovascular repair. MRI can be used to confirm the presence of aneurysm and define its morphology (saccular or fusiform), tortuosity, angulation, etc. It provides accurate and reproducible measurements of both luminal and wall-to-wall diameters by combining contrast-enhanced MRA with precontrast black-blood sequences or post-contrast SPGR. Multiplanar reformats or MIPs of 3D acquisitions offer the advantage of infinite spatial orientations to obtain true cross-sectional measurements, as diameters may be overestimated in 2D images if the vessel courses oblique to the imaging plane. The longitudinal extent of the aneurysm has important implications and can also be evaluated with MRI. Involvement of the suprarenal segment often contraindicates endovascular repair and increases the surgical risk. Similarly, it is important to determine distal extension into the iliac arteries. The number of branches included in the aneurysmal sac (for example accessory renal arteries) and their degree of patency are easily determined with MRA. Knowledge of the presence and extent of mural thrombosis, atheroma, or calcification is important before surgical clamping or stent deployment. MRI is unfortunately not well suited for the depiction of calcification, although it reliably visualizes the presence of clot or plaque (Figure 18.4). Additionally, MRI is useful in evaluating perianeurysmal anomalies, such as fibrosis or inflammation (Figure 18.6). Before endovascular repair, MRI can be used to assess the quality of proximal and distal landing zones (length, angulation, atheroma) and vascular accesses (iliac tortuosity, caliber, stenoses). The role of MRA is more limited in the post-operative follow-up of endovascular stents, particularly in the presence of materials such as stainless steel or cobalt that may be associated with severe artifacts. Nitinol-based stents are in general more suitable for evaluation with MRI. Although CT is normally preferred for the evaluation of endoleaks, preliminary results suggest a potential role of single-phase or time-resolved contrast-enhanced MRA, not only in the detection but also in the classification of endoleaks

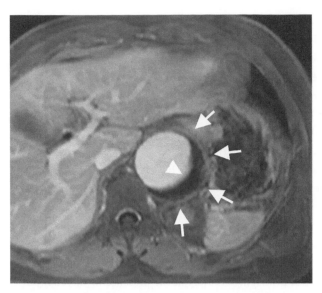

Figure 18.6 Axial T1-weighted post-contrast SPGR sequence showing a large abdominal aneurysm with extensive mural clot (arrowhead). Peri-aortic enhancement (arrows) is also noted, suggesting an inflammatory and/or fibrotic component.

(type 1=anastomosis site; type 2=retrograde flow through branches; type 3=graft defect including junctional leak and modular disconnect, and type 4=graft wall porosity).

Aortic dissection

Aortic dissection is determined by separation of the layers of the aortic wall with the creation of two separate channels (true and false lumen) divided by an intimal flap. The dissection may remain localized but most commonly propagates either retrogradely or anterogradely, often in a spiral fashion. In most instances (approximately 90% of cases) it is possible to identify one or more intimal tears connecting the true and false lumens (a situation known as *communicating dissection*). Occasionally, hemorrhage inside the vessel wall is present without noticeable intimal disruption. These cases of intramural hematoma are thought to originate from rupture of the vasa vasorum inside the vessel wall. Such hematomas may remain stable, be reabsorbed, or progress to aortic rupture or to an open dissection with a secondary intimal tear. The origin of an intramural hematoma or a communicating dissection may be an ulceration of the intima, usually in a region of atherosclerotic plaque.

Clinical considerations

An aortic dissection results in a much weakened aortic wall that may rupture, often with fatal consequences. Many additional clinical scenarios result from the hemodynamic relations between the true and false lumen. Although not always, blood flow tends to go preferentially into the true lumen. In other cases, the pressure can be higher within the false lumen, leading to compression of the true lumen. In cases of very slow flow, the false lumen may be completely obliterated by thrombotic material, a condition that has been correlated with better prognosis. However, blood supply to organs perfused by arteries originating from the false lumen may be compromised in such cases, resulting in severe ischemia. If there are multiple or large intimal tears, both lumens may have equalized pressures and flow. This leads to a higher risk for aortic expansion and aneurysm formation due to the relative frailty of the wall in the false lumen.

The combination of atherosclerotic disease and arterial hypertension is the most common predisposing factor for the development of aortic dissection. Others include connective tissue disorders (Marfan's syndrome, Ehlers–Danlos syndrome), congenital abnormalities (aortic coarctation, bicuspid aortic valve, Turner's syndrome), aortic inflammation (Takayasu's aortitis, giant cell arteritis), trauma (including iatrogenic origin), or drug use (cocaine). Isolated involvement of the abdominal aorta is uncommon and, more frequently, abdominal dissection represents the extension of a thoracic dissection affecting only the descending segment (Stanford type B), or also the ascending aorta (Stanford type A). Type A dissections have an extremely high mortality and require urgent surgical correction. In such cases, the ascending aorta is repaired, but the distal dissection is often left untouched. In type B dissection, the initial treatment of choice is medical management. In both cases, a dissection extending into the abdomen may still require intervention in cases of intractable pain, expanding aortic size, development of peri-aortic hematoma (a sign of imminent rupture), or ischemia in visceral organs or the lower extremities. The latter scenarios are associated with high mortality even with appropriate intervention, particularly if therapy is delayed. Interventions include surgery, percutaneous stenting (to seal an intimal tear and promote thrombosis of the false lumen), or fenestration (creation of new intimal communications to decompress the false lumen).

Role of MRI

MRI is highly accurate for the detection of aortic dissection and both sensitivity and specificity approximate 100%. In the acute setting MRI is not usually the preferred imaging modality because of less availability than transesophageal echocardiography or CT, contraindications in some patients with metallic devices, and safety concerns in subjects with high risk of hemodynamic decompensation. In this regard, it is currently possible to rule out the presence of dissection in less than 5 minutes using cine SSFP sequences or single-shot techniques that can be performed during free breathing. This may help overcome some of the earlier limitations associated with the use of MRI in acute dissection. In the chronic setting MRI is generally considered the imaging modality of choice because of high accuracy and reproducibility, large imaging fields, and lack of nephrotoxic contrast agents or ionizing radiation. This may be especially important in young individuals such as those affected with Marfan's syndrome. Serial imaging after an acute episode (regardless of the instituted therapy) is recommended at 1, 3, 6, 9, and 12 months, and yearly thereafter.

When evaluating an aortic dissection several features of the disease need to be addressed. The diagnosis relies on the visualization of an intimal flap separating both lumens. Although this is possible with single-shot spin echo sequences, it is usually more easily accomplished with bright-blood images such as SSFP or contrast-enhanced MRA. It is essential to determine both the proximal and distal extent of the intimal flap, which may progress past the aortic bifurcation. As in the case of the aortic aneurysms, the maximal cross-sectional dimension of the aorta (either luminal or wall-to-wall) has important therapeutic implications. Similarly, MRI can identify and measure the size of intimal tears connecting the true and false lumens, this representing an information that may determine the interventional approach.

It is crucial to distinguish the true from the false lumen, to evaluate the degree of flow within both, and to determine which one supplies the different aortic branches. The best way to differentiate the true lumen is to follow its course from the proximal origin of the flap. If this is not possible, additional imaging findings can be useful. The size of the false lumen usually tends to be larger and may compress the true lumen. The wall of the true lumen is composed of all three arterial layers, and therefore is thicker than the wall of the false lumen, formed only by the adventitia and remnants of the media. This may be visualized with high-resolution MRI images. Similarly, remnants of the media are sometimes seen as 'cobwebs' in the false lumen. The true lumen often receives preferential flow during systole, expanding during this cardiac phase and collapsing during diastole. The convexity of the intimal flap changes in parallel with these shifting pressure relationships. The dynamics of flow, luminal pulsatility, and flap mobility are best depicted using cine SSFP imaging. However, the presence or direction of flow through an intimal tear may be difficult to visualize with conventional cine sequences. In these cases, either in-plane or through-plane PC imaging with velocity encoding set usually at ≤50 cm/s can be useful to depict the characteristics of flow (frequently from true to false lumen in systole and reversed in diastole). Similarly, PC imaging can be employed to measure blood velocity and direction, with the false lumen displaying lower velocities and occasionally retrograde flow. The slower flow in the false lumen often results in high signal in black-blood techniques due to insufficient blood nulling. It is also important to determine whether the false lumen is partially or totally thrombosed. This may be difficult to accomplish with black-blood imaging, but it is easily achieved with bright-blood sequences, including T1-weighted SPGR and SSFP (Figure 18.7) images. With these techniques, thrombus is usually dark whereas flowing blood displays higher signal intensity because of the presence of moving spins or gadolinium molecules. In the case of MRA, enhancement in areas with little or slow residual flow may not be seen during the first but in

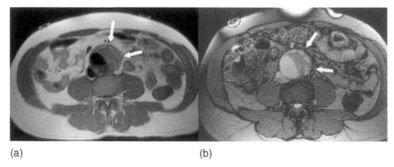

(a)   (b)

Figure 18.7   Dissection of the abdominal aorta as depicted by axial HASTE (a) and single-shot SSFP (b) images. The false lumen (arrows) is larger than the true lumen. With the HASTE sequence, there is high signal intensity within the false lumen and the degree of thrombosis cannot be ascertained. In the SSFP image residual flow in the periphery of the false lumen (bright signal; arrows) is clearly identified.

subsequent delayed acquisitions (Figure 18.8). PC imaging can also be useful in differentiating slowly moving blood from immobile clot. When assessing an abdominal dissection, the origin and patency of all main branches (celiac trunk, mesenteric, renal, and iliac arteries) needs to be assessed. In the abdominal aorta, the false lumen is often located posteriorly and to the left; thus, the left renal and left common iliac arteries are more commonly affected than their counterparts. The celiac trunk and superior mesenteric arteries frequently arise from the true lumen and have preserved blood supply, although malperfusion may occur if the pressure is high in the false lumen, with resulting compression and collapse of the true lumen. Malperfusion-related complications are also possible if a branch arises from a false lumen with slow flow or thrombosis or if the flap extends into the artery, dividing it into two lumens. Occasionally, a flap may be highly mobile and cover the ostium of an arterial branch like a curtain. Examples of branch involvement by a dissection are shown in Figure 18.9.

In cases of intramural hematoma, no obvious intimal tear is present. The diagnosis then relies on the visualization of an area of focal aortic wall thickening (>3 mm) which is

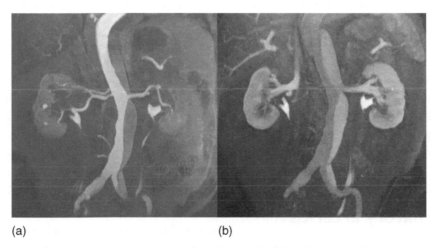

(a)   (b)

Figure 18.8 Arterial phase (a) and venous phase (b) of a contrast-enhanced MRA in a patient with abdominal aortic dissection. In the arterial phase (a) the preferential filling of the true lumen is well noted, although the degree of patency of the false lumen remains uncertain. The renal arteries are clearly visualized arising from the true lumen. In a later acquisition (b), the false lumen is noted to fill with contrast, confirming a 'communicating' dissection. Note also in both images the extension of the flap into the left common iliac artery.

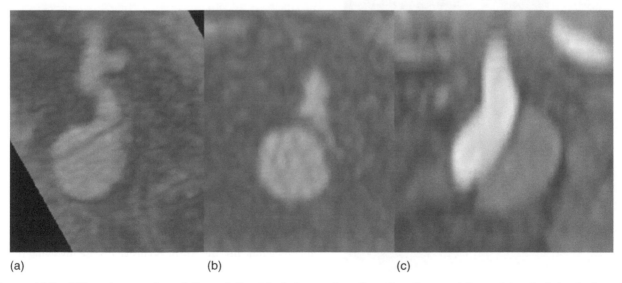

(a)   (b)   (c)

Figure 18.9 Different examples of the relationship between the dissection flap and the origin of abdominal aortic branches. (a) The intimal flap continues inside the celiac trunk, dividing it into a true and false lumen. (b) The superior mesenteric artery arises from the true lumen. However, the large false lumen compresses the true lumen, and this might lead to occlusion of the vessel ostium by the flap. (c) The dissection stops just at the ostium of the superior mesenteric artery, which arises from the true lumen.

usually smooth and crescent-shaped, although it may also be circumferential. An attractive feature of MRI is the ability to determine the tissue characteristics of a hematoma based on the paramagnetic characteristics of different hemoglobin compounds. Using T1-weighted spin-echo sequences, the presence of oxyhemoglobin in the acute phase may result in intermediate signal intensity. Subsequently, methemoglobin accumulates and causes shortening of T1 times and brighter signal. In the chronic phase the signal is reduced, and the presence of new areas of increased signal intensity may correspond to recurrent bleeding. It must, however, be mentioned that some of these data are derived from studies in subdural hematomas and extrapolations to the arterial wall may not necessarily be correct. Another aortic abnormality that can be readily visualized with MRI is the presence of penetrating aortic ulcers. Ulcers can be visualized both with black-blood or bright-blood techniques as protrusions of the lumen into the vessel wall (Figure 18.10). Concomitant intramural hematoma may be also observed. In these cases the distinction between a focal dissection versus an ulceration with extension into the arterial wall can be difficult.

Aortitis/inflammatory arteritis

Involvement of the abdominal aorta in the setting of vasculitis is relatively uncommon, although it may be seen in some

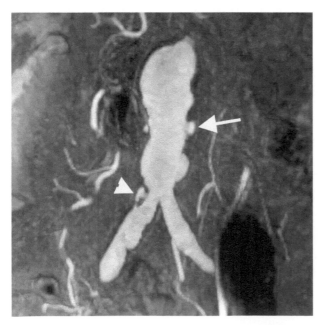

Figure 18.10 Maximum intensity projection (MIP) of a severely atherosclerotic infrarenal aorta, showing aneurysmal dilatation, multiple luminal irregularities, and ulcerations involving the aortic wall (arrow) and the origin of the right common iliac artery (arrowhead).

patients with giant cell or, in particular, with Takayasu's arteritis. Takayasu's arteritis is a granulomatous inflammatory process with mononuclear cells infiltrating all layers of the arterial wall. The etiology is unknown and the disease process is characterized by an early inflammatory phase followed by a late occlusive phase. Vascular wall thickening and edema are present in the active (early) phase. Subsequent intimal proliferation and fibrosis of the media and adventitia lead to areas of focal or diffuse luminal narrowing (even occlusion) and aneurysmal dilatations. Clinically, the disease may or may not display systemic inflammatory symptoms. It usually presents with absent or decreased pulses and manifestations of ischemia related to the specific vascular territories involved.

In the abdominal aorta, Takayasu's arteritis may result in diffuse stenosis, dissection, or aneurysm formation. Black-blood sequences are useful in evaluating wall thickness, which may be increased concentrically in focal areas or large segments. This may be noted even in cases of normal luminal appearance (Figure 18.11). T2-weighted double IR fast spin-echo images can reveal high signal intensity of the vessel wall, suggestive of mural edema. Similar T1-weighted sequences can be employed before and several minutes after contrast administration to depict enhancement of the arterial wall as a marker of disease activity. Contrast-enhanced MRA is useful in evaluating luminal irregularities, detecting significant stenoses and occlusions in abdominal branches (such as the renal arteries), or visualizing intimal flaps and aneurysmatic dilatations. In summary, MRI can be invaluable in the comprehensive assessment of inflammatory arteritis and obviates invasive angiography.

Aorto-iliac occlusive disease

Although an in-depth review of the uses of MRA for the evaluation of obstructive atherosclerosis in the lower extremities is discussed in another chapter of this book, we will briefly discuss aorto-iliac disease as this information is usually available during an MRA abdominal acquisition and is often valuable in making therapeutic decisions. Complete occlusion or high-grade occlusive disease involving the distal abdominal aorta and bifurcation usually occurs in older men with extensive atherosclerotic disease. Aortic occlusive disease involving the aortic bifurcation or distal abdominal aorta may also be seen in young women, typically smokers. The characteristic clinical triad of this disorder in males (Leriche's syndrome) includes intermittent claudication of the buttocks, hips, and thighs, erectile dysfunction, and atrophy of the lower extremities.

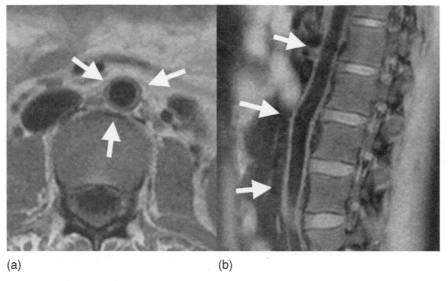

(a)   (b)

Figure 18.11   Abdominal axial T1-weighted (a) and sagittal proton density weighted (b) fast spin-echo images of a young woman with Takayasu's arteritis. Note the diffuse, concentric thickening of the aortic wall (arrows), with normal luminal appearance.

The occlusion develops progressively and is usually accompanied by extensive collateral circulation. The treatment includes general measures for the treatment of atherosclerosis, and often surgical revascularization.

Contrast-enhanced MRA is useful in depicting the site of occlusion, length of the occluded segment, and presence and degree of collateral supply. The imaged volume should include the main abdominal aortic branches, in order to identify the origin of collateral circulation (often the celiac or superior mesenteric arteries), and the presence of common concomitant stenoses of the renal or visceral arteries. It is also important to realize that collateral filling may be slow and delayed, and this should be taken into consideration when timing image acquisition. Additionally, distal patent vessels need to be identified as they may serve as targets for bypass grafting. MRI may be the only necessary test in the pre-operative evaluation in these patients.

Atherosclerotic plaque imaging

Another application of MRI is the in vivo detection and characterization of human atherosclerotic plaques in various vascular territories. Imaging of the abdominal aorta for this purpose is high yield, as this segment is commonly involved in atherosclerotic disease. Aortic plaques are usually evaluated using high-resolution, cardiac-gated, fat-suppressed, double IR fast spin-echo sequences. The size of individual plaques can be accurately measured and the extent of atherosclerotic disease in a large vascular segment quantified to derive indices of burden of atherosclerosis that correlate with traditional cardiovascular

risk factors. MRI can be employed to investigate the influence of various therapies on atherosclerotic burden, and may be used in the near future for detection of subclinical disease and estimation of cardiovascular risk. In addition, the combination of different image weightings (T1, T2, proton density) allows for the differentiation of various plaque components such as thrombus, lipid core, calcium, or fibrotic tissue. This ability may be exploited to identify those high-risk plaques that are more prone to the development of complications resulting in clinical events.

CONCLUSION

MRI and MRA techniques allow a comprehensive approach for the evaluation of diseases involving the abdominal aorta and its branches. Accurate detection of stenoses, precise and reproducible measurements of luminal dimension, evaluation of branch involvement, and characterization of the aortic wall and peri-aortic tissue may be obtained in one single setting. MRI is useful as an initial diagnostic tool and as a serial modality to track the evolution of various abnormalities, and for planning and follow-up of surgical or percutaneous vascular interventions. Current advances allow for data acquisition during brief periods of apnea and within reasonable total examination times ($\leq$30 minutes). In the near future, technical developments such as high-field imaging, improved coils, faster acquisition techniques, and novel contrast agents promise to further extend the clinical applications of MRI in the evaluation of systemic arterial disease.

PRACTICAL PEARLS

- It is preferable to employ phased-array surface coils for abdominal MRA, as they provide improved signal-to-noise ratio (SNR) and image quality when compared with the body coil.

- When possible, perform all acquisitions during breath holds to decrease motion artifacts and improve consistency in the position of imaged structures.

- The combination of black-blood and bright-blood sequences provides adequate differentiation between the vessel wall and the lumen.

- Precontrast images are useful to ensure adequate coverage and to perform subtractions during contrast-enhanced MRA.

- When setting the MRA, near-isotropic voxels result in better 3D reconstructions and are preferable to images with very high resolution in only one spatial direction and poor in another.

- Parallel imaging techniques should be employed whenever possible to reduce scanning time. The time saving can be employed to increase anatomic coverage or spatial resolution.

- The visceral and renal arteries should always be included in the imaged volume.

- Try to match the injection time to the scanning time, by modifying contrast dose and/or injection rate.

- Centric phase-encoding ordering results in more consistent acquisition of the center of k-space at the time of peak enhancement. If in doubt, it is better to start the acquisition slightly late than too early.

- Perform at least one additional 3D acquisition after contrast administration (venous phase).

- Always review the source images for diagnostic purposes, and the prescribed volume using a thick slab MIP to ensure adequate coverage of the anatomic structures and to rule out 'pseudostenosis' (partial arterial course outside of the prescribed volume).

FURTHER READING

Born M, Willinek WA, Gieseke J et al. Sensitivity encoding (SENSE) for contrast-enhanced 3D MR angiography of the abdominal arteries. J Magn Reson Imag 2005; 22: 559–65.

Choudhury RP, Fuster V, Badimon JJ et al. MRI and characterization of atherosclerotic plaque: emerging applications and molecular imaging. Arterioscler Thromb Vasc Biol 2002; 22: 1065–74.

Isselbacher EM. Thoracic and abdominal aortic aneurysms. Circulation 2005; 111: 816–28.

Maki JH, Chenevert TL, Prince MR. Contrast-enhanced MR angiography. Abdom Imag 1998; 23: 469–84.

McGuigan EA, Sears ST, Corse WR et al. MR angiography of the abdominal aorta. Magn Reson Imag Clin N Am 2005; 13: 65–89, v–vi.

Mukherjee D, Eagle KA. Aortic dissection–an update. Curr Prob Cardiol 2005; 30: 287–325.

Murray JG, Manisali M, Flamm SD et al. Intramural hematoma of the thoracic aorta: MR image findings and their prognostic implications. Radiology 1997; 204: 349–55.

Nastri MV, Baptista LPS, Baroni RH et al. Gadolinium-enhanced three-dimensional MR angiography of Takayasu arteritis. Radiographics 2004; 24: 773–86.

Pereles FS, McCarthy RM, Baskaran V et al. Thoracic aortic dissection and aneurysm: evaluation with nonenhanced true FISP MR angiography in less than 4 minutes. Radiology 2002; 223: 270–4.

Petersen MJ, Cambria RP, Kaufman JA et al. Magnetic resonance angiography in the preoperative evaluation of abdominal aortic aneurysms. J Vasc Surg 1995; 21: 891–8; discussion 899.

Prince MR, Narasimham DL, Stanley JC et al. Gadolinium-enhanced magnetic resonance angiography of abdominal aortic aneurysms. J Vasc Surg 1995; 21: 656–69.

Ruehm SG, Weishaupt D, Debatin JF. Contrast-enhanced MR angiography in patients with aortic occlusion (Leriche syndrome). J Magn Reson Imag 2000; 11: 401–10.

Upchurch GR, Elliason JL. Abdominal aortic aneurysms: management. In: Rajagopalan S, Mukherjee D, Mohler E, eds. Manual of Vascular Diseases. Philadelphia, PA: Lippincott Williams & Wilkins; 2005: 156–72.

Van Hoe L, De Jaegere T, Bosmans H et al. Breath-hold contrast-enhanced three-dimensional MR angiography of the abdomen: time-resolved imaging versus single-phase imaging. Radiology 2000; 214: 149–56.

Venkataraman S, Semelka RC, Weeks S et al. Assessment of aorto-iliac disease with magnetic resonance angiography using arterial phase 3-D gradient-echo and interstitial phase 2-D fat-suppressed spoiled gradient-echo sequences. J Magn Reson Imag 2003; 17: 43–53.

19

MR angiography of the renal circulation with imaging protocols

Santo Dellegrottaglie

INTRODUCTION

A number of different diagnostic modalities, such as invasive renal angiography, duplex ultrasound, CT angiography (CTA), and magnetic resonance angiography (MRA), may be employed for the evaluation of the renal vasculature. MRA combines several important advantages that may be relevant while imaging patients with renal vascular disease. These include: (1) high spatial resolution (submillimeter resolution in the x–y plane with current state of the art magnets and gradients); (2) hemodynamic information; (3) information on contiguous vascular beds; (4) evaluation of the renal parenchymal size; (5) renal vein and collecting duct information; (6) safety in patients with pre-existent renal insufficiency. The assessment of renal artery stenosis (RAS) represents the main indication for renal MRA. RAS is the most common cause of secondary hypertension ('renovascular hypertension') and is not infrequently responsible for renal impairment. The vast majority of RAS cases are attributable to atherosclerotic involvement of the renal arteries, while fibromuscular dysplasia (FMD) represents a less common cause of RAS (preferentially in young females). Additional applications for renal MRA may be encountered in patients with suspected vasculitis, renal artery aneurysms, aortic diseases potentially involving the renal arteries, or other conditions directly or indirectly affecting the renal circulation (Table 19.1).

FUNDAMENTALS OF RENAL MRA

Techniques

An understanding of basic concepts related to MRA techniques is required for a full appreciation of their role in renovascular disease (Chapter 12). The pulse sequences used, are for the most part similar to those utilized for the evaluation of the thoracic and abdominal aorta and the reader is referred to Chapter 12 for a complete overview of these techniques.

Time-of-flight angiography (TOF-MRA)

TOF angiography is based on the phenomenon of flow-related enhancement of spins entering into a partially saturated imaging section. In the selected section slice, the unsaturated spins of the flowing blood are detected as a bright signal against the dark signal generated by the stationary spins of the background. Images can be acquired as multiple two-dimensional (2D) slices or as a single 3D volume. Since the advent of gadolinium-based techniques, TOF-MRA is not used as a primary technique, in the evaluation of the renal arteries, as it is hampered by a number of

Table 19.1   Clinical indications to renal MRA

- Atherosclerotic renal artery stenosis
  - Main renal artery
  - Accessory renal artery
  - Transplant renal artery
  - Post-bypass grafting (aorto-renal, spleno-renal, gastroduodenal-renal bypasses)
  - Post percutaneous intervention
- Non-atherosclerotic renal artery stenosis (fibromuscular dysplasia, vasculitis, etc.)
- Renal artery aneurysm
- Aortic diseases involving the renal circulation (aortic dissection, aneurysm, etc.)
- Others (screening for kidney donors, renal vein evaluation, etc.)

drawbacks such as turbulence-induced signal loss at stenotic areas, in-plane saturation (saturation of signal in vessels that are flowing in the same plane as that of the slice), and inadequate visualization of distal segments. TOF-MRA may be occasionally used as a secondary technique to characterize severity of stenosis.

Phase contrast angiography (PC-MRA)

PC-MRA is typically performed using gradient echo techniques that employ special bipolar gradients ('flow-encoding gradients') to take advantage of phase shifts in the flowing blood. The magnitude of the measured phase shift is proportional to the flow velocity and, as a consequence, an approximate velocity of the blood may be derived. The amplitude of the bipolar gradients determines the degree of velocity encoding (Venc) and can be arbitrarily set. Flow encoding is typically performed in three axes yielding three data sets (performed in an interleaved fashion). A fourth data set is acquired without flow encoding (mask data set). These four data sets are then combined into an image using either a phase subtraction or complex difference techniques, to reconstruct both magnitude and phase images (phase map). PC-MRA can be implemented as a 2D or 3D sequence. Two-dimensional PC-MRA is based on the EKG-gated acquisition of multiple 2D images in a single plane, perpendicular to the long axis of the renal artery. The series of images acquired at high temporal resolution shows the cross-sectional renal blood flow over the cardiac cycle. On the generated time-resolved velocity profile, typical changes associated with significant renal artery stenosis include flattening of flow profile with delay or loss of the early systolic peak. Conflicting data have been reported

about the detection of significant renal artery stenosis using quantitative analysis of 2D PC flow curves alone. However, when used in conjunction with gadolinium-enhanced MRA, 2D PC-MRA appears to reduce the interobserver variability in grading renal artery stenosis associated with both the techniques.

When used in conjunction with gadolinium-enhanced MRA, 3D PC-MRA may also be very useful in estimating the hemodynamic severity of renal artery stenosis. Turbulent flow destroys signal phase coherence, causing 'dephasing' of the signal, which is especially prominent on 3D PC-MRA. In the presence of a severe stenosis (>75% narrowing), flow becomes disorganized and turbulent. On the other hand though, mild stenoses usually appear less severe because increased flow creates a 'blooming' effect.

Contrast-enhanced angiography (CE-MRA)

The high-resolution depiction of renal arteries obtained with CE-MRA allows an accurate characterization of renal artery diseases in most cases (Figure 19.1). Furthermore, delayed images can provide an assessment of renal veins and the status of the excretory system. For all these reasons, the other MRA approaches such as TOF serve an adjunctive role. The high-performance gradient systems currently employed for clinical MRA allow the acquisition of high quality images with reduced scan time. The use of phased-array coils for signal transmission and reception is crucial for adequate depiction of small or distal branches in the renal circulation. CE-MRA is commonly performed using a fast 3D T1-weighted spoiled gradient-echo sequence and is dependent on the effects of gadolinium-based contrast agent

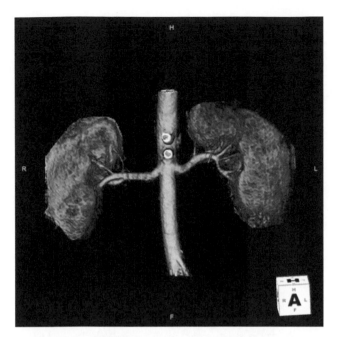

Figure 19.1   3D volume-rendered reconstruction of renal CE-MRA in a subject with normal renal arteries.

on blood magnetization (T1 shortening) for the generation of intravascular signal. Parallel imaging modalities (SMASH-like and SENSE-like techniques) are used widely and result in a doubling of spatial resolution and shortening of acquisition time. Correct timing, administration, and dosing of gadolinium is critical when imaging the renal arteries. The dose of gadolinium contrast agent is one of the most important determinants of image quality. Furthermore, the short parenchymal phase of contrast passage through the kidney makes accurate bolus timing for renal CE-MRA important to avoid venous contamination.

INTEGRATED APPROACH TO RENAL MRA

An integrated approach that combines a number of MRA techniques in a single study, provides for a comprehensive evaluation of the renal vessels parenchyma, and excretory system. Furthermore, a combination of techniques (CE-MRA and PC-MRA), when applied to RAS, may provide a better strategy to evaluate stenosis severity than either technique alone. The protocols described in this section are generally applicable to a 1.5 T imaging system (with high performance gradients and with the use of dedicated phased-array coils to enhance signal reception. After iv (20–22 gauge) placement in an antecubital vein, the patient is positioned within the magnet in the supine position (feet first). EKG gating or pulse

gating is not necessary, but may need to be turned on if one anticipates performing 2D PC-MRA.

MR scan protocol

The following sequences may be considered as part of an integrated imaging protocol for a comprehensive evaluation of renal vascular diseases:

(1) Localizer images

(2) Morphologic images: HASTE sequences with fat suppression in the three planes followed by single-shot SSFP in the axial and sagittal planes

(3) Bolus timing

(4) CE-MRA

(5) PC-MRA

The scan parameters applied for each sequence are reported in Table 19.2.

Localizer and morphologic images. A standardized protocol for renal MRA should begin with large field-of-view sequences (covering the entire region of interest) to plan subsequent acquisitions. These are also independently useful for gross morphologic characterization of kidneys and contiguous structures, including assessment of ascitis and organomegaly. A quick morphologic survey includes black-blood prepared HASTE (with fat suppression) in the three planes followed by single-shot bright-blood imaging (SSFP) in the axial and sagittal planes. If necessary, a T2-weighted turbo spin-echo sequence may be performed to further delineate abnormal anatomy (cysts, tumors, etc.).

Bolus timing. An empiric delay may be used between the beginning of the injection and the start of acquisition and may work in a number of patients, but is not recommended. Correct timing of the injection can be accomplished using the test bolus technique or an automatic triggering. With the test bolus technique, the time taken for a small amount of contrast material (2 ml) to travel from the injection site to the renal arteries is measured, using axial inversion pulse prepared fast low angle shot (FLASH) or steady-state free precession (SSFP) images (1 image/s), through the abdominal aorta at the level of the renal arteries, for a total period of 40–60 s. The measured time is then introduced as time delay for the actual CE-MRA scan, usually performed using a centric k-space acquisition mode. The second technique employs a contrast detection pulse sequence (specific for each scanner vendor) that automatically detects contrast arrival at the

Table 19.2 Scan parameters

	Black-blood HASTE	T2 Weighted TSE	Single-shot SSFP	Test bolus	CE-MRA	Post-contrast SPGR
Acquisition	2D	2D	2D	2D	3D	3D
Repetition time (TR, ms)	1100	5350	4.3	1000	3.1	3.2
Echo time (TE, ms)	25	102	2.1	1	1.2	1.4
Inversion time (TI, ms)	N/A	N/A	N/A	300	N/A	N/A
Flip angle (degrees)	160	180	79	50	25	15
Band width (Hz/pixel)	781	260	488	980	500	590
Fat saturation	Yes	Yes	Yes	No	No	Yes
Slice thickness (mm)	6	6	6	20	1.3	2.5
Gap (%)	30	30	30	N/A	N/A	N/A
Partitions/slices	20–30	20–30	20–30	1	72	120
Orientation	Axial/sagittal/coronal	Axial	Axial/sagittal/coronal	Axial	Coronal	Axial
Typical field-of-view (mm)	360×270–360	360×270–360	360×270–360	360×360	360×360	360×270
Phase direction	a-p/r-l	a-p	a-p/r-l	a-p, r-l	r-l	a-p
Matrix (lines)	256×125–166	256×106	256×144–192	128×100	320×275	256×146
Typical pixel size (mm)	2.2×1.4	2.5×1.5	1.9×1.4	2.8×2.8	1.3×1.1	1.8×1.4
Averages	1	1	1	1	1	1
Partial Fourier	4/8	off	off	off	Slice direction (6/8)	6/8
Parallel imaging	No	Yes	Yes	No	Yes	Yes
Duration (s)	22–33	20–25	11–13	45–60	19	17

HASTE: half-Fourier acquisition single-shot turbo spin-echo; TSE: turbo spin-echo; SSFP: steady-state free precession; SPGR: spoiled gradient-echo.

vessels of interest (abdominal aorta at the level of the renal arteries). CE-MRA sequence is started when a significant signal increase is detected. The contrast injection does not need to last for the entire duration of the image acquisition and a duration that equals the acquisition of a substantial portion of the central k-space information during the peak arterial contrast concentration should suffice (usually 2/3 of the acquisition time is sufficient.).

CE-MRA. The sequence for the 3D CE-MRA is performed in the coronal plane positioned to include the aorta and the renal arteries. To ensure adequate coverage of the relevant structures, particular attention needs to be paid to positioning the image volume. The abdominal aorta should be imaged from the portion above the celiac trunk to the

bifurcation, being careful to include the ventral aortic border and the origin of the main branches. To minimize the occurrence of image aliasing, the field-of-view should be set to approximately the width of the patient's torso (the skin fold may be used). The image acquisition is performed during breath holding with adjustments in spatial resolution that results in changes in image acquisition time approximate the breath holding capacity of the patient. Wherever possible, the resolution is increased to an approximate isotropic voxel resolution of 1 mm. Thus image parameters (section thickness, number of sections, and number of phase-encoding steps) should be adjusted to ensure that the acquisition is short enough for the patient to suspend breathing for the entire data acquisition (15–20 s), without a significant reduction in the image quality. Usually, we apply a

SMASH-based algorithm for parallel imaging to reduce acquisition time with an acceleration factor of 2. In ideal circumstances, a spatial resolution of $0.8 \times 0.8 \times 1.0$ mm can be obtained while keeping the scan time below 25 s. Isotropic spatial resolution has to be sought whenever possible to allow for superior multi-planar reformatting. A centric k-space algorithm is used to reduce venous contamination. After estimation of the timing delay (if a timing sequence is used), a 3D CE-MRA sequence is repeated three times: (1) before contrast injection (to check sequence appropriateness and for subsequent background subtraction); (2) after contrast injection during the arterial phase (to evaluate arterial circulation to the kidneys); and (3) during the equilibrium post-contrast phase (to assess venous circulation and parenchymal contrast uptake). The most used contrast agent is represented by gadolinium-DTPA (diethylenetriamine penta-acetic acid). Commonly, using an automated infusion pump, a dose of 30–40 ml of contrast agent (0.2–0.3 mmol/kg; injection rate of 2–3 ml/s) is given, followed by 20 ml of saline solution.

PC-MRA. A PC-MRA technique should be included in the protocol to help in the evaluation of the hemodynamic significance of RAS. It may be convenient to perform the PC acquisition after gadolinium contrast imaging because of the extra signal-to-noise ratio produced by the contrast agent. The Venc should be adjusted in each single case (range, 30–60 cm/s) to avoid aliasing. An axial 3D PC acquisition to cover the renal arteries may be prescribed routinely after performance of CE-MRA. This may be helpful for the visualization of flow dephasing at the level of a significant stenosis and can provide useful additive information for stenosis severity assessment. Two-dimensional cine PC-MRA may also be used for the quantification of stenosis severity at the level of the renal artery, but requires EKG or pulse gating. Two-dimensional PC-MRA images may be obtained with both high spatial and temporal resolution (<40 ms). A scan plane perpendicular to the renal artery is planned approximately 1cm distal to the ostium or 1–2 cm distal to a stenosis.

Image analysis and interpretation

For the correct identification and characterization of renal vascular disease, the images obtained should be analyzed systematically on a dedicated workstation. In order to reduce background signal and improve the contrast-to-noise ratio, background digital subtraction from the arterial phase

data set can be automatically obtained using precontrast mask images. The source images should be viewed initially as one may have artifacts related to the subtraction process. Tortuous renal artery anatomy can be unfolded by scrolling the 3D volume in the coronal and axial planes using multi-planar reformations (MPRs). With this technique, renal artery ostia are thoroughly evaluated and eccentric plaques easily identified. Additionally, the construction of maximal intensity projection (MIP) images allows the accurate evaluation of arterial lumen on oblique planes. A comprehensive renal artery imaging study should ideally strive to provide the following facets of information: localization and enumeration of the renal arteries, including accessory branches, assessment of hemodynamic and functional significance of stenosis, indirect cues indicating compromised renal function (e.g., reduced cortical thickness, reduced kidney size, and asymmetric concentration of contrast media in the collecting system, etc.) and identification of associated conditions (e.g. solitary kidney, abdominal aortic aneurysm, peripheral arterial disease, etc.) that might impact on treatment planning.

The degree of stenosis at the level of the renal artery can be calculated by measuring the ratio between the diameter (or area) of the narrowest segment and the diameter (or area) of a 'normal' segment of the same artery used as reference. However, a grading of the stenosis as mild, moderate, or severe is more practical than calculating percent stenosis as delineation of a true 'normal' segment is difficult. The presence and number of accessory renal arteries should also be assessed. Stenosis grading of accessory arteries is frequently difficult and can usually be performed only on a binary basis (present or absent). Additional indirect signs of a hemodynamically significant stenosis include post-stenotic dilatation, delayed renal enhancement, and asymmetric concentration of gadolinium in the collecting system during the equilibrium phase imaging. Other indirect signs include loss of cortical–medullary differentiation (particularly evident on post-contrast T1-weighted images) or reduction in kidney length and parenchymal thickness (from the HASTE images).

On 3D PC-MRA imaging, the artifactual loss of signal at the stenosis level owing to loss of phase coherence at the site of flow turbulence can be useful for characterizing the hemodynamic significance of a stenosis (Table 19.3). On the 2D PC-MRA images, a region of interest may be manually drawn along the margins of the vessel cross-section in each image obtained at different time frames and a velocity–time curve is derived from the flow data. Characteristic changes

Table 19.3 Estimation of the severity of renal artery stenosis combining information provided by CE-MRA and 3D PC-MRA

Stenosis grading	CE-MRA	3D PC-MRA
<75%	Stenosis	Absent/minimal dephasing
>75%	Stenosis	Severe dephasing
Occluded	Non-visualized renal artery	Non-detected renal artery

of the velocity flow profile have been documented in patients with RAS (Figure 19.2).

CLINICAL APPLICATIONS

Detection and characterization of RAS undoubtedly represents the main application of renal MRA (Table 19.1). The preponderance of commonly encountered cases of renal artery disease in practice is due to atherosclerosis, while the remainder are caused by less common conditions, such as FMD, aortic dissection, arteritis, congenital disease, embolization, and trauma.

Atherosclerotic renal artery stenosis

Atherosclerotic RAS represents the most common pathologic condition involving the renal arteries. Prompt detection and treatment (by medical therapy, surgery, or percutaneous angioplasty with stenting) of hemodynamically significant renal stenoses may improve hypertension, preserve kidney function, and positively affect patient prognosis. Clinical clues during the review of the patient's history and the physical examination, such as onset of hypertension <30 years or >55 years, malignant or accelerated hypertension, azotemia induced by ACE inhibitors, systolic/diastolic epigastric bruit, etc., may lead the clinician to suspect the presence of a RAS. MRA may be considered as a first-line screening modality for the presence of RAS in light of the fact that it is safe in renal insufficiency and provides excellent additional information that may be helpful in therapeutic decision-making (Figure 19.3). MRA can also be used as a confirmatory study before intervention in patients at high risk for angiographic complications such as contrast nephrotoxicity. A meta-analysis of 12 old studies (499 patients; period 1985–2001) evaluated the accuracy of CE-MRA in detecting significant renal stenosis and reported a sensitivity and specificity of 97%

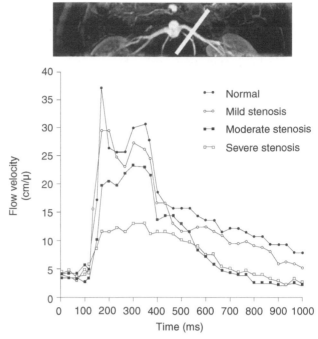

Figure 19.2 Schematic representation of typical velocity–flow curves obtained by 2D cine PC-MRA in subjects with a normal vessel or with various levels of renal artery stenosis. For the PC image acquisition, an image volume orthogonal to the imaged renal artery is defined on an axial reconstruction from CE-MRA images. A normal velocity curve is characterized by a high early-systolic peak and a lower mid-systolic peak separated by an incision. A low-grade stenosis (< 50% of vessel lumen diameter) produces a partial loss of the early-systolic peak. A moderate stenosis (50–75%) is associated with a significant loss of the early-systolic peak and decrease of the mid-systolic peak. Finally, a flattened flow profile, with lack of discernible systolic velocity components, is produced by severe stenosis (>75%).

and 93%, respectively. Of note, all these studies included a preponderance of patients with a final diagnosis of atherosclerotic RAS. These positive data have been subsequently confirmed in numerous studies. However, recent multicenter trials involving community sites seem to suggest that performance may not be as good as previously thought, especially when allcomers (FMD and atherosclerotic RAS) are included in the analysis (discussed below).

Accessory RAS. While hypertension can result from the stenosis of an accessory renal artery, the therapeutic impact of successful identification of such a lesion remains unclear, as these stenoses cannot be easily addressed by vascular interventions. Accessory renal arteries are often missed by Duplex ultrasounds but can be easily identified using CE-MRA (Figure 19.4). However, no large studies are available addressing the evaluation of the diagnostic accuracy of MRA in detecting accessory RAS.

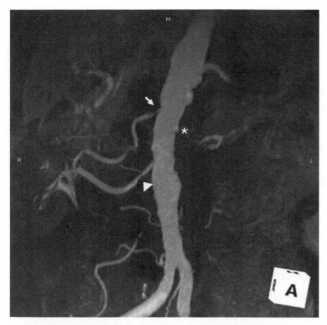

Figure 19.3 Renal CE-MRA in a patient with hypertension and moderate renal dysfunction. The main left renal artery has a mild stenosis (arrowhead), while a significant ostial stenosis involving an accessory right renal artery is seen (arrow). The left renal artery is occluded (asterisk).

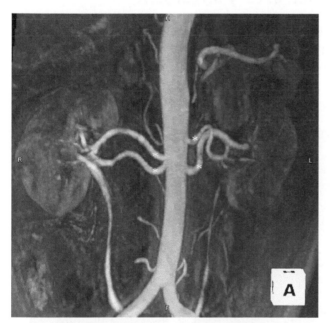

Figure 19.4 Renal MRA obtained during the injection of a bolus of gadolinium-DTPA (0.2 mmol/kg). Two renal arteries are visualized on both sides (asterisks), with no evidence of significant stenosis.

Transplanted RAS. Vascular complications associated with renal transplantation merit urgent investigation since they are often correctable and timely intervention can help save the graft kidney. Three-dimensional CE-MRA is particularly attractive for patients with kidney transplants in view of its safety in the setting of renal dysfunction. Transplanted kidneys are preferentially located extraperitoneally in the right iliac fossa. The donor artery is typically anastamosed to the recipient ipsilateral external or common iliac artery. Typically, stenosis/occlusion may occur at the anastamotic site between the transplanted renal artery and the iliac artery (Figure 19.5). For an adequate visualization of the transplanted kidney in its ectopic location, particular attention needs to be paid to the correct positioning of the acquisition volume. An additional sequence that is useful in the post-transplant kidney is axial fat suppressed T2-weighted fast spin echo. The transplanted kidney is typically hyperintense. This sequence allows the accurate delineation of peritransplant fluid collections.

Post-revascularization evaluation

After surgical renal revascularization it is recommended that patients have follow-up evaluations of the graft. Duplex ultrasonography followed by MRA are preferred techniques on account of their safety and accuracy. MRA is superior though, as it can provide simultaneous information on the inflow and outflow vessels and the aorta. The clinical imaging protocol described above may be conveniently adapted to the study of patients with renal revascularization. Knowledge of the specific surgical graft (e.g., aorto-renal, spleno-renal, and gastroduodenal-renal bypass), is necessary to ensure their inclusion in the CE-MRA volumes. The integrated renal MRA protocol may also be applied with good results in cases of suspected post-revascularization complications (renal artery thrombosis, renal infarction, aneurysms of bypass grafts, and recurrent stenosis of the renal artery). The common occurrence of susceptibility artifacts (from surgical clips or intra-vascular stents) in post-revascularization studies, is a main limitation for the MRA evaluation of these patients. In most cases, patency of the stent can be indirectly inferred from the presence of contrast medium in the artery distal to the stent, however no determination of restenosis can be made. Using PC-MRA, in-stent stenosis can also be diagnosed by the quantification of flow beyond the stent, but this requires additional time on the magnet.

Non-atherosclerotic renal artery stenosis

Non-atherosclerotic RAS may have multiple etiologies such as fibromuscular dysplasia (FMD), arteritis, embolization, trauma, etc. Although FMD represents a rare disorder, it constitutes the most common cause of RAS in young adults (especially women <40 years old). Medial fibroplasia is the histologic form that is most frequently observed. Because of a preferential involvement of the distal two-thirds of the renal arteries (typically with a series of stenosis with intermittent aneurysmal out pouchings, so-called 'string-of-beads' appearance), the diagnosis of FMD may be particularly challenging (Figure 19.6). High spatial resolution at the level of the distal main renal arteries is required to demonstrate subtle irregularities associated with FMD. The distal renal arteries are more prone to motion artifact and venous overlay, and MRA may therefore miss cases of FMD. This was demonstrated in the RADISH trial that prospectively evaluated the accuracy of CE-MRA (and CTA) in diagnosing RAS compared with invasive angiography as a gold standard. This multi-center study involved a total of 356 patients with hypertension and suspected RAS. Of the patients who had a significant stenosis (20% of the total), 38% had FMD, reflecting the young profile of the study cohort (mean age 52 years). An intrinsic bias owing to trial design involved exclusion of patients with renal insufficiency. The latter population has a higher prevalence of atherosclerotic RAS and lower prevalence of FMD. In this study, the overall sensitivity and specificity of CE-MRA were 62% and 84%, respectively. Furthermore, the value of sensitivity dropped to extremely low values (22%) when only patients with a final diagnosis of FMD were considered in the analysis.

The main renal arteries may present stenotic and/or aneurysmal lesions in patients with vasculitis involving the large-medium arteries (e.g., Takayasu's disease, polyarteritis nodosa, etc.). In these subjects, renal MRA can provide information on vessel wall thickening (even before lumen changes become apparent), luminal narrowing, and luminal dilatation, as well as provide a convenient non-invasive modality for repeated imaging follow-up.

Renal artery aneurysm

Aneurysms can be found at the level of the renal arteries with a prevalence of 0.01–0.1%. Atherosclerosis represents the most common cause, whereas less frequent are FMD, arteritis, and mesenchymal diseases (e.g., neurofibromatosis,

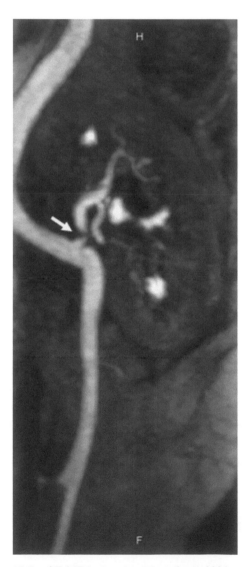

Figure 19.5   CE-MRA showing transplanted kidney in the right iliac fossa with the transplant artery anastomosed to the external iliac artery with a significant proximal stenosis (arrow).

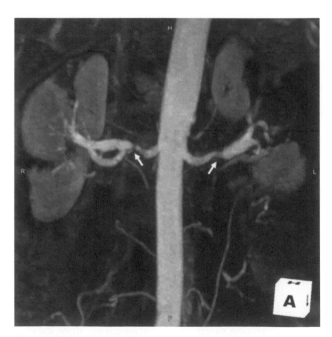

Figure 19.6   Renal MRA in a patient with a diagnosis of fibromuscular dysplasia. Significant stenoses (arrows) involve the mid-segments of the right and left renal arteries, while the distal arterial segments are moderately dilated.

Ehlers–Danlos syndrome, etc.) (Figure 19.7). Most patients are asymptomatic and the aneurysm may be incidentally discovered during imaging. MRA techniques are helpful in describing the location, number, size, type (saccular, fusiform, etc.), and possible complications of renal aneurysms. Renal artery aneurysms often contain mural thrombus and may give rise to emboli of the kidney. The risk of rupture is small, particularly when rimlike calcification is present in the wall of the aneurysm. Although hypertension is commonly present in patients with renal artery aneurysm, a causal relationship has not been well demonstrated.

Aortic diseases involving the renal circulation

Various pathologic conditions of the aorta may secondarily involve the renal circulation. MRA may depict the severity of aortic dissection, allowing a clear delineation of the intimal flap, the differentiation between the true and the false lumen, and the possible extension to the renal arteries (Chapter 18). In patients with aortic dissection, the renal artery flow may be compromised because of a direct extension of the dissection into the renal artery or in cases with a markedly reduced perfusion pressure in the true lumen (Figure 19.8). A kidney may still be perfused off the false lumen, if the latter has a communication with the true

lumen. In the event of renal artery aneurysm, careful assessment of the renal parenchyma for renal infarcts is indicated. Moreover, the patients will have clinical evidence of pain, hematuria, and rapidly deteriorating renal function.

The infrarenal abdominal aorta is the most common site of atherosclerotic aneurysms. CE-MRA allows assessment of the aneurysm and the renal arteries (by aneurysm or its complications), and may provide information on the suitability of the patient for surgical or percutaneous repair. Aortic coarctation is usually observed in the thoracic aorta (distal to the left subclavian artery), and may rarely be responsible for a reduction in renal perfusion pressure resulting in renovascular hypertension. In case of suspected coarctation, a large field-of-view (including the descending thoracic aorta) should be prescribed on MRA sequences. Rarely, aortic coarctation may involve the abdominal aorta and narrowing of the renal artery ostia is commonly observed in these cases.

Other clinical applications

Renal vein thrombosis. Thrombosis of the renal vein is more frequently caused by an underlying hypercoagulable state or renal neoplasm. Renal vein thrombosis is more common on the left side, presumably because of the longer length of the left renal vein. In patients receiving renal transplantation it can

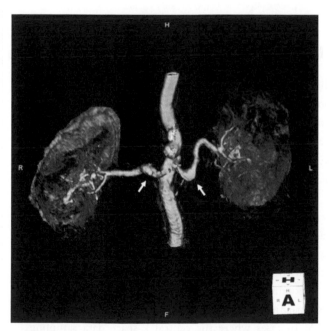

Figure 19.7 Patient with multiple vascular lesions and diagnosis of neurofibromatosis. The 3D MRA shows large aneurysms (arrows) involving the right and left renal arteries.

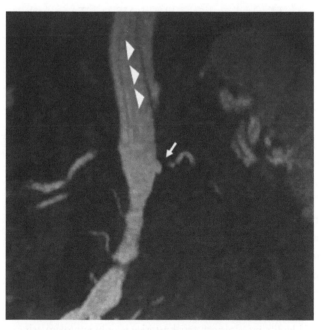

Figure 19.8 Dissection of the abdominal aorta (arrowheads) with evidence of extension to the left renal artery (arrow).

occur as a complication within the first week, in up to 4% of patients. When associated with tumor, it is frequently caused by direct tumor extension from the inferior vena cava and occurs most commonly in cases of renal cell carcinoma. The venous phase of a renal CE-MRA is usually helpful in demonstrating a thrombus with or without extension into the inferior vena cava. Additional imaging sequences such as inversion recovery prepared spoiled gradient-echo (SPGR) or FLASH sequence can be additionally helpful in delineating thrombus.

Evaluation of kidney donors. Careful evaluation of the renovascular anatomy for living kidney donors is essential to optimize donor and recipient outcomes. MRA is used widely for this application. In particular, MRA may be extremely helpful in these subjects for the identification of the number and location of accessory renal arteries prior to transplantation.

DIAGNOSTIC PERFORMANCE OF RENAL MRA

CE-MRA has been shown to compare extremely favorably with digital subtraction angiography in determining presence, location, and severity of stenosis in the renal arteries. Although selective intra-arterial angiography is still considered the 'gold standard' for the diagnosis of RAS, it is increasingly relegated to confirmation of the diagnosis in a patient who is a candidate for percutaneous revascularization. In cases with suspected FMD (in view of lower diagnostic yield with MRA), CTA or rarely DSA may required for the diagnosis. The contrast load in such patients is usually not a major consideration as most are young and have normal renal function. Duplex ultrasonography is a reasonable first-line imaging modality that may be used in lieu of MRA in certain centers. The ready availability, rapidity of the exam, physiologic information (including renal size assessment), and its ability to follow the degree of stenosis post-revascularization (especially after stents) make Duplex ultrasonography attractive as the test of choice in centers that are skilled in this modality. However, its clinical applicability is somewhat tempered by the need for experienced operators and by a number of potential limitations, including patient anatomy (size and girth of the patient), vessel anatomy (course of the artery, branches), pathophysiology (extensive calcification), and the ability to provide information on adjacent vascular beds, such as the aorta and mesenteric arteries. Moreover, the sensitivity of identifying accessory renal arteries is only approximately 60–70% with ultrasound. As reviewed in Chapter 9, CTA has substantially improved with the availability of multi-detector row CT systems. A number of studies have demonstrated high diagnostic accuracy of CTA for the detection of significant RAS. Compared with MRA, CTA may be better at evaluating stents. However, the applicability of CTA to the evaluation of renal artery stenosis is seriously limited by the risks associated with the use of ionizing radiation and iodinated contrast media.

LIMITATIONS

Although 3D CE-MRA images provide for a high degree of accuracy in atherosclerotic renal artery disease, this technique is not free from reduced accuracy. Recent studies have revealed important limitations in patients with distal vessel involvement such as FMD. Motion of the renal artery in these segments may be an important factor that precludes accurate assessment of distal RAS. A second problem, which has been well documented recently by a number of authors, is the high interobserver variability of the technique in grading the severity of RAS. Review of axial source images and of PC-MRA data may be helpful in reducing the variability in the interpretation of renal MRA. A relevant limitation is in the assessment of stents, as these preclude evaluation of the vascular lumen owing to susceptibility artifacts. These artifacts seem to be minimal with the nitinol and platinum alloy stents which may allow better evaluation of stent patency and diameter. Finally, high cost and limited scanner availability may restrict the use of MRA to select centers with the appropriate expertise and equipment.

PITFALLS AND ARTIFACTS

The most common pitfalls noted in CE-MRA are related to poor-quality images caused by failure to suspend breathing, poor timing of bolus injection, or inadequate setting for the image field-of-view. Especially in these instances, additional CE-MRA runs and PC imaging may represent a crucial back-up in evaluation of the renal arteries.

Breath holding is extremely critical in preventing the occurrence of motion artifacts, especially at the level of distal renal branches and accessory renal arteries. For this reason, any attempt to make tolerable the period of breath hold for each patient (by reducing the scan time) is worthwhile.

Suboptimal timing of image acquisition relative to contrast opacification is a common source of artifact with CE-MRA. In cases where the central k-space data sampling occurs during inadequate arterial opacification of contrast, or when contrast concentration is changing rapidly, truncation or Gibbs artifacts can create pseudodissection artifacts (Chapter 13). Venous overlay artifact may occur frequently in the renovascular territory. This is because the arteriovenous transit time at the level of the renal circulation is particularly short. This may compromise complete evaluation of the renal arteries. Inappropriate positioning of the imaging volume may frequently produce pseudostenosis. A small field-of-view in relation to the body size may generate aliasing artifacts at the lateral margin of the images. Finally, phase artifacts appear as ghost images with high signal intensity and when they are juxtaposed to vessels may result in mistaken diagnosis.

CONCLUSIONS

MRA is an important and first-line imaging modality for the comprehensive evaluation of patients with renovascular disease as it can provide information on renal and vascular anatomy, physiology, and function in a single examination. The major advantage of renal MRA is represented by the fact that this modality is virtually free of risk for the patient.

The main application for CE-MRA is in the evaluation of patients with suspected atherosclerotic RAS. A protocol combining CE-MRA and PC-MRA techniques may result in higher diagnostic accuracy in defining the location and severity of RAS. In addition, MRA is a valuable modality for preintervention planning in patients scheduled for renal revascularization.

Continuing evolution of pulse sequences, hardware, and contrast agents will allow optimization of renal MRA and help in establishing this technique as the gold standard for the evaluation of suspected RAS of any etiology.

PRACTICAL PEARLS

- Breath holds in expiration may allow more reproducible positioning of the visceral organs. Instructing the patient to regulate their breath holds to the same degree may be valuable.

- The differing positions of the viscera between different breath holds may generate artifacts when these image sets are used for subtraction. In case of limited patient compliance, subtraction from a precontrast image should be avoided.

- When imaging in the coronal plane (as for renal CE-MRA) remember to have the patient's arms elevated over the head to allow for a smaller field-of-view without aliasing artifacts.

- In post-stent implantation studies, better visualization of the intrastent lumen with reduced incidence of susceptibility artifacts can be obtained by using higher flip angles.

- Always review source images. MIP reconstruction may result in an overestimation of the degree of stenosis and can also obscure small intraluminal filling defects such as dissection flaps.

- Centric k-space acqusition schemes may provide for better studies and prevent venous overlay. Timing for such acquisitions should be performed as close to the renal arteries as possible.

FURTHER READING

Bakker J, Beek FJ, Beutler JJ et al. Renal artery stenosis and accessory renal arteries: accuracy of detection and visualization with gadolinium-enhanced breath-hold MR angiography. Radiology 1998; 207(2): 497–504.

Dellegrottaglie S, Sanz J, Rajagopalan S. Technology insight: clinical role of magnetic resonance angiography in the diagnosis and management of renal artery stenosis. Nat Clin Pract Cardiovasc Med 2006; 3(6): 329–38.

Hany TF, Debatin JF, Leung DA, Pfammatter T. Evaluation of the aortoiliac and renal arteries: comparison of breath-hold, contrast-enhanced, three-dimensional MR angiography with conventional catheter angiography. Radiology 1997; 204(2): 357–62.

Kim D, Edelman RR, Kent KC, Porter DH, Skillman JJ. Abdominal aorta and renal artery stenosis: evaluation with MR angiography. Radiology 1990; 174(3): 727–31.

McCauley TR, Monib A, Dickey KW et al. Peripheral vascular occlusive disease: accuracy and reliability of time-of-flight MR angiography. Radiology 1994; 192(2): 351–7.

Prince MR. Renal MR angiography: a comprehensive approach. J Mag Reson Imag 1998; 8(3): 511–16.

Schoenberg SO, Knopp MV, Bock M et al. Renal artery stenosis: grading of hemodynamic changes with cine phase-contrast MR blood flow measurements. Radiology 1997; 203(1): 45–53.

Schoenberg SO, Knopp MV, Londy F et al. Morphologic and functional magnetic resonance imaging of renal artery stenosis: a multireader tricenter study. J Am Soc Nephrol 2002; 13(1): 158–69.

Schoenberg SO, Rieger J, Johannson LO et al. Diagnosis of renal artery stenosis with magnetic resonance angiography: update 2003. Nephrol Dial Transplant 2003; 18(7): 1252–6.

Tan KT, van Beek EJ, Brown PW et al. Magnetic resonance angiography for the diagnosis of renal artery stenosis: a meta-analysis. Clin Radiol 2002; 57(7): 617–24.

Thornton MJ, Thornton F, O'Callaghan J et al. Evaluation of dynamic gadolinium-enhanced breath-hold MR angiography in the diagnosis of renal artery stenosis. AJR 1999; 173(5): 1279–83.

Vasbinder GB, Nelemans PJ, Kessels AG et al. Accuracy of computed tomographic angiography and magnetic resonance angiography for diagnosing renal artery stenosis. Ann Intern Med 2004; 141(9): 674–82.

Volk M, Strotzer M, Lenhart M et al. Renal time-resolved MR angiography: quantitative comparison of gadobenate dimeglumine and gadopentetate dimeglumine with different doses. Radiology 2001; 220(2): 484–8.

Willmann JK, Wildermuth S, Pfammatter T et al. Aortoiliac and renal arteries: prospective intraindividual comparison of contrast-enhanced three-dimensional MR angiography and multidetector row CT angiography. Radiology 2003; 226(3): 798–811.

Zhang HL, Prince MR. Renal MR angiography. Magn Reson Imag Clin N Am 2004; 12(3): 487–503.

Zhang HL, Schoenberg SO, Resnick LM, Prince MR. Diagnosis of renal artery stenosis: combining gadolinimum-enhanced three-dimensional magnetic resonance angiography with functional magnetic resonance pulse sequences. Am J Hypertens 2003; 16(12): 1079–82.

20

MR angiography of the mesenteric circulation with imaging protocols

Mushabbar A Syed, Gopi KR Sirineni, and Diego Martin

INTRODUCTION

The mesenteric circulation consists of arterial, venous, and lymphatic vessels of the abdominal organs. This vascular territory can be affected by a variety of vascular pathologies, most of which are asymptomatic, but can be occasionally catastrophic. Therefore, early diagnosis of mesenteric vascular disease requires a high degree of clinical suspicion and use of appropriate imaging techniques.

Catheter-based invasive angiographic techniques have been considered the gold standard for the diagnosis of abdominal vascular disease. In the acute setting, abdominal ultrasonography and computed tomography are routinely employed as the first-line imaging modality. Magnetic resonance imaging (MRI) and magnetic resonance angiography (MRA) with their excellent image quality, absence of ionizing radiation, and lack of significant nephrotoxicity of gadolinium-based contrast agents represent an attractive alternative to invasive angiography or computed tomography. These characteristics also make MRI/MRA ideally suited for follow-up examinations.

In this review, the relevant arterial and venous anatomy of the mesenteric circulation is described and practical aspects of MRI/MRA techniques for the diagnosis of mesenteric pathology are summarized (Table 20.1). The mesenteric MRA techniques described below are similar to the imaging sequences used in MRA of the abdominal aorta that are addressed in detail in Chapter 16.

MESENTERIC VASCULAR ANATOMY

The gastrointestinal tract is supplied by three major arteries (i.e., the celiac trunk, the superior mesenteric artery [SMA] and the inferior mesenteric artery [IMA]), all of which originate from the anterior aspect of the abdominal aorta. The celiac trunk originates at the level of T12 or L1 and after 1–2 cm divides into the common hepatic, splenic, and left gastric arteries. The common hepatic artery gives origin to the gastroduodenal artery and then divides into the right and left hepatic arteries. The SMA is located 10–20 mm below the celiac artery, around the level of the L1 vertebral body, and immediately turns inferiorly, running anterior and parallel to the abdominal aorta. The SMA supplies the pancreas, duodenum, jejunum, and the right half of the colon, up to the splenic flexure. The IMA originates from the anterior or left anterolateral aspect of the aorta below the renal arteries, around the level of the L3 vertebral body, and supplies the left half of the colon and rectum.

The mesenteric venous drainage follows a similar pattern to the arterial circulation, with the vena recta forming a venous arcade that drains the small bowel and proximal colon through the ileocolic, middle colic, and right colic veins to form the superior mesenteric vein. The superior mesenteric vein and splenic vein join to form the portal vein, which divides into the left and right branches at the porta hepatis.

Table 20.1 Major indications to MRA of the mesenteric circulation

- Chronic mesenteric ischemia
- Acute mesenteric ischemia
- Mesenteric venous thrombosis
- Portal hypertension
- Pre- and post-liver transplant evaluation
- Presurgical planning in patients with abdominal neoplasm
- Others (e.g., aneurysms, vasculitis, fibromuscular dysplasia, etc.)

The majority of the intestinal blood supply is delivered via the SMA, while the celiac trunk and IMA serve as minor contributors in normal subjects. However, in patients with mesenteric vascular occlusive disease these vessels assume a much greater significance due to extensive collaterals opening up to the gut normally supplied by the SMA.

Two mesenteric areas ('watershed areas') are especially vulnerable to ischemia during low flow states due to dependency on simultaneous nutrient blood supply contribution from two major arterial vascular beds. These are the hepatic flexure of the colon, receiving a blood supply from the ileocolic and middle colic branches of SMA, and the splenic flexure, supplied by the combination of the middle colic and left colic arteries. The sigmoid colon is vulnerable to ischemia due to dependency on the small caliber IMA. The rectum is relatively resistant to ischemic injury due to multiple vascular sources arising from the combination of the IMA in addition to the systemic pelvic floor vessels, arising from the left and right internal iliac arteries.

FUNDAMENTALS OF MESENTERIC MRA

A complete evaluation of mesenteric vessels includes visualization of the mesenteric arterial as well as the venous system. The primary goals of mesenteric imaging are delineation of anatomy and assessment of lumen patency, therefore MRI techniques used in mesenteric imaging involve sequences that are particularly suitable for this purpose.

After the initial localizer images, our protocol usually begin with anatomic imaging by using single-shot black-blood sequences (i.e., half acquisition Fourier-transformed turbo spin echo [HASTE] or single-shot fast spin echo), which can be performed within a single breath hold (Chapters 12 and 13). Alternatively, the single-shot steady-state free precession (SSFP) technique can provide rapid and good delineation of vascular anatomy.

The initial images are used to identify anatomic landmarks for planning of three dimensional (3D) MRA. The contrast enhanced 3D MRA allows very accurate evaluation of vascular anatomy. The first MRA acquisition is timed to coordinate with the maximum contrast concentration in the mesenteric arteries. A second MRA acquisition is subsequently repeated for visualization of the mesenteric and portal veins (venous phase imaging). Generally, we do not employ EKG or pulse-wave gating for black-blood or MRA imaging.

Additional optional sequences include axial T1 and T2 with fat saturation to evaluate the liver and other abdominal organs, and phase-contrast angiography (PC-MRA). In particular, measurement of fasting and post-prandial blood flow in the superior mesenteric vessels by PC-MRA flow imaging may be helpful in the diagnosis of chronic mesenteric ischemia (Chapter 13). Time-of-flight techniques are no longer favored for body imaging applications as these non-contrast techniques provide only limited visualization of the arterial system, particularly for the detection of disease in smaller vessels, and require long acquisition times, which prevent image acquisition in one breath hold and thus suffer from a higher susceptibility to motion artifacts.

CLINICAL IMAGING PROTOCOL

Hardware

An MRI scanner with high gradient performance and dedicated surface coils are essential for the successful acquisition of 3D mesenteric MRA. With this setting, the use of very short values of repetition time (TR) and echo time (TE) enables image acquisition within a comfortable breath hold period and also minimizes the signal from surrounding abdominal tissues. In our Institution, a 1.5 Tesla magnet (Magnetom Avanto, Siemens, Erlangen, Germany) with gradient performance of 45 mT/m maximum amplitude and 200 T/m/s slew rate, is employed. A body coil can provide adequate image quality. However, should it be preferred, a dedicated phased-array coil that provides a higher signal-to-noise ratio may be used to image with higher resolution and/or with shorter scan time.

Patient preparation

Patients are screened for any MRI contraindications, instructed about the procedure, and provided with breathing instruction before the examination is started. A peripheral intravenous access (20 gauge catheter) is placed in a large forearm or antecubital vein. In patients with small veins a 22 gauge catheter may be used and gadolinium contrast should be prewarmed to body temperature to reduce its viscosity. If a patient is claustrophic, we use Ativan 0.5–1 mg or Valium 5–10 mg orally. The patient is then placed supine on the MRI table in feet-first or head-first position (we prefer feet-first because of better tolerance by claustrophobic patients). The arms are raised above the head to avoid wrap-around artifacts in coronal acquisitions. The landmark for the center-scanner bore is positioned just below the tip of the xyphoid and the patient is then advanced into the magnet bore.

Contrast material

For adequate image contrast enhancement, we use gadopentate dimeglumine (Gd-DTPA) at 0.2 mmol/kg dose. In patients with low cardiac output, a dose of 0.3 mmol/kg (triple dose) may be preferable. The contrast is administered with a power injector at the rate of 2 ml/s, followed by a saline flush of 20 ml at the same injection rate as the contrast. Correct timing is of critical importance with rapid, short duration contrast injections and is facilitated by a timing bolus or an automated bolus tracking technique. We use a real time fast 2D sequence for bolus tracking in the coronal plane. The sequence is initiated at the same time as the contrast injection and monitors the arrival of contrast in the abdominal aorta at the level of the renal arteries. After contrast arrives at the level of the renal arteries, the patient is instructed to hold breath and the operator triggers the MRA acquisition manually. A delay of 3–5 s between contrast arrival and MRA acquisition is used to allow for the maximum contrast concentration to arrive in the imaged vessels and to develop images with maximum signal intensity in the mesenteric arteries.

Imaging protocol

The imaging protocol for mesenteric MRA is similar to MRA of the abdominal aorta and the reader is advised to review Chapter 18 for a detailed discussion. The most commonly used approach at our Institution is the 3D contrast-enhanced technique with gradient-echo (GRE) imaging. Non-contrast angiographic techniques such as time-of-flight (2D and 3D) and PC-MRA are rarely used.

Our scan protocol starts with three plane localizer images in the axial, sagittal, and coronal planes, which are low-resolution images and are only used to plan further image acquisitions. The localizer images are acquired without breath holding while all subsequent images are acquired during breath hold, with breathing held in end-expiration for each scan. The localizer scan is followed by HASTE images in a coronal plane, extending from the dome of the liver to below the aortic bifurcation to display the abdominal aorta anatomy. The coronal HASTE images are used to prescribe anatomic coverage of 3D MRA, which extends from the dome of the liver to below the aortic bifurcation in the superior–inferior direction and from 4–5 cm anterior to the portal vein bifurcation to mid-kidney in the anterior–posterior direction (Figure 20.1).

The next step is to set up the scanning parameters for mesenteric MRA (Table 20.2). A coronal orientation is generally used for 3D abdominal aorta imaging, which aids in the assessment of the abdominal aorta and renal arteries in addition to the mesenteric arteries. We routinely employ the parallel imaging technique with an acceleration factor of 2, which significantly speeds up the image acquisition. The field-of-view is reduced as much as possible, avoiding the wrap-around artifacts with a right-to-left phase-encoding direction for the coronal imaging plane. TR and TE are typically set at the minimum possible, in order to have the shortest total scan time and to minimize susceptibility effects. We aim for the highest spatial resolution possible (around 1–1.5 mm) with isotropic or near isotropic voxels for optimum 3D image reconstruction. We make sure that the acquisition time is short enough for a single breath hold. To make the scan shorter if needed, we decrease the phase-encoding steps with or without increasing slice thickness and decreasing the number of slices to maintain the same volume coverage.

A precontrast acquisition is initially obtained and serves as a mask for subsequent subtraction of soft tissues from post-contrast images. The mask image is also used to assess the adequacy of anatomic coverage and the absence of significant wrap-around artifacts. The pre- and post-contrast images need to be acquired with identical scanning parameters for successful subtraction. After the precontrast image acquisition, Gd-DTPA is injected and the abdominal aorta is imaged with a fast 2D real-time sequence for contrast arrival followed by 3D MRA acquisition as described above (Figure 20.2). Accurate timing of data acquisition in relation to contrast injection is essential in depicting the vascular structures of greatest interest. After the first MRA (arterial phase), the patient is allowed 3–4 quick breaths and the MRA is repeated to acquire the venous phase for portal vein imaging (Figure 20.3). Additional delayed acquisition after several breaths may be acquired at the equilibrium phase.

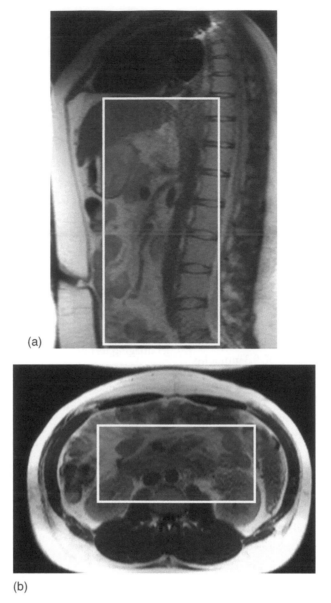

Figure 20.1   Sagittal (a) and axial (b) HASTE images showing the prescription box for the anatomic coverage for mesenteric MRA.

An alternative technique, called time-resolved MRA, displays multiple phases of contrast transit by acquiring very fast 3D volumes as the contrast is being injected. This technique provides multiple high-resolution images of blood vessels with a high temporal resolution and without the need for timing image acquisition over contrast injection.

Image analysis

The images are generally reviewed on a dedicated workstation where the 3D image data set can be manipulated in the axial, coronal, or sagittal planes as needed. The importance of first reviewing the MRA unsubtracted source images cannot be

overstated. The process of subtraction can remove important information from the data set or introduce errors that can be avoided by reviewing the source images. Stenoses of mesenteric artery primarily affect the ostium or the proximal portion of the vessels and a sagittal view is ideal for the display of source images and evaluation of disease. Additionally, axial images can display the ostium of mesenteric vessels very well. After source image review, further assessment can be performed by 3D image reconstructions. The three major types of image reconstructions used are volume rendering (VR), maximum intensity projection (MIP), and multi-planar reconstruction (MPR). VR reconstruction provides a 3D image of the abdominal aorta and its branches in relation to surrounding structures (Figure 20.4). However, this format is not very use-

Table 20.2 Imaging parameters for mesenteric contrast-enhanced MRA

Parameters	Description
Superior–inferior coverage	Dome of liver to below the level of iliac bifurcation
Anterior–posterior coverage	4–5 cm anterior to portal vein bifurcation to mid-kidney
Plane orientation	Coronal
Mode	3D
TE (ms)	Minimum
TR (ms)	Minimum
Flip angle (degrees)	20
Band width (Hz/pixel)	810
Matrix – Frequency	384
Matrix – Phase	269
Typical spatial resolution (mm)	1.9×1.3×1.5
Averages	1
Acceleration factor	2
Field-of-view	32–40
Slice thickness (mm)	1.5 mm
Slices (n)	60
Gd-DTPA dose and infusion rate	0.2 mmol/kg at 2 ml/s

ful for clinical assessment of vascular stenosis. For clinical diagnostic purposes, thin- or thick-slab MIP is preferable. MIP images can display limited or extended vascular segments by adjusting the slice thickness (Figure 20.2). Although MIP images provide high contrast between vessel and surrounding tissues it may overlook an eccentric plaque or focal stenosis, particularly if thick MIP images are used. As a rule, concurrent evaluation of the corresponding source thin section and MRP images is essential for optimal study interpretation.

CLINICAL APPLICATIONS

All diseases and conditions that affect the arteries in general have been reported to affect the mesenteric arteries, including atherosclerosis, arteritis, aneurysms, emboli, thrombosis, dissections, infections, and fibromuscular dysplasia. The most common vascular problem affecting the intestines is ischemia, which can be acute or chronic in presentation.

Chronic mesenteric ischemia

Chronic mesenteric ischemia, also called 'intestinal angina', is an uncommon but well described disorder in patients with

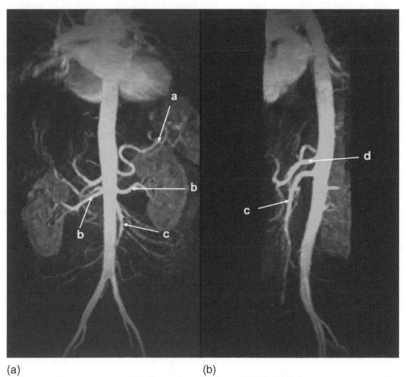

(a)   (b)

Figure 20.2 Coronal (a) and sagittal (b) maximum intensity projection (MIP) images derived from coronal 3D GRE source data set showing the abdominal aorta and its major branches (a: splenic artery, b: renal arteries, c: superior mesenteric artery, d: celiac axis).

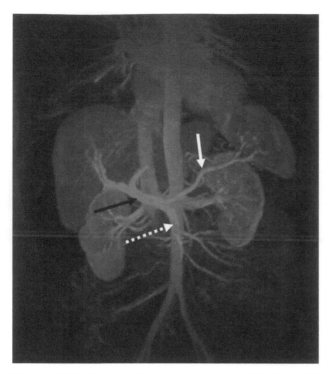

Figure 20.3 Portal vein anatomy demonstrated on 3D GRE images in the late vascular phase. The splenic vein (solid white arrow) joins the superior mesenteric vein (dashed white arrow) to form the portal vein (solid black arrow).

mesenteric atherosclerotic disease. Patients are often female (70%) and have recurrent episodes of abdominal pain, usually within the first hour after eating and subsiding over the course of the next 2 hours, food phobia, and weight loss. The typical patient has risk factors or established vascular disease, with the majority of patients having peripheral vascular disease or coronary artery disease. Symptoms are often progressive and some patients may develop acute mesenteric ischemia due to plaque rupture and thrombosis. Physical findings are usually non-specific and may include an abdominal bruit in 50% of patients.

The celiac, SMA, and IMA are all extensively interconnected and therefore under usual circumstances proximal occlusion of one artery is well tolerated. The classical syndrome requires occlusion of at least two of the three intestinal arteries. However, there are well-documented cases of intestinal ischemia as a result of only SMA stenosis. The typical lesions are located at the origin of vessels from the aorta and in most cases are in the form of protruding aortic plaques. Duplex ultrasonography for the detection of high-grade stenosis of celiac and SMA can be accomplished in the majority of patients with >90% accuracy in highly experienced laboratories. Both contrast-enhanced MRA and CT angiography are well suited for visualizing the typical plaques at the

origin of intestinal arteries. In particular, the use of gadolinium-enhanced MRA has been found to be very promising in patients with suspected chronic mesenteric ischemia with high values of sensitivity and specificity when compared to invasive angiography (Figures 20.5 and 20.6). In some cases, measurement of fasting and post-prandial blood flow in the superior mesenteric vessels by PC-MRA may be helpful in the diagnosis of chronic mesenteric ischemia. The usefulness of MRA and CTA is less reliable in detecting more distal lesions. Invasive arteriography provides the definitive diagnosis of intestinal lesions and in selected patients a percutaneous endovascular treatment of intestinal arterial stenosis can be performed at the same time.

Acute mesenteric ischemia

Acute intestinal ischemia is an abdominal emergency with an in-hospital mortality of 60–80%. Acute mesenteric ischemia commonly occurs either as a result of embolism, acute thrombosis on a pre-existing atherosclerotic plaque, or a low flow state due to systemic illness (non-obstructive mesenteric ischemia). Embolic mesenteric occlusion is commonly associated with a cardiac or proximal aorta source of embolism. The presence of pre-existing SMA atherosclerosis with a history of chronic abdominal pain and weight loss is a risk factor for the development of acute SMA thrombosis. In most cases, a non-obstructive acute mesenteric ischemia is reported. This generally affects elderly patients with low cardiac output states or those with sustained mesenteric vasoconstriction. Patients with acute mesenteric ischemia usually present with sudden onset of severe abdominal pain that is out of proportion to the abdominal examination findings. If the ischemia progresses, patients can develop abdominal distension, gastrointestinal bleeding, and signs of peritoneal irritation. Rapid diagnosis is essential to avoid the catastrophic outcome associated with bowel infarction. Plain abdominal X-rays are usually of very low diagnostic yield for most of the important causes of acute abdomen. Late findings may include thumb printing due to bowel edema or hemorrhage and the presence of pneumatosis or portal vein gas consistent with bowel infarction. Duplex scanning is potentially useful but is highly user dependent and can be technically difficult in these patients due to body habitus, presence of bowel gas and ascites, or tortuous and deeply located intestinal arteries. CT may reveal bowel wall thickening, ascites, pneumatosis, portal vein air, atherosclerotic disease of intestinal arteries, or obvious thrombosis of proximal intestinal arteries. However, most of these signs are non-specific and appear in late stages of

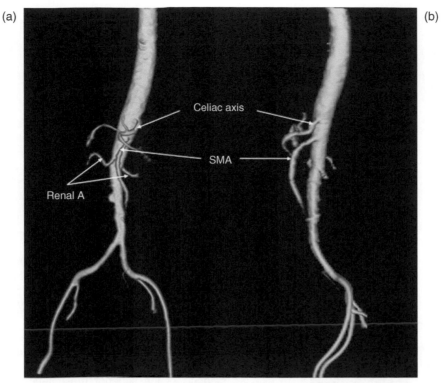

Figure 20.4 Coronal (a) and sagittal (b) 3D volume rendering reconstructed from a 3D GRE data set showing the celiac axis, superior mesenteric artery (SMA), and the renal arteries.

the disease. Additionally, administration of intravenous iodinated contrast material may affect the results of later angiography.

MRA can provide much more detailed information about the mesenteric vessels and the small bowel. However, human data comparing the sensitivity and specificity to conventional angiography are lacking. Typical early MRI features of ischemic bowel include bowel wall thickening and edema, best appreciated on T2-weighted, single-shot echo-train fat suppressed images. There is typically fluid accumulation along the serosal margins of the involved bowel. Although these features may overlap with other etiologies, the diagnosis may be suspected based on the combination of imaging features and clinical presentation. In addition, patients with underlying atherosclerotic disease will demonstrate mural plaque on vascular imaging obtained with dedicated mesenteric MRA. It has yet to be determined whether non-invasive studies can accurately detect the presence of small thromboemboli, early reversible ischemia, or non-occlusive ischemia. Selective mesenteric angiography and digital subtraction angiography are still considered the gold standard in the setting of suspected acute mesenteric ischemia. Apart from diagnosing occlusive mesenteric disease and differentiating from non-obstructive mesenteric ischemia, angiography also provides important

pre-operative information for mesenteric bypass surgery. Furthermore, catheter-based intervention of arterial stenosis is also possible in some patients. However, its use in the emergency setting is controversial and some experts feel that performing angiography will delay surgical treatment for critically ill patients and recommend taking patients directly to surgery.

Mesenteric venous thrombosis and portal hypertension

Thrombosis of the mesenteric veins accounts for approximately 5–15% of the episodes of acute mesenteric ischemia. On the other hand, chronic mesenteric venous thrombosis is usually asymptomatic and is often discovered on abdominal imaging performed for some unrelated reason. Mesenteric venous thrombosis has multiple causes, including hypercoagulable state, abdominal malignancies, cirrhosis, abdominal infections, blunt abdominal trauma, pancreatitis, prior abdominal operations, oral contraceptive use, and inflammatory bowel disease. Approximately 20% of cases may be idiopathic. Abdominal ultrasound can diagnose portal vein thrombosis and show ascites and intestinal edema. However, superior mesenteric and splenic

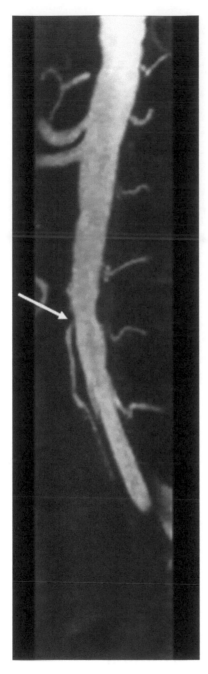

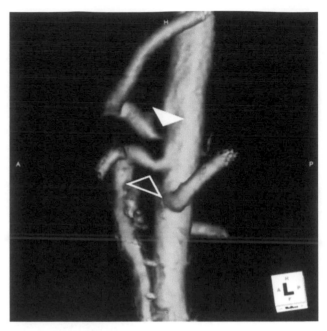

Figure 20.6 Volume-rendering image from 3D contrast-enhanced GRE images showing a severe ostial stenosis of the celiac trunk (closed arrow head) and a mild ostial stenosis of the superior mesenteric artery (open arrow head).

Figure 20.5 Oblique MIP images reconstructed from coronal 3D GRE images showing a narrowing at the origin of inferior mesenteric artery (arrow).

and superior mesenteric veins. Determining the venous flow characteristics with PC techniques can also complement 3D MRA.

Accurate assessment of portal venous system anatomy and patency is essential for management decisions in patients with hepatic cirrhosis and portal hypertension. The ability of MRA to display the portal venous system in axial and coronal planes may be helpful in planning a transjugular intrahepatic portosystemic shunt.

Pre- and post-liver transplant evaluation

MRA is routinely used for mesenteric vascular imaging in patients with chronic liver disease. Abdominal MRI and mesenteric MRA help in pre-liver transplant planning, liver and tumor surveillance in patients waiting for liver transplantation, and assessment of vascular complications after liver transplantation, e.g. transplant hepatic artery stenosis.

CONCLUSIONS

Three dimensional MRA techniques allow a comprehensive and accurate evaluation of mesenteric arteries and veins

venous thrombosis is difficult to diagnose on ultrasound. CT is considered a test of choice and can show thrombosis in the portal, superior mesenteric, and splenic veins with or without mucosal edema or pneumatosis.

The value of MRA as an alternate non-invasive technique for diagnosing mesenteric venous thrombosis is increasingly being recognized (Figure 20.7). The use of 3D MRA has been found to have 90% agreement with intra-arterial angiography for the evaluation of portal, splenic,

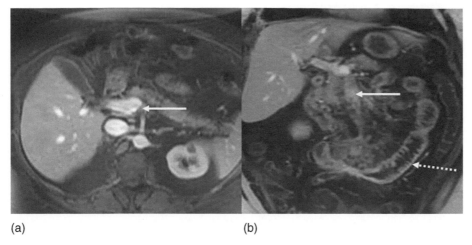

(a)   (b)

Figure 20.7 Superior mesenteric vein (SMV) thrombosis. Axial post-contrast 3D GRE images in the late vascular phase showing SMV thrombosis (solid arrow, a). In the same patient, coronal post-contrast GRE images in the late vascular phase show the SMV thrombosis (solid arrow, b) and secondary edematous bowel wall thickening (dotted arrow, b).

using a single gadolinium injection and in one setting. A variety of disease states directly or indirectly affecting the mesenteric vascular anatomy and patency can be readily identified and serially followed. Technical advances have allowed for data acquisition with high spatial resolution within a comfortable breath hold time, making MRA a method of choice for studying the mesenteric circulation.

PRACTICAL PEARLS

- A complete evaluation of mesenteric vessels always includes visualization of the mesenteric arterial as well as the venous system.

- The mesenteric arteries originate from the anterior aspect of the abdominal aorta and particular attention needs to be paid to avoiding their accidental exclusion from the acquired 3D volume.

- Concurrent evaluation of the source thin section images is essential for optimal study interpretation in addition to thin- or thick-slab MIP reconstruction.

FURTHER READING

Batellier J, Keny R. Superior mesenteric artery embolism: eighty two cases. Ann Vasc Surg 1990; 4: 112–16.

Bradbury AW, Brittenden J, McBride K, Ruckley CV. Mesenteric ischemia: a multidisciplinary approach. Br J Surg 1995; 82: 1446–59.

Dalman RL, Li KC, Moon WK, Chen I, Zarins CK. Diminished postprandial hyperemia in patients with aortic and mesenteric arterial occlusive disease. Quantification by magnetic resonance flow imaging. Circulation 1996; 94 (Suppl 9): II206–10.

Hagspiel KD, Leung DA, Angle JF et al. MR angiography of the mesenteric vasculature. Radiol Clin North Am 2002; 40: 867–86.

Hirsch AT, Haskal ZJ, Hertzer NR et al. Peripheral Arterial Disease: ACC/AHA 2005 Guidelines for the Management of Patients With Peripheral Arterial Disease (Lower Extremity, Renal, Mesenteric, and Abdominal Aortic): A collaborative Report From the American Association for Vascular Surgery/ Society for Vascular Surgery, Society for Cardiovascular Angiography and Interventions, Society for Vascular Medicine and Biology, Society of Interventional Radiology, and the ACC/AHA Task Force on Practice Guidelines (Writing Committee to Develop Guidelines for the Management of Patients With Peripheral Arterial Disease). J Am Coll Cardiol 2006; 47: 1239–312.

Holland AE, Goldfarb JW, Edelman RR. Diaphragmatic and cardiac motion during suspended breathing: preliminary experience and implications for breath-hold MR imaging. Radiology 1998; 209: 483–9.

Kim AY, Ha HK. Evaluation of suspected mesenteric ischemia: efficacy of radiologic studies. Radiol Clin North Am 2003; 41: 327–42.

Laghi A, Iannaccone R, Catalano C, Passariello R. Multislice spiral computed tomography angiography of mesenteric arteries. Lancet 2001; 358: 638–9.

Laissy JP, Trillaud H, Douek P. MR angiography: noninvasive vascular imaging of the abdomen. Abdom Imag 2002; 27: 488–506.

Meany JF, Prince MR, Nostrand TT et al. Gadolinium enhanced magnetic resonance angiography in patients with suspected chronic mesenteric ischemia. J Magn Reson Imag 1997; 7: 171–6.

Rodgers PM, Ward J, Baudouin CJ, Ridgway JP, Robinson PJ. Dynamic contrast enhanced MR angiography of the portal venous system: comparison with X-ray angiography. Radiology 1994; 191: 741–5.

Yasuhara H. Acute mesenteric ischemia: the challenge of gastroenterology. Surg Today 2005; 35: 185–95.

21

MR angiography of the lower extremity circulation with protocols

John Grizzard, Dipan J Shah, Igor Klem, and Raymond J Kim

INTRODUCTION

Peripheral arterial disease (PAD) is a common problem worldwide, with an estimated 20 million patients in the US alone. Although most patients with PAD are asymptomatic, it is common to present with lower extremity symptoms such as claudication and sometimes with atypical lower extremity symptoms. A much smaller percentage of patients may present with symptoms of critical limb ischemia. Although the initial assessment of the patient is performed with physical exam, often supplemented by lower extremity ankle brachial indices and segmental pressures, most patients will ultimately require imaging of the vasculature prior to definitive surgical or percutaneous therapy. Magnetic resonance angiography (MRA) has emerged over the last decade as a preferred modality in imaging PAD. Earlier time-of-flight techniques had significant limitations due to prolonged imaging times and image artifacts, contrast-enhanced MRA using a multi-station bolus-chase technique is now a rapid and robust technique that consistently allows comprehensive imaging from the level of the abdominal aorta to the proximal pedal vessels. Figure 21.1 is an example of the coverage and image quality now possible with MRA. In any MR exam, there are virtually an unlimited number of permutations of parameters such as scan duration, resolution, slice thickness, etc. The user can be easily overwhelmed by the variety of choices available. It is the goal of this chapter, therefore, to provide the reader with a practical approach to high-quality MR imaging of the lower extremity arteries. The physics will be discussed as it relates to practical issues related to imaging this vascular bed. For other details the reader is referred to Chapters 12 and 13. Protocols and their application in lower extremity disorders as well as the rationales for those choices will be presented, so that the reader will have a sense of the options available, and will understand the relative advantages and disadvantages of each. Table 21.1 outlines the common indications for MRA of the abdominal, pelvic, and lower extremity vessels in individuals presenting with lower extremity symptoms. Atherosclerotic PAD is by far the commonest indication for imaging and MRA and is usually indicated in the evaluation of the symptomatic patient presenting with either intermittent claudication or critical limb ischemia (rest pain, ulceration, or both).

ANATOMIC CONSIDERATIONS

The anatomic considerations pertinent to imaging are covered in Chapter 11. The reader is requested to refer to this chapter for these details.

FUNDAMENTALS OF LOWER EXTREMITY ARTERIAL IMAGING

The physics of MR angiographic sequences is discussed in detail in Chapter 13. The selection of sequences used in

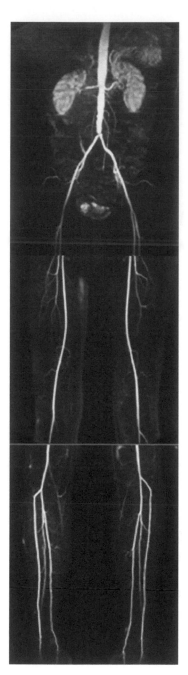

Figure 21.1   Three station MRA demonstrating the coverage and scan quality now available on a routine basis.

Table 21.1   Indications for MRA of the lower extremity
Diagnosis

• Atherosclerotic PAD (claudication and chronic critical limb ischemia)
• Arteritis and inflammatory disorders
  – Buerger's disease
  – Giant cell arteritis
  – Systemic lupus erythematosis
  – Pseudoxanthoma elasticum, Ehlers–Danlos syndrome
  – Takayasu's arteritis
• Embolization
  – Proximal aneurysm (popliteal/femoral/abdominal)
  – LV thrombus
  – Ulcerated atherosclerotic plaques
• Dissection
• Congenital
  – AV malformations
  – Hypoplasia and acquired coarctation of the abdominal aorta ('mid-aortic syndrome')
• Miscellaneous
  – Fibrodysplasia (external iliac artery)
  – Popliteal etiologies (adventitial cystic disease, entrapment)
  – Persistent sciatic artery

peripheral MRA is based on their ability to fulfill a specific imaging purpose. As in any MR sequence, the user must weigh the relative advantages and trade-offs between improved spatial resolution and prolongation of imaging time, but these issues take on special importance in imaging of the lower extremities. In the lower extremities, the need to image small structures with adequate resolution must be balanced with the need to image these arterial structures before venous filling contaminates the image. As a general rule, the resolution used and the slice thickness will vary such that the lower leg station is performed with the highest resolution and the thinnest slices. Automated table movement along with dedicated peripheral phased-array coils is required for covering the abdomen, pelvis, and lower extremities in one single exam. The table movement between stations should allow for overlap of the imaged anatomy, so that no gaps in coverage occur. For example, for a scanner with a 400 mm field-of-view, the table movement should be 375 mm between stations (5 cm overlap). In cases where a short patient is imaged on a large field-of-view scanner, the degree of overlap can be increased (Tables 21.2–21.5).

Pulse sequences in MRA of the lower extremities

Localization sequences

Localizers should allow a global overview of the anatomy of the abdomen and lower extremities, and should facilitate easy identification of vascular structures within the imaged

Table 21.2 Acqusition parameters for localizer sequences

Sequence	Localizer coronal	Localizer sagittal	Localizer transverse
TR (ms)	3	3	3
TE (ms)	1.5	1.5	1.5
Flip angle (degrees)	64	64	64
Slice thickness (mm)	8	8	8
Number of slices	15	18	20
Field-of-view (mm)	500×500	500×500	500×500
Matrix (lines)	256×180	256×180	256×180
Averages	1	1	1
Acceleration factor	0	0	0
Band width (Hz/pixel)	900	900	900
Scan duration (s)	23	23	23

Table 21.3 Acquisition parameters for 3D contrast-enhanced MRA (Siemens, Avanto)

	Abdomen/pelvis	Thigh	Calf	Calf time-resolved
TR (ms)	2.9	3.51	3.51	2.91
TE (ms)	1.1	1.25	1.25	1.07
Flip angle (degrees)	20	25	25	30
Slice thickness (mm)	1.4	1.4	1.2	1.3
Number of slices	88	80	104	60
Field-of-view (mm)	500×375	500×406	500×406	500×400
Matrix (lines)	384×245	512×291	512×291	448×186
Spatial resolution (mm)	1.4×1.3×1.4	1.4×1.0×1.4	1.4×1.0×1.2	1.9×1.1×1.3
Averages	1	1	1	1
Acceleration factor	2	2	2	2
Band width (Hz/pixel)	500	360	360	470
Scan duration (s)	15	21	26	8.5
k-Space acquisition	Linear	Linear	Centric	Centric

Table 21.4 Traditional 3D contrast-enhanced MRA (Siemens Symphony, without IPAT)

	Abdomen/pelvis	Thigh	Calf
TR (ms)	3.6	3.8	4.8
TE (ms)	1.5	1.7	1.8
Flip angle (degrees)	20	25	25
Slice thickness (mm)	1.5	1.4	1.1
Number of slices	64	56	80
Field-of-view (mm)	500×333	500×344	500×406
Matrix (lines)	384×182	512×194	512×291
Spatial resolution (mm)	1.8×1.3×1.5	1.7×1.0×1.4	1.4×1.0×1.2
Averages	1	1	1
Acceleration factor	NA	NA	NA
Band width (Hz/pixel)	450	490	270
Scan duration(s)	19.8	19	43
k-Space acquisition	Linear	Linear	Centric

Table 21.5 Traditional 3D-contrast-enhanced MRA (GE SIGNA 1.5 T ECHOSPEED)

	Abdomen/pelvis	Thigh	Calf
TR (ms)	5	5	5
TE (ms)	MIN (2)	MIN (2)	MIN (1)
Flip angle (degrees)	30	30	30
Slice thickness (mm)	3.6	3.6	3
Number of slices	34	36	32
Field-of-view (mm)	440×296	440×296	440×296
Matrix (lines)	256×160	256×160	256×192
Spatial resolution (mm)	1.7×1.8×3.6 (Interpolated to appear 1.8)	1.7×1.8×3.6 (Interpolated to appear 1.8)	1.7×1.5×3.0 (Interpolated to appear 1.5)
Averages	1	1	1
Acceleration factor	NA	NA	NA
Band width (MHz)	62.5	31.25	31.25
Scan duration (s)	20	19	29
k-Space acquisition	Centric	Centric	Elliptic centric
Interpolation	ZIP2	ZIP2	ZIP2

volume. Low-resolution steady-state free precession images (True-FISP/FIESTA/Balanced FFE) images are ideal for this purpose and can be acquired in three planes in less than 30 seconds (Table 21.2). These allow bright-blood imaging of the vascular system and usually suffice for vessel localization. In occasional circumstances, black-blood half Fourier acquisition single-shot turbo spin-echo (HASTE) sequences can be obtained to improve vessel conspicuity, as can two-dimensional time-of-flight images, but these are not usually necessary.

3D Gradient-echo angiographic sequences

The contrast-enhanced three-dimensional angiographic data set is acquired using a heavily T1-weighted spoiled gradient-echo sequence obtained in the coronal plane (3D Turbo FLASH or SPGR). This sequence is the cornerstone of 3D contrast-enhanced MRA, and is repeated at every imaging station. It is T1 weighted in order to visualize the intra-arterial contrast, which produces shortening of the T1 of blood from 1200 ms to approximately 150 ms. Spoiling is used to destroy any residual transverse magnetization and to accentuate the T1 weighting. The flip angle used is variable, but is usually in the range of 20 to 35°. (Note: Older texts may make reference to techniques using higher flip angles; however, this was usually done because older gradient systems were limited in the minimum TR achievable, and thus required higher flip angles for adequate tissue

suppression (Tables 21.2–21.5). These are not necessary for the more recent generations of scanners.) The sequences can be performed with fat saturation in the abdomen/pelvis and upper leg stations, but with an increase in imaging time, and a decrease in signal-to-noise ratio. Additionally, subtraction of the post-contrast images from the precontrast mask images also results in improved vessel conspicuity and may be sufficient.

Supplementary sequences

Often, additional imaging to characterize the vessel wall may be desired, particularly in the abdomen, to better delineate the interface between thrombus, atheroma, and lumen. Sequences that may be chosen for this purpose include black-blood HASTE images or a fat-saturated volumetric T1 gradient-echo sequence such as the volumetric interpolated breath hold examination (VIBE) imaging. This sequence is a gradient-recalled-echo sequence similar to that of a 3D sequence used for MRA, with two main differences. The echo read-out for a VIBE sequence is symmetric, in contrast to an asymmetric echo for a dedicated MRA sequence. In addition, the flip angle is reduced to 12° to 15°. The purpose of these two changes is to improve the signal from the background tissue structures. These can be added to the standard protocol with only a minimal increase in scan time. They are particularly useful in characterizing aneurysms, and may be obtained in regions where these are prevalent, such as the abdomen, inguinal regions, and popliteal fossae, to screen for aneurysms that could be missed on luminographic images alone. In addition to allowing improved characterization of the vessel wall, these sequences can also be helpful in evaluating other abdominal and pelvic structures seen on the scans (Chapter 18).

Parallel imaging

The addition of parallel imaging (IPAT/SENSE /ASSET) technology has made peripheral run-off MRA significantly more robust, with fewer failed studies and with improved image quality (Chapter 12). In its most common implementation, an acceleration factor of 2 is used, resulting in a decrease in imaging time by slightly less than half or increased spatial resolution (up to 2-fold). Most often, the improved efficiency is used to obtain some combination of both decreased time and improved resolution. The cost of this improvement relative to the non-accelerated technique is a decrease in signal-to-noise ratio by a factor of 1 divided by the square root of the acceleration factor (in this case 2). That is, for a 2-fold increase in speed, the signal-to-noise drops to approximately 70% of the non-accelerated technique, not 50%. Gadolinium-enhanced 3D MRA is usually a signal-rich imaging study, and the trade-off is advantageous. At facilities having this capability, MRA is almost always performed using parallel imaging technology. The parameters used for the coronal 3D acquisition will depend on a variety of factors and specific recommendations for various scanners will be given in following sections. Imaging choices represent compromises between competing priorities of spatial resolution and time available to complete the acquisition.

CLINICAL PROTOCOL CONSIDERATIONS

Patient preparation and scan set-up

Prior to scanning, the procedure must be explained to the patient, and emphasis should be placed on the need to remain still during the exam. This is particularly important given the multiple subtractions that will be required and will frequently reduce the patient's anxiety, making the experience easier for the patient. If the patient has rest pain, or skin ulceration, they should be reassured that appropriate care will be taken of the affected limb. An IV is required,

and 20 gauge is preferred, although a 22 is acceptable given the low rate of contrast infusion. An antecubital vein is preferred; hand veins may be used if necessary, although transit times will be prolonged. The patient should be placed on the table entering the gantry feet first, and the phased-array extremity coils placed, with attention to the patient's comfort. Additional body coils will often be placed over the lower abdomen, just above the extremity coil assembly. The patient should be notified that the table will move intermittently during the exam, and that compressive devices may be placed about the thighs to minimize venous contamination. A dual head power injector with the capability of multiphase bolus administration is preferred. Saline flush should be loaded along with the contrast in the injector prior to scan initiation.

Scanning

The scan protocol will vary somewhat depending on the protocol selected (see below). In general, the scan sequence will be initiated with low-resolution scout true FISP images at the abdominal station, the upper leg station, and the lower leg station. Depending on user preference, additional localizers using either HASTE images or phase contrast images can also be used to localize the vessels of interest to ensure that they are enclosed in the imaging volume. Subsequently, higher resolution non-contrast images are obtained in all three stations, beginning at the lower leg and proceeding cephalad to the upper leg and the abdomen/pelvis station. Subsequently, the scan is initiated, either following a timing bolus or using fluoroscopic triggering. High-resolution angiographic images are obtained with the identical scan protocol used for the precontrast data set, and in-line subtraction can be preprogrammed, as can the creation of MIP images. The patient initiating a breath hold at the start of the scan improves image quality at the abdomen/pelvis station. The table is then moved sequentially such that the upper leg and lower leg stations are sequentially acquired. Two acquisitions at the lower leg level may be performed, to insure that if there is significant disparity in flow, both legs will be adequately imaged with arterial contrast present.

Field of view. In general, the field-of-view should be maximized in order to obtain the maximum anatomic coverage for any given scanner, and to minimize the number of table movements required to encompass the desired anatomy. Newer scanners with a 500 mm field-of-view allow scanning from the diaphragm to the pedal vessels in three stations in virtually all patients, but on scanners with a 400 mm field-of-view, four stations will often be needed in taller patients (Tables 21.3–21.6).

Slab thickness (partition thickness). The slab thickness must be sufficient to cover the vessels of interest, and the slice thickness, number of slices, and the desired resolution are selectable parameters that can be varied to achieve the desired blend of spatial resolution, signal-to-noise, and imaging speed (Tables 21.3–21.6). As can be seen in Figures 21.2 and 21.3, changes in imaging resolution, slice thickness, and number of slices all have an impact on scan duration.

Various other manipulations, including half-scanning techniques (useful if parallel imaging is not available, but should not be used with acceleration), use of a rectangular field-of-view, and zero-filling interpolation are available in most modern scanners, and will be considered in the protocol selection.

k-Space ordering schemes. An additional important parameter to be considered is the ordering of k-space acquisition. Centrically ordered acquisitions are useful when the user wishes to acquire the central k-space data containing contrast information right at the start of image acquisition, such as when imaging the lower leg as the last station in a bolus chase acquisition. At that point, contrast will already be present in the arteries, and the user will wish to rapidly fill the central lines of k-space prior to venous filling (Tables 21.3–21.6). This is also useful when using a bolus-triggered technique, as will be described below.

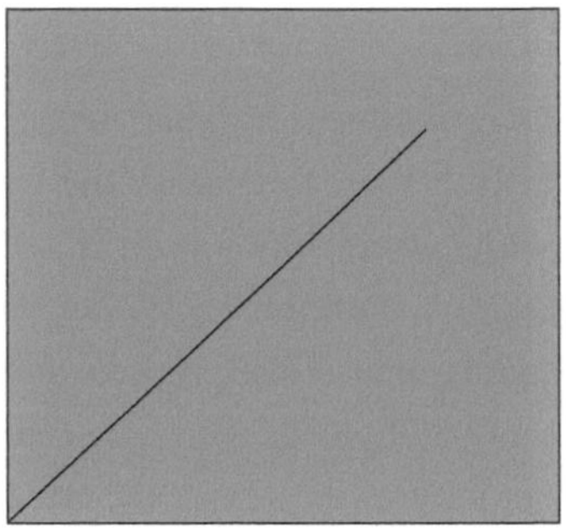

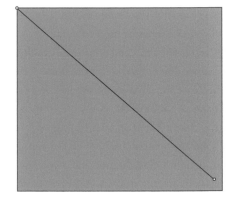

Figure 21.2 For a given region of coverage, as the slice number or resolution increases, the scan duration increases.

Figure 21.3 For a given slab of coverage, as the slice thickness decreases (better spatial resolution), the number of slices and the imaging time increase.

Table 21.6 Traditional 3D contrast-enhanced MRA (Philips Intera 1.5 T Scanner)

	Phillips Intera 1.5 T	Software V11.1	
	Abdomen/pelvis	Thigh	Calf
TR (ms)	5.7	5.7	5.7
TE (ms)	1.6	1.6	1.6
Flip angle (degrees)	35	35	35
Slice thickness (mm)	1.5	1.5	1.5
Number of slices	70	70	70
Field-of-view (mm)	430×302	430×302	430×302
Matrix (lines)	512×512	512×512	512×512
Spatial resolution (mm)	1.5×0.8	1.5×0.8	1.5×0.8
Averages	1	1	1
Acceleration factor	N/A	N/A	N/A
Band width (Hz/pixel)			
Scan duration (s)	40	40	40
k-Space acquisition	Linear	Linear	Linear

Contrast and timing issues

Although timing is critical in all implementations of contrast-enhanced MRA, this is especially true in multi-station bolus-chase MRA, where mistakes in timing may have a cumulative effect. Two imperatives must be remembered regarding timing in run-off MRA:

(1) As always, the acquisition of the central lines of k-space must be synchronized to the presence of contrast in the arterial system.

(2) The acquisitions need to be completed before venous filling occurs, particularly at the lower leg level.

Synchronization of the image acquisition with the arterial phase of contrast passage can be performed with use of a timing bolus or with the bolus triggering technique.

Timing bolus. A timing bolus acquisition consists of a series of one per second T1-weighted image acquisitions obtained in the axial plane through the region of the vessel of interest, for example the abdominal aorta at the level of the renal arteries. A 1 cm thick axial FLASH or SPGR acquisition is initiated simultaneously with the injection of 1 to 2 ml of contrast and 25 ml of flush, all administered at 2 ml/s. The image with maximal opacification (not the first image with contrast) can be determined visually or by using a region of interest placed in the aorta with subsequent computer calculations. The appropriate time for the initiation of the scan is then calculated using the formula (assuming linear ordering of k-space data):

Scan delay = circulation time + (the injection duration/2)
          − (the scan duration/2)

For example, an MR angiogram of the abdominal aorta that takes 18 s to acquire might be performed using 20 ml of contrast administered at a rate of 2 ml/s. The injection duration is 10 s, and the scan duration is 18 s. The circulation time obtained from visual evaluation of the axial images of a small test bolus is 19 s. Therefore, 19 + 5 − 9 equals 15 s is the appropriate time for the scan delay. Thus, the contrast injection is initiated, and 15 s later the scan is initiated. This results in the mid-way point of the arterial phase of the contrast injection and the mid-way point of the image acquisition both occur simultaneously at 24 s after the start of the contrast injection. In actuality, it is desirable to have contrast present and at a relatively stable level throughout the scan. The foregoing formula represents 'conventional wisdom' regarding the use of a timing bolus, and the dynamics of the bolus passage are not addressed; specifically, the degree to which the bolus 'spreads out' during its passage. One could

argue that the reason this technique works is due to this prolongation of bolus duration, which allows far greater contrast 'presence' than is called for by the formula, and more nearly approximates the ideal. One could also argue that timing might actually be done most easily by simply choosing the start time of the scan to equal the circulation time (defined above as the time of maximum opacification). No calculations are then necessary, and the scan will be obtained with contrast present in a steady state.

One advantage of the test bolus technique as outlined above is that the scan will actually start simultaneously with the arrival of the maximum plateau phase of the contrast, with no time lost switching from scan monitoring to image acquisition, and the arterial phase of contrast passage will coincide with the center of k-space acquisition. Therefore, this scan will finish and the next position can be obtained more rapidly than when using a bolus triggering approach.

Bolus triggering. With a bolus triggering technique, the contrast is administered as intended for the scan, and multiple one per second images of the abdominal aorta are obtained in the coronal plane and displayed in real time on the scanner console. Scan triggering is then usually performed by the technologist based on the visualization of arterial contrast in the vessels of interest. Automated triggering can also be performed using measurement of a region of interest, with scan initiation occurring when the specified region of interest exceeds a predetermined signal intensity threshold. When using the bolus triggering technique, since contrast is already present throughout the vasculature at scan initiation, centric ordering of k-space acquisition is advised. The main advantage of the bolus triggering technique is the ease of use; most technologists feel very comfortable with fluoroscopically-monitored bolus-triggered techniques. Also, variation from the patient's baseline for any number of reasons is accounted for by the real-time nature of the scan initiation.

Contrast administration. Various studies have evaluated bolus optimization strategies. Given the prolonged scan times when viewed in aggregate, and the desire to minimize venous opacification, most often a biphasic contrast administration is chosen with an initial rate of approximately 1.2 to 1.5 ml/s for half the bolus administration followed by 0.4 to 0.5 ml/s for the remainder of the injection. This latter rate approximates the tissue extraction rate, which would allow arterial opacification with theoretically no venous filling. This results in a prolonged arterial phase of injection, with slow and delayed filling of the venous structures. For combined imaging of the abdomen, pelvis, and lower extremities, typically 35 to 40 ml of contrast are administered.

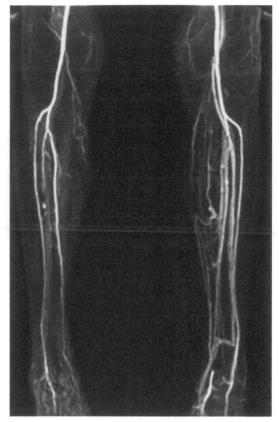

Figure 21.4 Standard image at calf station showing venous contamination on the left, while timing on the right is appropriate.

Minimizing venous contamination. The presence of venous contamination in run-off studies ranges in severity from being a nuisance that minimally complicates image interpretation (see Figure 21.4) to rendering an interpretation nearly impossible. In any case, the desire to minimize its presence drives much of the selection of imaging parameters and bolus administration techniques used. Venous contamination can be minimized by:

(1) Completing imaging in less than 45–60 s (as a general rule) after study initiation as, beyond these times, there is a high likelihood of venous contamination. Venous circulation times however show considerable interindividual variation. The presence of critical limb ischemia may increase the likelihood of venous contamination, while the presence of diminished cardiac output (typified by the patient with myocardial infarction) may result in reduced venous contamination due to a prolongation of the arterial phase.

(2) Using a biphasic administration of gadolinium with a lowered rate of injection for the second bolus (e.g 1.5 ml/s for the first phase and 0.8 ml/s for the second phase), along with a slow prolonged infusion flush.

(3) Using venous compression devices at the level of the thighs (with pressures set to less than or equal to 50 mmHg) to delay venous filling. Note: this technique should be used with caution in patients with bypass grafts, as the grafts are often superficial in location and subject to compromise by the compression device. Use of this technique has been recently reported in a series of 32 patients, and was demonstrated to slow down arterial transit times, increase arterial signal-to-noise, and reduce venous contamination.

Alternative and supplementary techniques

Despite the optimization of imaging and contrast administration parameters, the frequent presence of venous contamination in the lower legs has stimulated the search for alternative techniques that can minimize this problem. In addition, although most patients tolerate the venous compression techniques well, some patients find them objectionable, and, as above, patients with prior bypass grafts should probably not undergo thigh compression. Therefore, alternative techniques have been sought that can minimize the problem of venous contamination in the lower leg station. Hybrid imaging techniques along with time-resolved angiographic techniques have been utilized for this purpose.

Time-resolved MRA in conjunction with 3D contrast-enhanced MRA

This is a common supplementary sequence typically performed before 3D MRA acquisition detailed above. Time-resolved techniques are based on the use of shared echo lines, where data are shared from one 3D data set to the other (Chapter 13). While the center of k-space is repetitively sampled, the periphery of k-space is only intermittently sampled. This allows a reduction in sampling time and thereby improvement in the temporal resolution. This technique enables rapid updating of 3D data sets in several seconds, eliminating the need for timing acquisitions or triggering methods. Each acquisition is typically performed with the matrix size of 448×192 (acquisition time for the first measurement (used as the background mask) that involves sampling k-space in its entirety, takes longer then subsequent measurement owing to preparatory pulse sequences). Sequential acquisitions are obtained during administration of 8 ml of contrast at 1 ml/s followed by 30 ml of flush, with up to 15 sequential acquisitions obtained. Each acquisition is subtracted from the mask image, and only the resulting MIP image in the coronal plane is saved. The 15 MIP images generated are subsequently viewed as a movie loop.

Following the performance of the time-resolved sequence the study is performed in the conventional fashion, with sequential table movement into the upper leg and abdomen–pelvis stations for procurement of the mask images. The antegrade bolus-chase technique is then used in the conventional fashion using the remainder of the contrast administration previously described. This technique has the advantage of being able to successfully image the arteries of the lower leg free of venous contamination, and also allows for visualization of discrepant flow if one leg is more severely diseased and has slower flow than the other (Tables 21.7 and 21.8). Figures 21.4 and 21.5 show how this technique can be helpful in obtaining images free of venous contamination.

Hybrid imaging

A newer strategy that may be used to solve the problem of venous contamination in the calf vasculature is the use of a dedicated high-resolution imaging study at the lower leg level performed prior to imaging of the abdomen and pelvis. In this technique, initial mask images of the lower legs are obtained, followed by a timing bolus acquisition centered on the popliteal arteries. Using this timing bolus, appropriate imaging delay is instituted, and 15 ml of contrast at a rate of 1 ml/s with flush also administered at 1 ml/s for 25 ml. Two sequential 3D high-resolution coronal image acquisitions are then obtained. Subsequently, the abdomen–pelvis and upper legs are imaged in the standard fashion as previously described using approximately 25 ml of contrast. Standard imaging triggering techniques are used, and the table is moved one time. This technique was found to yield diagnostic images free of venous overlay in 95% of studies, and has demonstrated good agreement with selective DSA. Other groups have reported similar findings, with a significant improvement in diagnostic accuracy at the calf level compared with standard bolus-chase methods.

Post-processing/image interpretation

In-line subtraction of the post-contrast images from the pre-contrast mask image can be programmed in advance to be automatically performed, along with creation of MIP images in various imaging planes. Typically, post-processing will also include a series of coronal MIP images that are rotated through 360°. The full volume MIP image provides a quick review of the arterial structures, but review of the source images is required as well, as the MIP algorithm can result in obscuration of important findings. Since a MIP is created by

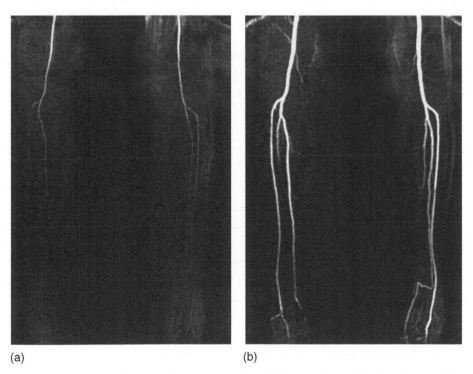

(a)   (b)

Figure 21.5 Time-resolved images with early (a) and then optimal (b) arterial opacification, (same patient as Figure 21.4).

Table 21.7   Sequence of steps for 3D contrast-enhanced MRA (Siemens Avanto) without time-resolved angiography

1. Patient placed in magnet feet first, and centered at mid-abdomen
2. Abdomen true–FISP scout localizers (3 planes) – 20 s
3. Table moves 375 mm (pt <5'10") or 420 mm (pt >5'10") – 2 s
4. Upper leg 3 plane scout – 20 s
5. Table moves (see above) – 2 s
6. Lower leg 3 plane scout – 20 s
7. 3D standard angio non-contrast acquisition at lower leg (26 s)
8. Table moves to upper leg station – 2 s
9. 3D standard angio non-contrast acquisition – 21 s
10. Table moves to abdomen/pelvis station – 2 s
11. 3D standard angio non-contrast acquisition – 15 s
12. Contrast indicator clicked ON (VERY IMPORTANT)
13. CARE-Bolus acquisition (in coronal plane centered on aorta) started
14. Contrast injected at 1.4 ml/s for 18 ml, then at 0.4 ml/s for remainder with flush at 0.4 ml/s
15. 3D angio data set of abdomen/pelvis post-contrast acquisition triggered when contrast seen in abdominal aorta – 15 s. (in-line subtraction from precontrast mask preprogrammed, along with SAG and COR MIPs)
16. Table moves to upper leg level –2 s
17. Upper leg 3D post-contrast angio data set obtained –21 s (with in-line subtraction, MIPs preprogrammed)
18. Table moves to lower leg station – 2 s
19. Lower leg 3D angio data set acquired × 2 – 26 s each (sub/MIPs etc prepprogrammed)
20. Additional VIBE post-contrast sequences at abdomen, femorals, popliteals

Note: For venous studies following arterial studies, simply rerun the sequence in reverse order – wait approximately 30 s and re-acquire the lower leg, then the upper leg, then the abdomen/pelvis

a ray-tracing algorithm through a volume of tissue, it may miss lesions that are adjacent to high signal structures along the ray path. For example, in Figure 21.6 the full-volume MIP image shows an irregularity of the proximal right common iliac artery that might easily be interpreted as atherosclerotic plaque. However, review of the source images in thin sections clearly demonstrates the presence of clot. Therefore, complete analysis of the angiographic data sets requires simultaneous interrogation of the axial, sagittal, and coronal imaging planes using the source data reviewed in multi-planar reformation mode on a commercially available workstation. Review of the unsubtracted data set at the abdominal station is recommended, as it allows visualization of the vessel wall, and not just the lumen, as may be the case on subtracted images. In addition, other abdominal structures included in the study but poorly depicted by MIPs can also be better seen. Figure 21.7 demonstrates a renal cell carcinoma that is better visualized on thin MIPs and axial reformatted images than on standard MIP images. Sliding thin submaximal MIP images also allow visualization of the arteries without overlap of overlying structures, and are often

useful as well. Multi-planar curved reformations can be performed as needed.

Modern workstations can also create images using the volume-rendering technique, as well as endoscopic views of the images. The volume-rendered 3D images can be impressive and are well received by clinicians (Figure 21.8). They are, however, not well suited for diagnostic purposes due to their tendency to either overestimate or underestimate lesions depending on the algorithm and thresholds used.

Automated evaluation of stenoses and MR angiographic data sets would simplify image interpretation, and potentially allow a more accurate, quantitative evaluation of the cross-sectional areas of stenosis. A study looking at the accuracy of semi-automated analysis of 3D contrast-enhanced MR angiographic data sets for the detection and quantification of aorto-iliac stenoses using commercially available software found that the overall sensitivity for the detection of stenosis was approximately 89%, with a specificity of 88%. Further studies are needed to validate this concept, but it certainly has intuitive appeal.

Table 21.8 Sequence of steps for 3D contrast-enhanced MRA (Siemens Avanto) with time-resolved angiography

1. Patient placed in magnet feet first, and centered at mid-abdomen
2. Abdomen true–FISP scout localizers (3 planes) – 20 s
3. Table moves 375 mm (pt <5'10") or 420 mm (pt >5'10") – 2 s
4. Upper leg 3 plane scout – 20 s
5. Table moves (see above) – 2 s
6. Lower leg 3 plane scout – 20 s
7. Contrast injected at 1 ml/s for 8 ml total, with 25 ml flush at 1 ml/s
8. Time-resolved dynamic acquisition
9. 3D standard angio non-contrast acquisition at lower leg (26 s)
10. Table moves to upper leg station – 2 s
11. 3D standard angio non-contrast acquisition – 21 s
12. Table moves to abdomen/pelvis station – 2 s
13. 3D standard angio non-contrast acquisition – 15 s
14. Contrast indicator clicked ON (VERY IMPORTANT)
15. CARE–Bolus acquisition (in coronal plane centered on aorta) started
16. Contrast injected at 1.4 ml/s for 18 ml/s then at 0.4 ml/s for remainder with flush at 0.4 ml/s
17. 3D angio data set of abdomen/pelvis post-contrast acquisition triggered when contrast seen in abdominal aorta – 15 s (in-line subtraction from precontrast mask preprogrammed, along with SAG and COR MIPs)
18. Table moves to upper leg level – 2 s
19. Upper leg 3D post-contrast angio data set obtained – 21 s (with in-line subtraction, MIPs preprogrammed)
20. Table moves to lower leg station – 2 s
21. Lower leg 3D angio data set acquired × 2 – 26 s each (sub/MIPs, etc. preprogrammed)
22. Additional VIBE post-contrast sequences at abdomen, femorals, popliteals prn*

Note: For venous studies following arterial studies, simply rerun the sequence in reverse order – wait approximately 30 s and re-acquire the lower leg, then the upper leg, then the abdomen/pelvis
*VIBE images may be obtained at the femoral and popliteal levels on an 'as needed (prn) basis'

CLINICAL APPLICATIONS

Atherosclerotic peripheral vascular disease

This is the most common indication for MRA of the lower extremity circulation. This section will address the more common presentations of atherosclerotic peripheral arterial disease, recognizing that significant overlap occurs. In addition, given that such imaging is usually performed prior to either surgical or percutaneous intervention, emphasis will be placed on a discussion of findings relevant to planned interventions. In short, we will address what the surgeon or interventionalist needs to know.

Aorto-iliac disease. High-grade occlusive disease of the terminal aorta or proximal iliac arteries often results in Leriche syndrome, a clinical entity characterized by the triad of diminished or absent femoral pulses, gluteal or thigh claudication, and impotence in males. Pallor and wasting of the lower extremities may also be seen in extreme cases. The aortic or proximal iliac occlusive disease may be total, as in Figure 21.9, or may be partial, as seen in Figure 21.1. Distal disease involving the femoral and tibio-peroneal circulation may frequently coexist.

In analyzing MRA images in such patients, note should be made of the degree of stenosis, as well as the status of collateral vessels. The anatomic extent of stenosis or occlusion and the level at which the native circulation is reconstituted are quite important, as this will determine the feasibility of percutaneous or surgical approaches. Specifically, the status of the more distal iliac and femoral arteries becomes extremely important. For example, the length of iliac or femoral occlusion often determines whether or not the

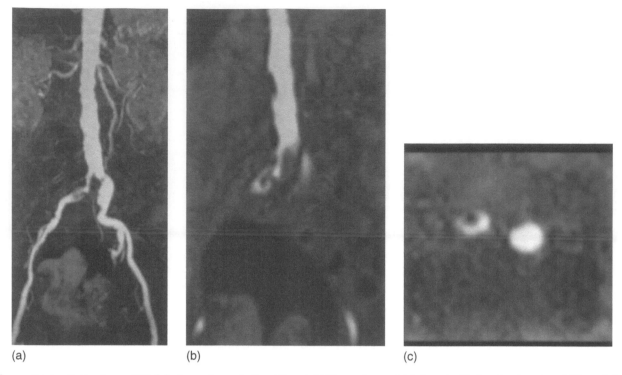

(a)   (b)   (c)

Figure 21.6 Full-volume MIP (a) shows irregularity of the right iliac artery, which is noted to be due to a focal filling defect on thin-section MIP (b), and is shown to be clot on axial image (c).

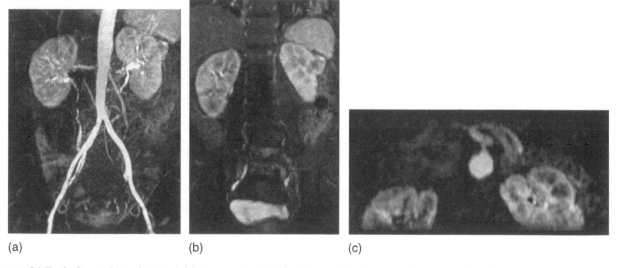

(a)   (b)   (c)

Figure 21.7 Left renal carcinoma (a) better seen on subvolume MIP (b) and axial reformation (c).

patient is a candidate for percutaneous treatment, or will require some open surgical therapy. In the treatment of long segment bilateral iliac occlusions or stenosis in conjunction with aneurysmal disease, aorto-bifemoral bypass grafting may be preferable due to its superior patency in the long term (> 95% patency rates at 5 years). For short segment iliac disease, even if bilateral, endovascular therapy is preferable (Figures 21.10 and 21.11).

Superficial femoral artery (SFA) disease. Occlusive disease of the superficial femoral artery is often surprisingly symmetric bilaterally. High-grade occlusions often result in claudication of the calf musculature on walking, and if accompanied by severe run-off disease, may progress to rest pain (Figure 21.12).

Analysis of MR angiographic images in this circumstance requires attention again to the length of the occluded

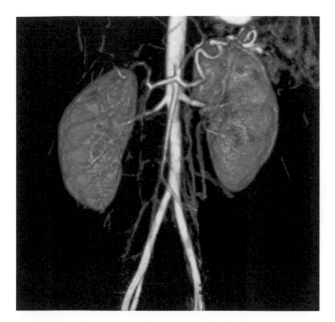

Figure 21.8 Volume-rendered MRA in color.

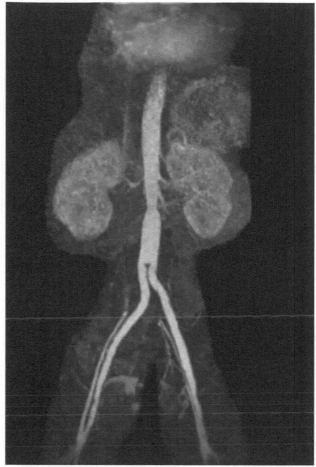

Figure 21.10 MRA demonstrating an aortobifemoral graft.

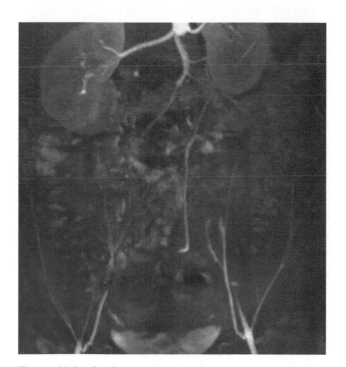

Figure 21.9 Aortic occlusion just distal to the renal arteries.

or narrowed segment, as short segment occlusions are capable of percutaneous treatment while longer segment occlusions more often require grafting. Particular attention should be paid to the level of reconstitution.

The level of resumption of a normal vessel caliber and its extent are quite important as it serves as the likely site of distal anastamosis. Also, if the anastomosis can be made proximal to the articular portion of the popliteal artery, synthetic graft material remains a viable choice, sparing the patient's native veins for future use if necessary. However, if it is necessary to traverse the knee joint, synthetic material is usually not advised, and native veins are preferred.

Percutaneous treatment of infrainguinal atherosclerotic disease continues to evolve and the reader is referred to the recent literature. Percutaneous treatment may prove to be quite helpful for patients who are poor operative candidates. Percutaneous treatment of SFA disease is plagued by higher rates of restenosis, but may still be an option in patients who are poor operative candidates. Additionally this is often first-line therapy in individuals presenting with critical limb ischemia, patients who often have substantial multi-segment multi-level disease and usually benefit from therapy aimed at improving distal limb flow. Subintimal recanalization techniques have been developed in such patients, which often allow limb salvage (Figure 21.13).

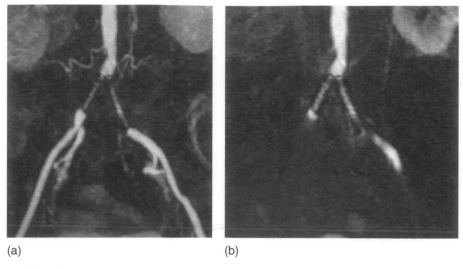

(a)   (b)

Figure 21.11   Thick (a) and thin (b) MIP images from a patient with bilateral iliac artery stents.

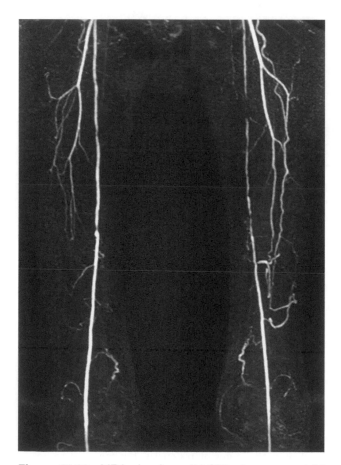

Figure 21.12   MRA showing mild SFA plaques on right and multisegmental occlusive disease on the left.

Distal (tibio-peroneal) disease. The usual patient with infra-articular distal (run-off) disease often presents with critical limb ischemia (rest pain, lower extremity ulceration, or both). Diabetics in particular are at risk for distal small vessel involvement (Figure 21.14). Early venous filling and

arteriovenous shunting is not uncommon in patients with severe run-off disease, particularly in those with cellulitis, and coexisting soft tissue infection may complicate image interpretation (Figure 21.15). In fact, if the patient is known to have a foot or lower leg ulcer, steps to shorten image acquisition are recommended, which implies that the final (distal station) acquisition on a bolus chase exam should be initiated well prior to 45 s. Thus this implies that the preceding stations are acquired rapidly. The use of a time-resolved angiographic acquisition in this circumstance in conjunction with the traditional 3D MRA is often very helpful and may be the only set of images procured without venous contamination.

The status of the popliteal artery, the tibio-peroneal trunk, and the vessels of the lower leg often determine whether or not the patient is a candidate for possible revascularization, or whether amputation is likely in the presence of rest pain. Given the multi-segmental nature of atherosclerotic disease, improvements in inflow alone (e.g. iliac or common femoral disease) may sometimes result in limb salvage, with more targeted intervention targeting the distal circulation planned at a later date, provided this is possible.

The status of the distal vasculature is important. The study should demonstrate which, if any, vessels are patent in a continuous fashion from the knee to the ankle. In addition, likely sites of possible anastomosis should be identified, as should the caliber of the vessel distal to that point. It is often helpful to prepare unsubtracted images for demonstration of bony landmarks for the referring physician, in order that the angiographic images may be correlated to the patient's anatomy. Using thin section MIP images to eliminate venous overlap can minimize venous contamination if present.

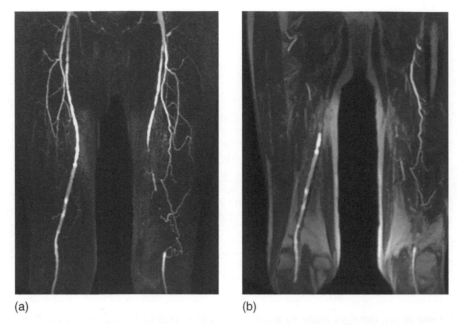

(a)　　　　　(b)

Figure 21.13 Thick (a) and thin (b) MIP images from a patient status post right SFA nitinol stent placement. Note also the left SFA occlusion.

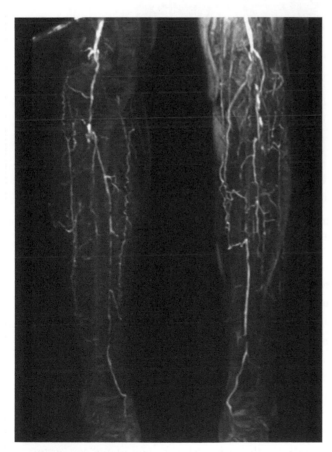

Figure 21.14 Diabetic patient with severe bilateral run-off disease. Note that no single vessel extends in continuity from the knee to the ankle.

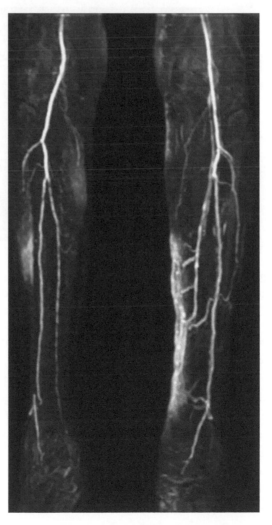

Figure 21.15 Patient with cellulitis of the medial aspect of the left leg and the lateral aspect of the right leg.

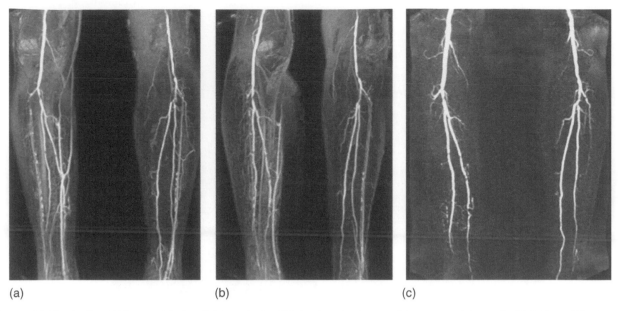

(a) (b) (c)

Figure 21.16 In the AP image (a), the right posterior tibial artery is obscured by an overlying vein. Rotation of the image (b) offsets the vein, revealing significant posterior tibial artery disease, which is confirmed on the time-resolved image (c).

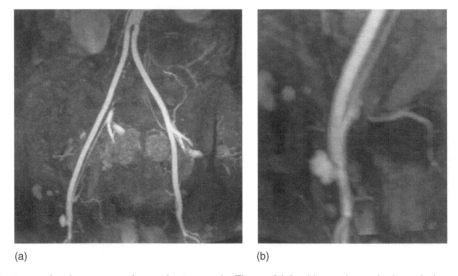

(a) (b)

Figure 21.17 Postoperative images on the patient seen in Figure 21.9 with aortic occlusion s/p bypass grafting with a pseudoaneurysm at the anastomosis. Pelvic MRA (a) and magnified view (b) of the anastomosis.

In addition, rotating the imaging to various obliquities can also sometimes help (Figure 21.16).

Imaging of the pedal vessels may sometimes be required, and they may or may not be adequately imaged on the standard multi-station bolus-chase angiography. In individual circumstances, 2D time-of-flight images can be used at the time of the initial study as this is felt to be a clinical consideration. Alternatively, a dedicated high-resolution stationary exam of the pedal circulation can be performed at a separate time.

Graft surveillance. Ultrasound imaging is most commonly used for graft surveillance. Prompt identification of graft disease and progression of lesions in the inflow vessels can lead to appropriate graft revision and salvage. Aortobifemoral grafts (Figure 21.10) are widely used for the treatment of long segment iliac artery occlusions. Synthetic graft materials do not present a problem for MR imaging, but occasionally clips at the site of the surgical anastomosis may produce artifact. Anastamotic complications including pseudoaneurysm formation can be well visualized. Figure 21.17 a and b depicts images from the patient shown in Figure 21.9 with aortic occlusion, now status post-aorto-bifemoral surgery, and a resultant pseudoaneurysm at the right femoral anastamosis. In addition, because of the capability of reformatting the images into virtually any plane,

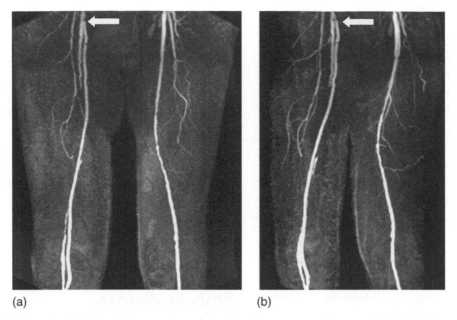

Figure 21.18   Mild stenosis at origin of fem-pop bypass graft better seen on oblique projection (b), than on AP image (a).

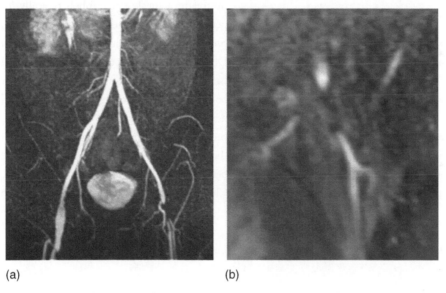

Figure 21.19   Apparent left femoral artery occlusion (a) is actually due to stent artifact (b).

rotation of the data set allows improved visualization of the surgical anastomosis. In Figure 21.18, note that in this patient with a right femoropopliteal bypass, the straight AP view of the anastomosis at the femoral site is poorly rendered due to overlap. However, upon rotation, a mild to moderate stenosis is unmasked.

Stents. Endovascular stent placement is frequently performed to increase the long-term patency of percutaneous interventions. These are commonly placed in the iliac region (Figure 21.11), but placement into the femoral vessels is also commonly performed (Figure 21.13). As can be seen from these examples, visualization of luminal contrast in the presence of stents may be possible depending on the composition of the stent. Specifically, nitinol-containing stents (as seen in Figure 21.13) usually produce minimal if any artifact. However, stainless steel stents, particularly the Palmaz stent, usually result in such significant signal drop-out that luminal visualization is not possible. In fact, the appearance often suggests the presence of a short segmental occlusion (Figure 21.19). However, the true nature of the abnormality is easily clarified if radiographs are available. If not, recognition of the sharply marginated border and the absence of collaterals should make one suspicious that a stent is present rather than a true occlusion. In addition, review of thin section multi-planar images from the unsubtracted source images will often allow depiction of the stent artifact. Patients who are status post-endovascular stent graft treatment of an abdominal aortic aneurysm may subsequently present for run-off imaging as well. It should be noted that most of the current versions of the stent grafts produce minimal if any artifact. MRA has been well studied in evaluation of patients status post-covered stent graft repair of abdominal aortic aneurysm, and has been found to be superior to CT for the detection of endoleak. In this setting, delayed imaging through the aorta is necessary, and is often best performed with a T1-weighted, fat-saturated, 3D volume technique (VIBE). Figure 21.20 is from a patient who is status post-endograft repair of an abdominal aortic aneurysm. Note the excellent depiction of the vessel lumen with minimal artifact. No evidence of delayed endoleak is seen on the accompanying 3D volumetric acquisition (Figure 21.20b).

Buerger's disease and arteritis

Buerger's disease, also known as thromboangiitis obliterans, is a disorder predominantly affecting young male smokers. However, the disorder is increasingly being recognized in women smokers, and so the disorder is not exclusively limited to male patients. This disorder produces an obliterative arteritis of the medium and small vessels of the peripheral extremities, affecting both the upper and lower extremities. The characteristic angiographic hallmark that allows accurate recognition is the presence of extensive distal occlusive

disease accompanied by the development of 'corkscrew collaterals'. In Figure 21.21, an illustrative case is presented. Note the characteristic absence of distal run-off arteries, and the presence of multiple, irregular collaterals. It can often be differentiated from the more common atherosclerotic disease by the relative preservation of the proximal vessels. Arteritis such as Takayasu's and other collagen vascular disease involves the proximal iliac arteries and the abdominal vasculature predominantly. In these disorders there is often evidence of vessel wall thickening and gadolinium uptake on post-contrast T1-weighted images. Thus if there is clinical suspicion, careful evaluation of the abdominal, visceral, and renal arteries is indicated.

Embolic disease

Peripheral arterial emboli affecting the lower extremity circulation typically originate either in the heart or the aorta upstream of the lesion. Emboli typically lodge in the more peripheral vessels, where their size precludes further migration, or at sites of pre-existing stenosis (see Figure 21.6). Depending on the abundance of collaterals, the degree of ischemia that results can be quite profound and MRA, if it is to be performed, must be performed urgently. Figure 21.22 demonstrates the presence of a popliteal clot in a patient who presented with the acute onset of lower leg ischemia on the left. One can see from these images the excellent correlation between the MR appearance and the angiographic appearance. Clot lysis was performed with intra-arterial thrombolytics and

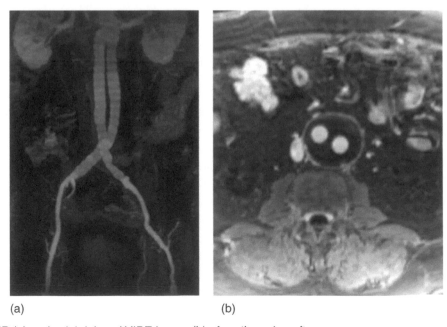

(a)   (b)

Figure 21.20   MIP (a) and axial delayed VIBE image (b) of aortic endograft.

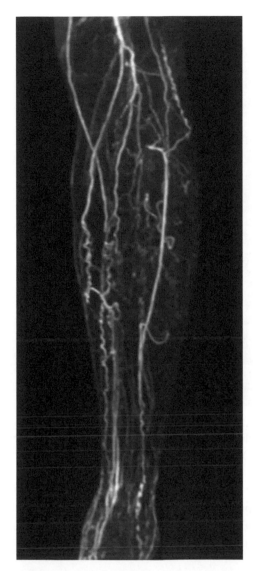

Figure 21.21 Buerger's disease. Note the characteristic 'corkscrew' appearance of the collateral vessels, and the occlusive disease of the trifurcation vessels.

restoration of patency was achieved, as can be seen in the accompanying figures. In such cases, detailed attention should be paid to the evaluation of the more proximal aorta, and a cardiac imaging study to exclude intraventricular thrombi may also be helpful. Figure 21.23 is a thin section image reconstruction from an MR angiogram of the thoracic aorta performed to evaluate for the source of recurrent peripheral embolism, and demonstrates a left atrial thrombus. Cardiac MR imaging may be superior to echocardiography for the detection of ventricular thrombi, and dedicated cardiac MR evaluation should be considered in such patients.

Aneurysms and dissection

Although atherosclerotic aneurysms predominately involve the infrarenal abdominal aorta, they can be seen in any of the vessels in the pelvis and lower extremity circulation. A general rule of thumb for labeling a segment as an aneurysm is that it should exceed the native reference vessel diameter by 150%. Therefore, a 1.2 cm segment of dilatation in a vessel that in adjacent normal segments measures 8 mm would represent a localized aneurysm. Abdominal aneurysms are often associated with femoral and popliteal aneurysms. These latter aneurysms are particularly prone to thrombosis and distal embolization. Thus every patient with an abdominal aortic aneurysm should be evaluated for the presence of femoral and popliteal aneurysms. Evaluation for aneurysms should include review of the source images and additional complementary sequences (e.g. VIBE, as outlined earlier) so as not to miss the vessel wall pathology.

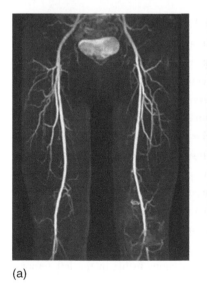

(a)

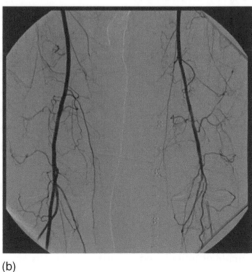

(b)

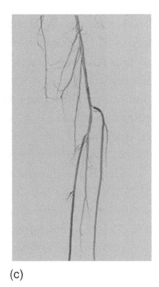

(c)

Figure 21.22 Clot occludes the left popliteal artery on MRA (a), and is confirmed on DSA (b). After intra-arterial thrombolysis, restoration of patency is demonstrated (c).

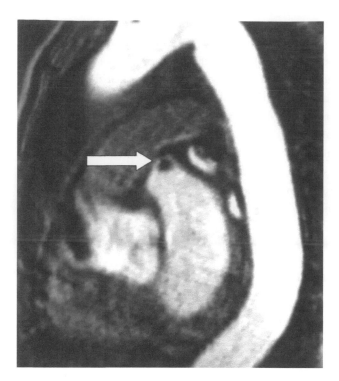

Figure 21.23 Left atrial clot seen on thin-section review of thoracic MRA.

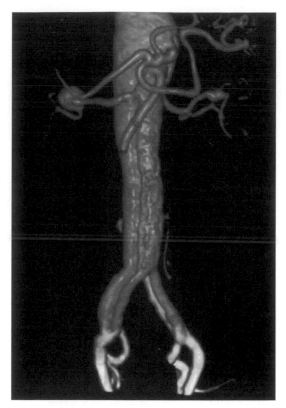

Figure 21.24 Color volume-rendered image of aortic dissection extending into the iliac arteries. Note the incidental renal artery aneurysms.

Spontaneous abdominal and/or iliac dissection is relatively less common than propagation of a dissection originating in the thoracic aorta. Figure 21.24 demonstrates the appearance of an aortic dissection extending from the thoracic aorta into the iliac vessels. Note the excellent depiction of the filling pattern of the various vascular structures on this volume-rendered MR angiographic image. The delineation of true and false lumen in addition to the origin of visceral or limb vessel branches from these is an important piece of information to be gleaned from an MR angiographic study of dissection cases. Relative contributions of the true and false lumens to the supply of the abdominal and pelvic vasculature are extremely important, and close attention should be paid to the relative perfusion patterns of the visceral organs. In particular, disparate perfusion of the kidneys is often evident in such patients and should be evaluated.

When spontaneous aortic or iliac dissections do occur, there is often an underlying connective tissue abnormality present, such as Ehlers–Danlos syndrome, as depicted in Figure 21.25. This patient had a spontaneous right common iliac artery dissection, which extended into the right external iliac artery. This was subsequently treated with a covered stent graft, with exclusion of the false lumen, resulting in resolution. Note that the stent graft is made of nitinol, and produces minimal artifact.

Pseudoaneurysms occur most often due to prior trauma, or may represent a complication of surgical therapy. For an example of a post-surgical pseudoaneurysm, please refer to Figure 21.10.

Arteriovenous malformations and fistulas

Both arteriovenous fistulas and arteriovenous malformations (AVMs) result in abnormal early opacification of venous structures. AVMs are congenital anomalies in which there are abnormal connections between the arterial and venous structures, without an intervening capillary bed (Figure 21.26, AVM of the mid-portion of the left foot). The abnormal early venous filling during the arterial phase of imaging identifies the AVM in the latter illustration. Time-resolved imaging may occasionally be helpful in such instances, but a rapid frame rate is necessary for this purpose. Arteriovenous fistulas are more commonly traumatic in origin, and may result from iatrogenic causes, especially following cardiac catheterization at the level of the common femoral artery. Figure 21.27 demonstrates a patient who has an arteriovenous fistula in the left femoral artery, resulting from a prior catheterization procedure.

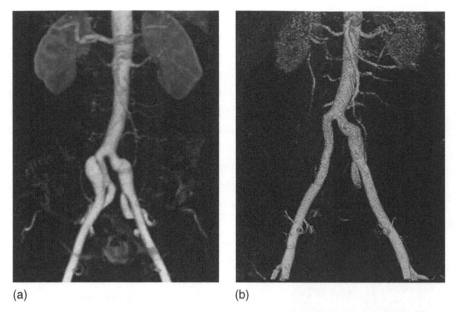

Figure 21.25 Pre-intervention (a) and post-intervention (b) images from a patient with right iliac artery dissection treated with a covered stent graft. Note the absence of stent artifact.

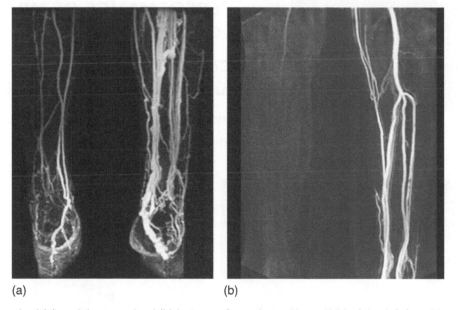

Figure 21.26 Standard (a) and time-resolved (b) images of a patient with an AVM of the left foot. Note the early venous filling on the left which cannot be mitigated even with time-resolved imaging.

Congenital disorders and miscellaneous

Uncommon causes of aortic narrowing include abdominal coarctation, also known as mid-aortic syndrome. This may be associated with other systemic arterial abnormalities as may be seen with Williams syndrome, or may occasionally be seen in association with neurofibromatosis. In this disorder, an area of constriction is present in the mid-portion of the abdominal aorta, and is often associated with bilateral renal artery stenosis. Figure 21.28 demonstrates a volume-rendered image as well as an angiographic imaging of such a patient.

Patients with Klippel–Trenaunay–Weber syndrome may occasionally present for angiographic imaging. In this disorder, abnormal arteriovenous connections may be present, and hemihypertrophy or hemiatrophy of the distal lower extremity is often seen. Abnormalities both of the arterial supply and of the draining veins may be present. (*Note*: some authors separate Klippel–Trenaunay syndrome

[KTS] from Parke–Weber syndrome [PWS], while others lump the two together as Klippel–Trenaunay–Weber syndrome. The distinction is that classic KTS has only anomalous venous structures and is a low-flow disorder, while PWS patients have AV fistulae and high-flow lesions and do

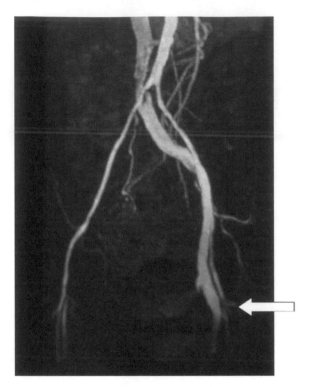

Figure 21.27   AV fistula secondary to prior catherization procedure.

less well.) Delayed imaging in the venous phase may be helpful in evaluation of such patients.

Popliteal entrapment syndrome is a disorder that results from abnormal medial placement of the medial head of the gastrocnemius muscle, resulting in compression of the popliteal artery in the popliteal fossa during exercise. This disorder may go unrecognized if imaging is not performed with the patient attempting plantar flexion. In cases where this disorder is suspected, dedicated imaging at the level of the popliteal arteries is suggested, both at rest and with provocative maneuvers.

Cystic adventitial disease is an uncommon disorder resulting in localized arterial narrowing that may progress to occlusion, often involving the popliteal arteries. It is characterized by the development of myxoid cystic changes of the adventitia, with resultant compression of the vessel lumen. Review of the axial source images is important in its recognition.

PERFORMANCE OF MRA OF THE LOWER EXTREMITIES

Comparison with digital subtraction angiography (DSA)

MRA has been well validated for the detection and quantification of stenoses and occlusions in the aortoiliac and

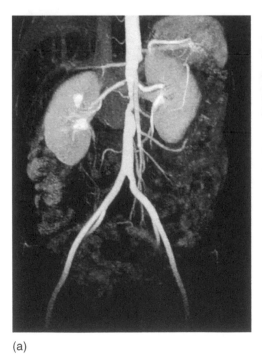
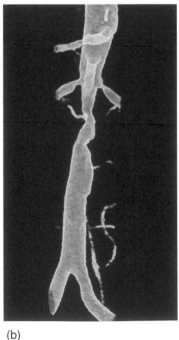

(a)   (b)

Figure 21.28   MIP (a) and VRT (b) images of mid-aortic syndrome. Note the bilateral renal artery stenoses which are frequent co-existing findings.

femoral vessels. Initial studies used 2D time-of-flight imaging, and demonstrated a high level of agreement with conventional angiography in the iliofemoral region. In the lower legs, 2D time-of-flight MRA detected all vessels identified by conventional angiography, and in addition demonstrated an additional 22% of run-off vessels that were not identified with conventional arteriography. The detection of these additional vessels altered the surgical management of the disorders in 17% of cases. Three-dimensional contrast-enhanced MRA has now superseded 2D time-of-flight imaging, and shows an improved sensitivity and specificity. Several studies have demonstrated the superiority of contrast-enhanced MRA over 2D time-of-flight angiography, with contrast-enhanced MRA demonstrating a significantly faster imaging time and a larger coverage area than did 2D time-of-flight angiography. The contrast-enhanced MR angiogram also allowed better visualization of the pedal vessels than 2D time-of-flight imaging. As expected, the 3D contrast-enhanced MR angiographic images were found to be significantly less prone to artifact. In particular, 3D contrast-enhanced MRA was able to visualize vessels with reversed diastolic flow, or if the flow extends in a retrograde fashion as is often the case with collateral vessels.

Multiple recent studies have demonstrated that contrast-enhanced MRA performed with a bolus-chase moving-table technique has a sensitivity and specificity greater than 95% when compared with catheter angiography.

MRA vs multi-slice CT angiography (MSCTA) for run-off imaging

MSCTA using multi-slice spiral acquisitions has emerged recently as a non-invasive alternative to MRA. In this technique, rapid thin section imaging is performed in the axial plane from the level of the renal arteries to the feet during the prolonged administration of contrast material, 16-slice scanners have made this technique feasible, and are becoming widely available. In addition, newer 64-slice scanners are now available, and also allow thinner slice acquisitions and more rapid scanning. In fact, timing of the arterial bolus becomes important due to the ability of the scanner to outrun the contrast bolus.

A study of 157 consecutive patients randomized to either MSCTA using a 16-slice scanner or bolus-chase MRA using a high-performance gradient system demonstrated a minimal difference in observer diagnostic confidence favoring MSCTA, which was not statistically significant, and which diminished with increased observer experience. The patients

in the MR angiogram group required slightly more follow-up vascular imaging, likely related to the slightly decreased confidence. However, the same researchers subsequently also demonstrated that the interobserver agreement for MRA was higher than that for MSCTA for evaluating the degree of arterial stenosis or occlusion. In particular, the presence of calcification significantly decreased the interobserver agreement of multi-detector MSCTA for the evaluation of stenosis. The small calf vessels with calcification present were the most problematic area. The authors did note that a high number of non-diagnostic segments were found on MRA, and speculated that performing an initial high-resolution sequence of the tibial vessels would reduce the number of non-diagnostic segments.

Other studies have demonstrated that in the aorto-iliac and renal arteries, the performance of MRA and MSCTA was essentially identical. Anecdotally, the image interpretation time required for MSCTA is significantly higher than that for MRA, largely due to the presence of calcification within the vessels of interest. Calcifications are not a problem in MR, nor are the bony structures, which are subtracted from the images.

At the present time, the choice of MRA or MSCTA for evaluation of peripheral vascular disease will depend largely on scanner availability, with MR preferred in general, and in particular in patients with pre-existing renal insufficiency or contrast allergy. MSCTA is an acceptable alternative, particularly in patients with pacemakers.

ARTIFACTS AND PITFALLS

Artifacts should always be considered in the differential diagnosis of a suspected MRA abnormality. Stent artifact has been previously discussed as a potential cause of apparent localized vascular occlusion. Stent artifact can be recognized by reviewing source images, where metal will usually have a characteristic MR appearance.

Indwelling metallic structures such as prosthetic joint replacements may also produce extensive artifact. These are usually easily recognized, but will usually result in extensive signal loss, with the resultant appearance of an occlusion, or a missing segment of vessel.

Additional artifacts may be seen as the result of poor timing of the arterial bolus. In particular, if triggering is performed too early, a ringing artifact (Gibbs or truncation artifact, Chapter 12) is frequently seen. In unusual circumstances this appearance can mimic a dissection. However, review of the source images and the characteristic appearance of this finding usually allow the correct assessment to

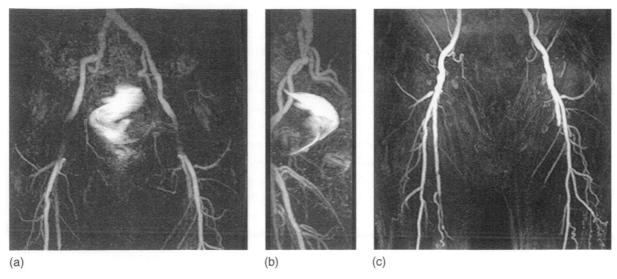

(a)   (b)   (c)

Figure 21.29   Apparent bilateral femoral artery occlusions (a) produced by incorrect positioning of the imaging slab, as seen on a sagittal image (b). Repeat exam with correct positioning (c).

be made. In unusual circumstances, repetition of the acquisition with improved timing may be necessary.

Inappropriate positioning of the acquisition slices (3D volume) may result in exclusion of the vessel of interest from the imaging slab, resulting in apparent stenosis/occlusion. Figure 21.29 demonstrates the appearance of an apparent area of occlusion in the femoral arteries. Review of the imaging slab position indicates that the vessels are actually not included in the image, explaining the resulting appearance. Repeat acquisition with appropriate positioning allows the proper evaluation to be made.

Image subtraction used in MRA demonstrably improves the contrast-to-noise ratio of the images, but can also lead to artifact. In particular, patient motion may result in such severe artifact as to limit the diagnostic value of the study.

Injection of undiluted contrast into veins may also result in a pseudostenosis appearance. This situation is most often encountered during thoracic MRA in the subclavian region, where the presence of high concentrations of gadolinium due to the intrinsic slower flow rates in veins results in significant T2 shortening, with a consequent susceptibility artifact involving the subclavian artery which lies in close proximity to the subclavian artery, at its entry into the thorax. Similar findings are possible in the abdomen, should a femoral venous catheter injection be performed.

NEW HORIZONS

MR angiographic imaging at 3 T has been recently reported. Given the increased signal-to-noise ratio inherent in

imaging at 3 T, submillimeter image resolution is possible, with markedly accelerated imaging acquisitions using extensively parallel imaging protocols. This has the simultaneous benefit of decreasing scan time, as well as diminishing the specific absorption rate (SAR) impact of the higher field strength. Encouraging preliminary results have been reported.

A novel angiographic MR imaging technique is that of global coherent free precession imaging. In this technique, spins passing through a preselected region of interest acquire signal, while the background is suppressed, resulting in an angiographic appearance. The slab can be positioned freely, resulting in dynamic image acquisitions. This manipulation can be performed in real time from the scanner console. Possible future applications include real-time evaluation of the coronary arterial flow, as well as guidance of interventional procedures.

CONCLUSIONS

MRA of the abdomen, pelvis, and lower extremities is easily and rapidly performed and is ideal for the evaluation of peripheral arterial disease. The technique is robust, reproducible, and results in images that are equivalent and sometimes superior to X-ray digital subtraction angiographic images, without the complications of radiation or arterial puncture. Continued improvements in scan hardware and software will no doubt enable further refinements in spatial resolution.

PRACTICAL PEARLS

- Positioning the 3D angiographic slab is critically important. This is important in the abdomen/pelvis station and in the upper leg. The smaller the slab, the shorter the scan time, and the quicker imaging is accomplished. BUT, you must not exclude relevant vessels.

- In the upper leg, the arteries course posteriorly as they descend toward the knee; therefore, the slab should be tilted in the sagittal plane such that the front of the slab encompasses the skin along the anterior aspect of the thigh at the top, and extends posterior to the back of the knee at the bottom.

- At the abdomen/pelvis level, remember that the iliac arteries can dip quite far posteriorly, and should be the marker for the most posterior aspect of the slab. The anterior margin of the slab must include the skin anterior to the femoral heads, which can serve as the marker for the front of the slab. If these regions are not included in the slab, you need to make the slab thicker (increase slice number or thickness).

- If you think a vessel is occluded, remember to look for a stent on thin section images.

- MIPs are not enough!! Multi-planar thin section review of the images is essential to avoid missing significant lesions.

- If the timing is off, or in case of technical glitches, consider rapidly repeating the acquisition, and using subtraction and thin section imaging review to salvage the study.

- If information about the venous structures is also desired, the sequence can be rerun in reverse order (feet to head) after the arterial acquisition, with a 30 s pause in between.

FURTHER READING

Ayuso JR, de Caralt TM, Pages M et al. MRA is useful as a follow-up technique after endovascular repair of aortic-aneurysms with nitinol endoprostheses. J Magn Reson Imaging 2004; 20(5): 803–10.

Barkhausen J, Hunold P, Eggebrecht H et al. Detection and characterization of intracardiac thrombi on MR imaging. AJR Am J Roentgenol 2002; 179(6): 1539–44.

Bertschinger K, Cassina PC, Debatin JF, Ruehm SG. Surveillance of peripheral arterial bypass grafts with three-dimensional MR angiography: comparison with digital subtraction angiography. AJR Am J Roentgenol 2001; 176(1): 215–20.

Binkert CA, Baker PD, Petersen BD, Szumowski J, Kaufman JA. Peripheral vascular disease: blinded study of dedicated calf MR angiography versus standard bolus-chase MR angiography and film hard-copy angiography. Radiology 2004; 232(3): 860–6.

Brothers TE, Greenfield LJ. Long-term results of aortoiliac reconstruction. J Vasc Interv Radiol 1990; 1(1): 49–55.

Cejna M, Loewe C, Schoder M et al. MR angiography vs CT angiography in the follow-up of nitinol stent grafts in endoluminally treated aortic aneurysms. Eur Radiol 2002; 12(10): 2443–50.

Costantini V, Lenti M. Treatment of acute occlusion of peripheral arteries. Thromb Res 2002; 106(6): V285–94.

de Vries M, de Koning PJ, de Haan MW et al. Accuracy of semiautomated analysis of 3D contrast-enhanced magnetic resonance angiography for detection and quantification of aortoiliac stenoses. Invest Radiol 2005; 40(8): 495–503.

Elias DA, White LM, Rubenstein JD, Christakis M, Merchant N. Clinical evaluation and MR imaging features of popliteal artery entrapment and cystic adventitial disease. AJR Am J Roentgenol 2003; 180(3): 627–32.

Hany TF, McKinnon GC, Leung DA, Pfammatter T, Debatin JF. Optimization of contrast timing for breath-hold three-dimensional MR angiography. J Magn Reson Imag 1997; 7(3): 551–6.

Herborn CU, Goyen M, Lauenstein TC, Debatin JF, Ruehm SG, Kroger K. Comprehensive time-resolved MRI of peripheral vascular malformations. AJR Am J Roentgenol 2003; 181(3): 729–35.

Huber ME, Kozerke S, Pruessmann KP, Smink J, Boesiger P. Sensitivity-encoded coronary MRA at 3T. Magn Reson Med 2004; 52(2): 221–7.

Klem I, Rehwald WG, Heitner JF et al. Noninvasive assessment of blood flow based on magnetic resonance global coherent free precession. Circulation 2005; 111(8): 1033–9.

Klemm T, Duda S, Machann J et al. MR imaging in the presence of vascular stents: A systematic assessment of artifacts for various stent orientations, sequence types, and field strengths. J Magn Reson Imaging 2000; 12(4): 606–15.

Lapeyre M, Kobeiter H, Desgranges P, Rahmouni A, Becquemin JP, Luciani A. Assessment of critical limb ischemia in patients with diabetes: comparison of MR angiography and digital subtraction angiography. AJR Am J Roentgenol 2005; 185(6): 1641–50.

Lee VS, Martin DJ, Krinsky GA, Rofsky NM. Gadolinium-enhanced MR angiography: artifacts and pitfalls. AJR Am J Roentgenol 2000; 175(1): 197–205.

Leng GC, Davis M, Baker D. Bypass surgery for chronic lower limb ischaemia. Cochrane Database Syst Rev 2000(3): CD002000.

Lenhart M, Volk M, Manke C et al. Stent appearance at contrast-enhanced MR angiography: in vitro examination with 14 stents. Radiology 2000; 217(1): 173–8.

Letourneau-Guillon L, Soulez G, Beaudoin G et al. CT and MR imaging of nitinol stents with radiopaque distal markers. J Vasc Interv Radiol 2004; 15(6): 615–24.

Lipsitz EC, Ohki T, Veith FJ et al. Does subintimal angioplasty have a role in the treatment of severe lower extremity ischemia? J Vasc Surg 2003; 37(2): 386–91.

Meissner OA, Rieger J, Weber C et al. Critical limb ischemia: hybrid MR angiography compared with DSA. Radiology 2005; 235(1): 308–18.

Morasch MD, Collins J, Pereles FS et al. Lower extremity stepping-table magnetic resonance angiography with multilevel contrast timing and segmented contrast infusion. J Vasc Surg 2003; 37(1): 62–71.

Muhs BE, Gagne P, Sheehan P. Peripheral arterial disease: clinical assessment and indications for revascularization in the patient with diabetes. Curr Diab Rep 2005; 5(1): 24–9.

Ouwendijk R, de Vries M, Pattynama PM et al. Imaging peripheral arterial disease: a randomized controlled trial comparing contrast-enhanced MR angiography and multi-detector row CT angiography. Radiology 2005; 236(3): 1094–103.

Ouwendijk R, Kock MC, Visser K, Pattynama PM, de Haan MW, Hunink MG. Interobserver agreement for the interpretation of contrast-enhanced 3D MR angiography and MDCT angiography in peripheral arterial disease. AJR Am J Roentgenol 2005; 185(5): 1261–7.

Owen RS, Carpenter JP, Baum RA, Perloff LJ, Cope C. Magnetic resonance imaging of angiographically occult runoff vessels in peripheral arterial occlusive disease. N Engl J Med 1992; 326(24): 1577–81.

Prince MR, Chabra SG, Watts R et al. Contrast material travel times in patients undergoing peripheral MR angiography. Radiology 2002; 224(1): 55–61.

Quinn SF, Sheley RC, Semonsen KG, Leonardo VJ, Kojima K, Szumowski J. Aortic and lower-extremity arterial disease: evaluation with MR angiography versus conventional angiography. Radiology 1998; 206(3): 693–701.

Raffetto JD, Chen MN, LaMorte WW et al. Factors that predict site of outflow target artery anastomosis in infrainguinal revascularization. J Vasc Surg 2002; 35(6): 1093–9.

Ramdev P, Rayan SS, Sheahan M et al. A decade experience with infrainguinal revascularization in a dialysis-dependent patient population. J Vasc Surg 2002; 36(5): 969–74.

Sharafuddin MJ, Stolpen AH, Sun S et al. High-resolution multiphase contrast-enhanced three-dimensional MR angiography compared with two-dimensional time-of-flight MR angiog-

raphy for the identification of pedal vessels. J Vasc Interv Radiol 2002; 13(7): 695–702.

Steffens JC, Schafer FK, Oberscheid B et al. Bolus-chasing contrast-enhanced 3D MRA of the lower extremity. Comparison with intraarterial DSA. Acta Radiol 2003; 44(2): 185–92.

Vosshenrich R, Kopka L, Castillo E, Bottcher V, Graessner J, Grabbe E. Electrocardio-graph-triggered two-dimensional time-of-flight versus optimized contrast-enhanced three-dimensional MR angiography of the peripheral arteries. Magn Reson Imaging 1998; 16(8): 887–92.

Wang Y, Chen CZ, Chabra SG et al. Bolus arterial-venous transit in the lower extremity and venous contamination in bolus chase three-dimensional magnetic resonance angiography. Invest Radiol 2002; 37(8): 458–63.

Willmann JK, Wildermuth S, Pfammatter T et al. Aortoiliac and renal arteries: prospective intraindividual comparison of contrast-enhanced three-dimensional MR angiography and multi-detector row CT angiography. Radiology 2003; 226(3): 798–811.

Willmann JK, Baumert B, Schertler T et al. Aortoiliac and lower extremity arteries assessed with 16-detector row CT angiography: prospective comparison with digital subtraction angiography. Radiology 2005; 236(3): 1083–93.

Wright LB, Matchett WJ, Cruz CP et al. Popliteal artery disease: diagnosis and treatment. Radiographics 2004; 24(2): 467–79.

Zhang HL, Ho BY, Chao M, et al. Decreased venous contamination on 3D gadolinium-enhanced bolus chase peripheral MR angiography using thigh compression. AJR Am J Roentgenol 2004; 183(4): 1041–7.

Zhang HL, Khilnani NM, Prince MR et al. Diagnostic accuracy of time-resolved 2D projection MR angiography for symptomatic infrapopliteal arterial occlusive disease. AJR Am J Roentgenol 2005; 184(3): 938–47.

22

MR venography: practical imaging techniques

Chanh D Nguyen, Mahesh R Patel, Young S Kang, and Robert R Edelman

INTRODUCTION

Ultrasonography, computed tomography (CT), and catheter venography have been historically used to evaluate venous pathology. Ultrasound offers the benefits of availability and low cost, but is operator dependent and may be limited by a patient's body habitus. Accurate venous mapping and evaluation of complex venous anatomy such as duplications can be challenging. Although CT venography of the lower extremities and pelvis can be performed in conjunction with CT pulmonary angiography for evaluation of pulmonary embolism, this requires additional radiation exposure and larger doses of iodinated contrast media, with the associated risks of extravasation, thrombophlebitis, allergic reactions, and nephrotoxicity. Catheter venography, is excellent in the depiction of venous anatomy, is invasive, and involves radiation and administration of iodinated contrast media with their attendant complications. Moreover, it can be technically challenging and has limitations while evaluating pelvic veins. Magnetic resonance venography (MRV) overcomes many of the aforementioned limitations while allowing for continuous imaging over longer periods of time. Gadolinium chelates have a better patient safety profile than iodinated contrast. Advances in MR techniques and instrumentation have made high-quality images of small, deep venous structures possible. This chapter will describe MRV with attention to common venous anatomic variants, existing MRV techniques, and current clinical applications (Table 22.1).

Table 22.1 Clinical indications for MR venography
• Thrombo-occlusive of lower extremity and inferior vena cava
• Thrombo-occlusive of upper extremities and superior vena cava
• Cranial vein thrombosis
• Renal vein and mesenteric thrombosis
• Portal venous imaging
• Pelvic and ovarian vein thrombosis
• Hemodialysis access and shunt evaluation
• Congenital vascular malformation

ANATOMIC CONSIDERATIONS

Variations in venous anatomy are very common and can be complex. For example, only one in six patients will have a lower limb venous system consisting of continuous, non-duplicated veins. Hence, knowledge of the normal peripheral venous anatomy will aid in interpretation of MRV. Common variations encountered in clinical practice are discussed below.

Lower extremity

Venous circulation in the lower extremities has two main pathways, the superficial saphenous system and the deep venous system, which are connected by perforating veins. The deep veins of the calf are often paired or duplicated, including the posterior tibial vein, which drains the deep plantar venous arch of the foot and joins the peroneal vein in the upper calf. The upward continuation of the dorsalis pedis vein is the anterior tibial vein, which passes between the fibula and tibia to unite with the posterior tibial vein to form the popliteal vein.

Within the popliteal fossa, the popliteal vein is usually superficial to the popliteal artery. The popliteal vein becomes the femoral vein (FV) superior to Hunter's adductor canal, with the FV usually assuming a medial position in the mid thigh. The FV is a deep vein that is also widely known as the superficial femoral vein (SFV), which introduces the possible and significant mistake of labeling it as part of the superficial saphenous system.

The major variations involve duplications that are often of variable length. In a retrospective study using catheter venograms, a third of patients had variations in the FV with the most common being duplication. The duplicated veins were often smaller and had an equal probability of being either medial or lateral to the main veins. The duplicated segment varied in length from 1 to 30 cm, with a mean length of 10 cm, and occurred most often in the mid thigh.

Duplication of the popliteal vein has been shown to occur in approximately one half of extremities. Calf veins are almost always duplicated. Other variations of the calf veins are usually seen with respect to the venous confluence that forms the popliteal vein. With respect to the greater saphenous vein and superficial venous system, duplication and multiple veins have been reported in up to a half of extremities. The presence of duplicated veins in one limb has a strong correlation with the presence of duplicated veins in the contralateral limb.

Upper extremity and superior vena cava

Venous drainage of the upper extremity also occurs via a superficial or deep system, with frequent and variable anastomoses. The superficial venous system includes the cephalic, basilic, and median antecubital veins. At the inferior margin of the teres minor muscle, the basilic vein (a superficial vein) becomes the axillary vein (a deep vein). The deep veins follow the course of the arteries and are generally paired. Deep vessels include the ulnar, radial, brachial, axillary, and subclavian veins. Near the inferior margin of the subcapularis muscle, the paired brachial veins join the axillary vein. The subclavian vein is then formed by the union of the cephalic and axillary veins.

Central venous anomalies are less common and are usually discovered incidentally in patients imaged for other reasons. A duplicated or left-sided superior vena cava (SVC) occurs when there is embryologic persistence of the left anterior cardinal vein. A duplicated SVC almost always drains into the coronary sinus. Direct drainage into the right atrium usually occurs in conjunction with congenital heart disease.

Inferior vena cava and pelvis

Common venous variants in the abdomen include duplication of the inferior vena cava (IVC), left-sided IVC, and left retroaortic or circumaortic renal vein. Less frequent IVC anomalies, such as interruption (with azygos or hemiazygos continuation) and abnormal insertion of the IVC, are associated with visceral heterotaxy syndromes including situs ambiguus with polysplenia or asplenia.

Gonadal venous anatomy is remarkably constant, with the left gonadal vein draining into the left renal vein and the right gonadal vein draining into the IVC. An occasional variant is drainage of the right gonadal vein into the right renal vein.

An anatomic variant with the pathologic consequence of chronic or recurrent deep venous thrombosis (DVT) is the May–Thurner syndrome. Compression of the left common iliac vein between the right common iliac artery and spine leads to stasis of flow or venous occlusion of the left lower extremity. Flow instead is rerouted to the heart via lumbar, pelvic, and abdominal collaterals.

FUNDAMENTAL TECHNIQUES

MRV techniques can be divided into three major categories: (1) non-contrast flow-dependent techniques such as time-of-flight (TOF) and phase contrast (PC); (2) dynamic three-dimensional (3D) contrast-enhanced MR venography (3D CE MRV); and (3) miscellaneous methods including non-contrast flow-independent techniques, direct thrombus imaging, and blood pool imaging. In addition to these acquisition techniques, post-processing such as maximum intensity projection (MIP) is integral to image interpretation.

Non-contrast flow-dependent techniques

Non-contrast techniques are performed without the need for injection of gadolinium chelates. They have been shown to be accurate with good sensitivity (100%) and specificity (96%) for the evaluation of the venous system compared to ultrasound (US) and catheter venography.

TOF MRV uses short repetition time (TR) gradient recalled echo (GRE) pulse sequences for flow-related enhancement (Chapter 13). The dominant signal on an image is generated by blood, which has recently moved into the imaging plane, whereas signal from stationary tissues is suppressed with repetitive radiofrequency pulses. Separation of venous from arterial signal can be achieved by placing a presaturation band in the upstream direction of the arterial flow to negate inflowing arterial spins (Chapter 13).

Two-dimensional (2D) and 3D TOF techniques are available to isolate vessels from the surrounding tissue (Chapter 13). The former acquires data from multiple thin sections separately, while for the latter the acquisition is from a volume of tissue. Compared to 3D TOF, 2D TOF is generally preferred for venous imaging because of its higher sensitivity for slow flow and its ability to cover a larger field of view.

PC MRV is a subtraction technique that takes advantage of flowing spins acquiring phase shifts under a gradient field (Chapter 13). Its advantages over TOF include absence of misleading shine-through artifacts as well as the potential ability to produce quantitative velocity maps with the signal intensity in a voxel proportional to the actual flow velocity in a particular direction. Flow sensitivity is affected by the chosen velocity-encoding value with suggested value of 20 cm/s for body venous imaging.

Non-contrast techniques, however, are not without limitations. Disadvantages of 2D TOF include respiratory artifacts, saturation of in-plane flow, and poor resolution. Both TOF and PC techniques are less accurate in evaluating vessels with very slow flow rates such as small, deep or superficial veins. Increasing the acquisition time in PC techniques can help evaluate such slow flowing vessels, but the increased sensitivity to motion artifacts which compromise image quality precludes their common usage. Disadvantages such as increased susceptibility effects, pulsation artifacts, and lengthy acquisition times have limited non-contrast techniques to specific clinical indications. 2D TOF is still commonly used for the evaluation of pelvic veins (Figure 22.1).

Contrast-enhanced techniques

The mainstay of MRV are dynamic 3D CE-MRV techniques that utilize gadolinium chelates to enhance venous signal. Compared to 2D TOF, the acquisition time of 3D CE-MRV is shorter, and images are produced with increased contrast-to-noise ratio and reduced flow-related artifacts (Figure 22.2). Due to the relatively short imaging time, images can be obtained in the venous phase in the plane of the vessel of interest with coverage of a large vascular territory such as the lower extremity. Dynamic T1-weighted 3D gradient-echo sequences, typically with breath hold, are performed via *direct* or *indirect* techniques.

Analogous to catheter venography, direct 3D CE-MRV relies on upstream access to the target vein of interest. Contrast medium diluted 1:20 with normal saline is continuously infused with imaging performed of the targeted venous system after 50–60 ml of diluted contrast medium have been injected. Compared to non-contrast and indirect CE-MRV techniques, the direct technique produces images of superior quality due to higher contrast-to-noise ratios and absence of superimposed enhancing vessels. Time-resolved acquisitions can also be easily performed. Disadvantages include the requirement for venous access of the extremity of interest, poor evaluation of the central system, and possible T2 shortening effects if the contrast dilution is insufficient.

Compared to the direct method, indirect 3D CE-MRV has gained widespread usage because selective venous access is not required. With indirect 3D CE-MRV, a large volume of contrast is injected in a peripheral vein analogous to contrast injection in a CT angiography study. Images are acquired during the recirculation phase, usually early in the equilibrium phase to avoid significant dilution due to redistribution to the extravascular space. Similar to the direct technique, time-resolved acquisitions of the entire 3D volume can be obtained. Data from the arterial phase can be subtracted from more delayed data to generate images with improved arterial-venous differentiation. Unlike the direct technique, any vein can be used for intravenous contrast administration. A disadvantage is the need for much larger volumes of contrast media.

Miscellaneous techniques

This category includes alternative techniques that have a limited role in clinical practice or are of an experimental nature.

Non-contrast flow-independent techniques take advantage of differences in T1, T2, and chemical shifts of blood versus static structures to produce vascular images. For lower extremity imaging and to visualize vessels with slow flow, sequences such as RARE (rapid acquisition relaxation

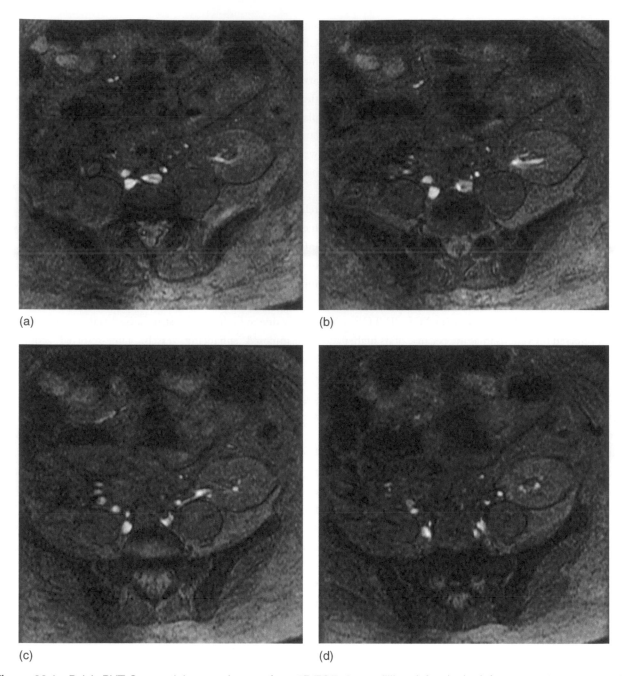

(a)

(b)

(c)

(d)

Figure 22.1   Pelvic DVT. Sequential source images from 2D TOF show a filling defect in the left common iliac vein consistent with pelvic deep venous thrombosis. Images courtesy of Charles E Spritzer.

enhancement) have been used. Because they do not depend on flow, these sequences can image very small vascular branches with relatively short acquisition times. However, reconstructed images such as MIPs are difficult to interpret due to the high number of vessels imaged. In addition, vessels with higher flow rates may not be properly depicted.

Steady-state free-precession (SSFP) sequences such as true FISP (fast imaging with steady-state precession) and FIESTA (fast imaging employing steady-state acquisition) are produced by favorable T2*/T1 properties that are nearly independent of flow, so flow-related artifacts can be suppressed. High spatial resolution images covering large regions of the body can be produced without the need for intravenous contrast (Figure 22.3). A disadvantage of SSFP involves sensitivity to patient-induced field inhomogeneities.

Direct thrombus imaging depicts thrombus in occluded blood vessels that may be missed by catheter venography (due to lack of filling) or by flow-sensitive non-contrast MRV techniques such as TOF and PC. In clinical practice, thrombus is often directly visualized on multiple sequences including those of standard MR (Figure 22.4). Visualization of a thrombus

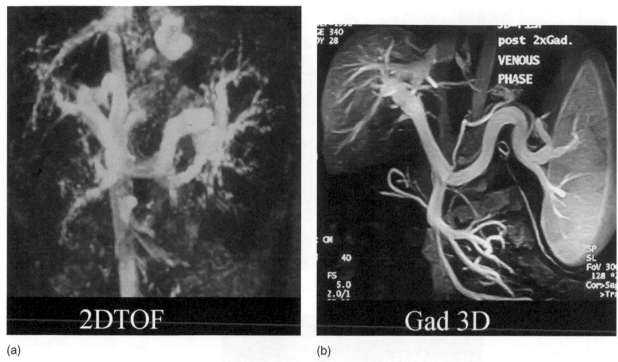

(a)   (b)

Figure 22.2 2D TOF versus 3D CE-MRV. (a) Maximum intensity projection image from a 2D TOF acquisition shows the limitation of TOF, mainly in-plane saturation and dephasing artifacts, compromising image quality and interpretation. (b) Acquisition performed with 3D gadolinium-enhanced MR venography with short TE in the same patient eliminates artifacts from saturation and dephasing. In-plane vessels such as branches of the superior mesenteric vein and portal vein are clearly depicted.

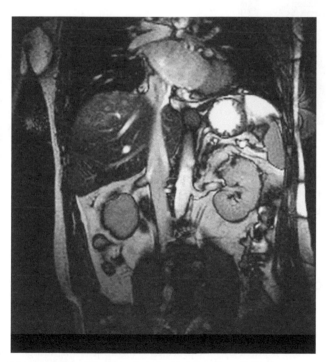

Figure 22.3 Steady-state free precession (SSFP) for MR venography. SSFP is a non-contrast flow-independent technique that can produce high spatial resolution images with little flow artifact, such as that depicted in this coronal image showing portions of the abdominal aorta and inferior vena cava.

depends on its relaxation times, which change with age. In the acute setting, thrombus is composed mostly of deoxyhemoglobin, which is hypointense or isointense compared with unclotted blood and thus may not be conspicuous on either T1-weighted or T2-weighted images. As the clot ages, degradation to methemoglobin produces T1 shortening, thereby increasing signal intensity on T1-weighted images. This T1 shortening usually occurs at the margin of the thrombus and progresses centrally. During the late stages, signal intensity on T2-weighted images diminishes due to the build-up of hemosiderin in macrophages, which also occurs at the periphery. The conspicuity of a thrombus can be further enhanced with an inversion recovery or chemical saturation sequence to suppress signal of unclotted blood or reduce background fat signal.

Blood pool imaging is an emerging technique, which attempts to improve on traditional contrast agents, as rapid redistribution of contrast into the extravascular space degrades image quality. Blood pool contrast media remain within the intravascular space. These agents work by binding to albumin when injected, or have a molecular structure which prevents diffusion from the intravascular space, thereby producing images acquired during the equilibrium phase with superior contrast-to-noise ratios (Chapter 14). The increased intravascular half-life may permit imaging of

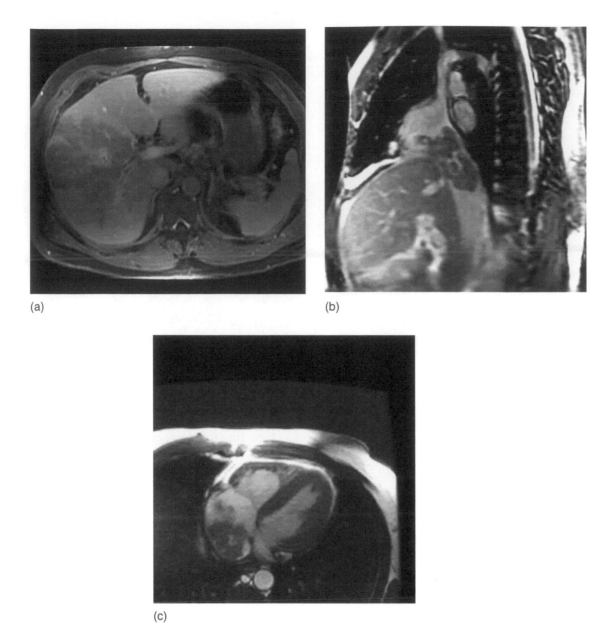

(a)

(b)

(c)

Figure 22.4 Direct visualization of a thrombus on multiple sequences. (a) Axial post-gadolinium T1-weighted image with fat saturation shows a heterogeneously enhancing mass in the right hepatic lobe representing a hepatocellular carcinoma. (b) Sagittal gradient recalled echo image shows tumor thrombus extension into the IVC and right atrium. (c) Oblique axial gradient recalled echo image shows the tumor thrombus producing a filling defect within the right atrium.

additional vascular sites and areas of delayed filling due to obstruction or post-inflammatory changes as seen in the post-thrombotic syndrome. Limited use has been made of blood pool agents such as ultrasmall superparamagnetic iron oxide (USPIO) particles. Ferumoxytol (Figure 22.5) has been shown to possess T1 relaxation times several-fold higher than standard gadolinium chelates, thereby improving both venous and arterial phase imaging at an equivalent injection rate. To date, these agents have not found their way into routine clinical practice (Chapter 14).

Post-processing

In addition to review of directly acquired MRV source images, the evaluation of complex vascular anatomy and pathology is aided by post-processing techniques including maximum intensity projection (MIP), image subtraction, volume rendering, and other 3D algorithms (Chapter 4). Gadolinium chelates and blood pool agents are present in both arteries and veins; hence, separation is necessary to produce pure venographic images.

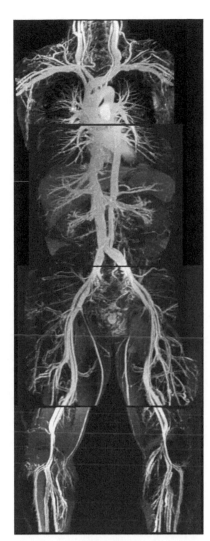

Figure 22.5 Blood pool imaging. Equilibrium-phase whole-body MR angiography/venography using ferumoxytol, an ultrasmall superparamagnetic iron oxide (USPIO) particle, was performed with total acquisition time of 5 minutes 45 s for 8 stations. Higher T1 relaxation times compared to gadolinium chelates produce higher contrast-to-noise ratio images at an equivalent injection rate. Post-processing with arterial venous subtraction would be necessary to produce venographic images.

CLINICAL APPLICATIONS WITH DETAILED CLINICAL PROTOCOLS

MRV is an accurate tool for evaluating deep venous thrombosis, pelvic and central venous pathology, and vascular anomalies such as venous malformations. It has an expanding role as a primary imaging modality or as a supplementary technique to US, CT, or catheter venography for evaluating hemodialysis access and for the diagnosis of portal vein thrombosis. The following sections will list specific clinical entities, outline common imaging techniques, and

discuss their MR venographic findings. Table 22.2 lists general parameters for commonly used MRV techniques.

Thrombo-occlusive disease of the lower extremities and inferior vena cava

The vast majority of deep venous thrombosis occurs in the lower extremities. DVT usually starts in the deep soleal calf veins and then propagates superiorly. A wide range of clinical presentations and consequences exist, from no symptoms to lethal outcome due to massive pulmonary embolism. Clinical exam is unreliable as DVT is often confused with other common lower extremity pathologies such as cellulitis, chronic venous insufficiency, and leg edema. Accurate diagnosis is paramount to avoid unnecessary exposure to or withholding of anticoagulant therapy. Permanent sequelae of DVT include vein and valve damage that can lead to post-thrombotic syndrome, which is characterized by chronic limb edema, hyperpigmentation, claudication, pain, and development of venous stasis ulcers months or years after the initial injury.

Although US is readily available and cost-effective, it is operator dependent, it cannot evaluate above the inguinal ligament, it is often limited in the assessment of Hunter's canal, it can be difficult in an obese patient, and it can produce false negative results in the presence of complex venous anatomy such as duplication. Evaluation by CT submits the patient to ionizing radiation and iodinated contrast media. Although acceptable in most patients, CT may not be ideal for children, or patients who are pregnant, have iodinated contrast allergy, or who have renal insufficiency.

Dynamic 3D CE-MRV is the technique of choice if high-resolution images of the peripheral vessels are a must. It will display all vessels containing contrast medium, regardless of the flow characteristics. Three-dimensional CE-MRV has also been used for evaluation of post-thrombotic change, varicosities, and anatomy of the greater saphenous vein prior to cardiac bypass surgery. The detection of a filling defect or occlusion of a deep vein with collateral flow is the basis for diagnosis of DVT.

Direct 3D CE-MRV has the advantage of detailed time-resolved evaluation of a selected vessel. Superficial varicosities and perforating veins that contain slow or even retrograde flow can be differentiated from thrombosed or partially occluded veins. Its major disadvantages are the need for distal access to the extremity of interest and the application of tourniquets for the exam to improve venous filling.

Table 22.2 Sample clinical protocols for MRV techniques used for imaging the extremities and pelvis on a 1.5 T MR scanner[a]

	General parameters									Comments		
	TR (ms)	TE (ms)	Flip angle	Slice thickness (mm)	FOV (cm)	Matrix	Plane	Flow comp	Fat sat	Lower extremity	Upper extremity	Pelvis and IVC
2D TOF MRV	30	10	45°	3	34	160×256	Ax	Yes	No	3 ml gadolinium mixed with every 57 ml saline (1:20 dilution). Dilution infused at 1 ml/s for total of 180 ml with acquisition starting at 60 s delay. Coil wrapped around lower extremities	Prone with arms extended above head. Coil wrapped around arms and thorax	Use 1:10 gadolinium:saline dilution if not imaging lower extremity
Direct 3D CE-MRV	4	1	30°	2	30	160×256	Cor	No	Optional	Tourniquet around ankle. Repeat without tourniquet if imaging superficial veins using additional bolus	Tourniquet around upper arm	If performed with lower extremity, image the IVC, pelvis, and thighs first
Indirect 3D CE-MRV	4	1	30°	2	30	160×256	Cor	No	Optional	0.2 mmol/kg gadolinium injected at 2–3 ml/s. Bolus-timing acquisition performed with 2–3 ml gadolinium to determine time delay		

[a]Note that specific parameters may vary for different MR vendors and with field strength. For 3D CE-MRV, repetitive acquisitions are performed. Post-processing of MRV data sets, which may include subtracted images, is performed at a workstation.

Ax, axial; Cor, coronal; TR, repetition time; TE, echo time; fov, field of view; flow comp, flow composition; fat sat, fat saturation.

Indirect 3D CE-MRV image acquisitions occur during the contrast-equilibrium phase following injection of undiluted contrast media. Venous access need not be in the symptomatic limb. The need to time the contrast bolus can be eliminated by using dynamic 3D CE-MRV with very short TR and TE, which makes possible the acquisition of multiple 3D data sets in a relatively short amount of time.

With indirect 3D CE, post-processing subtraction methods are necessary to create pure venographic images. In addition, whole-body indirect 3D CE-MRV with a single contrast injection can be achieved with the aid of the continuous moving table technique and surface coils to allow for ultrafast data acquisition. Further image quality improvement can be achieved by using blood pool agents such as USPIO particles (Figure 22.5).

Two-dimensional TOF has the advantage of not requiring venous access or intravenous contrast media. This technique has been shown in many studies to be highly accurate when compared to catheter venography. Evaluation of DVT from the popliteal vein to the IVC by 2D TOF has a sensitivity of 100%, specificity of 96%, positive predictive value of 90%, and negative predictive value of 100%. Evaluation of DVT in the infrapopliteal vessels using flow augmentation (compression and decompression) and ultrafast imaging has a sensitivity of 87% and a specificity of 97%. Two-dimensional TOF is limited by in-plane saturation effects, which will not depict veins that run parallel to the plane, poor image quality, and lengthy acquisition times (Figure 22.2).

Non-contrast flow-independent techniques such as heavily T2-weighted fast spin-echo (FSE) techniques or RARE can depict lower extremity veins with relatively high resolution, including vessels with slow flow such as in the calf, and with relatively short acquisition times. SSFP techniques can similarly improve thrombus visualization without the need for contrast.

Thrombo-occlusive disease of the upper extremities to the superior vena cava

Deep venous thrombosis of the upper extremity is less common than DVT of the lower extremity or pelvis. The upper extremity deep veins best evaluated by MRV include the axillary, subclavian, innominate, and superior vena cava.

The specific clinical entity of superior vena cava syndrome occurs with near-complete or complete occlusion of the SVC. The characteristic physical findings include cyanosis, facial swelling, venous distention of the neck, and upper extremity edema. Obstruction of the SVC is commonly caused by neoplastic invasion of the venous wall, extrinsic compression by tumor or mass, irritation by indwelling central venous catheters, hypercoagulable states, or anatomic causes. Anatomic causes that contribute to DVT include the presence of a cervical rib, post-traumatic deformity of surrounding osseous structures, and anomalous musculofascial bands.

The role of MRV is to demonstrate the presence of venous thrombosis, determine its extent, and possibly reveal the cause. An obstructed SVC will initiate collateral venous drainage to the heart via four main pathways, and it is these dilated collateral pathways that may be visualized on imaging. Most commonly, drainage to the heart occurs via the azygos venous system, which includes the azygos and hemi-azygos veins with interconnecting intercostal veins. Internal mammary veins and secondary communications to the inferior epigastric veins via the superior epigastric veins make up a second pathway. The long thoracic veins with their collateralization to the pelvic and vertebral veins make up the final two pathways.

Direct 3D CE-MRV of the upper extremities, as in lower extremity imaging, involves injection of 50 to 60 ml of diluted contrast into each extremity and image acquisition during first pass and the arteriovenous phase with breath hold 3D spoiled GRE sequences. Tourniquets may be applied to insure adequate venous filling. Unilateral injections do not allow for evaluation of the central veins due to mixing artifacts from unenhanced blood flow coming from the contralateral limb. Bilateral evaluation of the axillary, subclavian, and innominate veins necessitates simultaneous bilateral injections; even then, flow-related artifacts may result from unenhanced blood coming from the internal jugular veins.

Indirect 3D CE-MRV is another means of visualizing the upper extremity veins and SVC. As in the lower extremities, image acquisitions occur during the contrast-equilibrium phase following injection of contrast media. The need to time the contrast bolus can be eliminated by utilizing dynamic 3D CE-MRV using very short TR and TE to produce multiple data sets.

Two-dimensional TOF MRV is less commonly used, but has shown good agreement to catheter venography for imaging of thoracic veins. It was also shown to provide more comprehensive information than catheter venography for central venous anatomy and blood flow. But since data need to be acquired in perpendicular planes to the vessels going from the upper arm veins to the subclavian to the SVC, multiple acquisitions are needed; hence 2D TOF MRV is limited by long examination times and motion artifacts.

Renal vein imaging

MRI and MRV have emerged as the most accurate and sensitive modalities to assess renal vein thrombosis and its most common cause, renal cell carcinoma (RCC). The knowledge of tumor extent determines clinical staging and surgical approach, in addition to providing prognostification. Other causes for renal vein thrombosis include glomerulonephritis, trauma, dehydration, and extension of IVC thrombosis.

MRV using gradient-echo images has been shown to have a sensitivity of 100% and a specificity of 98% for characterization of venous involvement by RCC. Although full body staging of renal cell carcinoma is more accurately performed with CT due in part to CT's superior osseous and pulmonary parenchymal evaluation, local staging of RCC and its renal vein/IVC involvement is more accurate with MR. One study evaluating patients with RCC using a contrast-enhanced MRV technique found excellent sensitivity (100%) and specificity (96%) for the detection of venous thrombosis. A sensitivity of 89% and specificity of 96% was found when bland versus tumor thrombus was determined. Hence, MRI and MRV can be used as the primary modality for local staging of RCC.

Ovarian vein and pelvic vein imaging

The pelvis is an anatomic region where MRV has shown definite advantage over CT and US. A retrospective study identified DVT isolated to the pelvic veins in approximately 20% of patients with DVT, which is significantly higher than reported in prior studies using US or catheter venography. CT tends to underestimate the presence of pelvic vein thrombosis due primarily to the pelvic veins' oblique course relative to the plane of imaging, and because pelvic vein evaluation is more technically challenging.[2] MRV is recommended for patients with negative US study or non-diagnostic CT, but in whom the clinical suspicion for pelvic DVT remains high (Figure 22.6).

Another challenging diagnosis for US is gonadal or ovarian vein thrombosis, which can clinically mimick acute appendicitis, pyelonephritis, ureteral obstruction, and, in the post-partum female, endometritis. The ovarian veins arise from venules, which drain the ovaries, parametrium, and portions of the pelvic brim. Septic puerperal ovarian-vein thrombosis is a distinct clinical entity presenting on the second or third post-partum day, with a higher prevalence in cesarean sections than in vaginal births. Thrombosis usually occurs on the right in the post-partum female due to a variety of factors including physiologic dextroposition of the uterus compressing the right ovarian vein, and antegrade flow in the right ovarian vein compared with retrograde flow in the left ovarian vein. One prospective comparative study showed that MRV is superior to both CT and duplex-Doppler US with a sensitivity and specificity of 100%.

MR venographic evaluation of the pelvis is often performed in conjunction with lower extremity imaging; hence sequences used for lower extremity MRV can be applied to include the pelvis, not to mention the IVC. One modification occurs with direct 3D CE-MRV, for which a less dilute mixture (1:10) of gadolinium chelate is used than that for imaging the lower extremities and IVC due to dilution from draining unopacified veins. A dedicated vascular coil is recommended to produce superior contrast-to-noise ratio images.

Vascular malformation imaging

Congenital vascular malformations result from in utero insults, genetic factors, or environmental causes. They can present as small, isolated, circumscribed lesions to complex vascular masses. Various forms exist involving the venous, arterial, and/or the lymphatic system. Generally, vascular malformations are considered as *slow-flow* malformations (capillary, venous, lymphatic, capillary-venous, or capillary-lymphatic-venous malformations) or *high-flow* malformations (arteriovenous fistulas or arteriovenous malformations) (Figure 22.7). Venous malformations are the most common vascular malformations.

Treatment depends on the extent of the malformation and includes both surgical and catheter-based interventions. Optimal treatment stratifications, therefore, require a comprehensive characterization of the feeding and draining vessels as well as adjacent soft tissue and osseous structures. MRV offers a non-invasive modality for the evaluation of vascular malformations. MR evaluation of vascular malformations and involves utilization of conventional MRI with MRV. Dynamic 3D CE-MRV, through acquisition of different phases of flow, permits evaluation of the speed and signal intensities of blood flow over time. Comprehensive MR evaluation of vascular malformations also includes conventional sequences such as T1-weighted, T2-weighted,

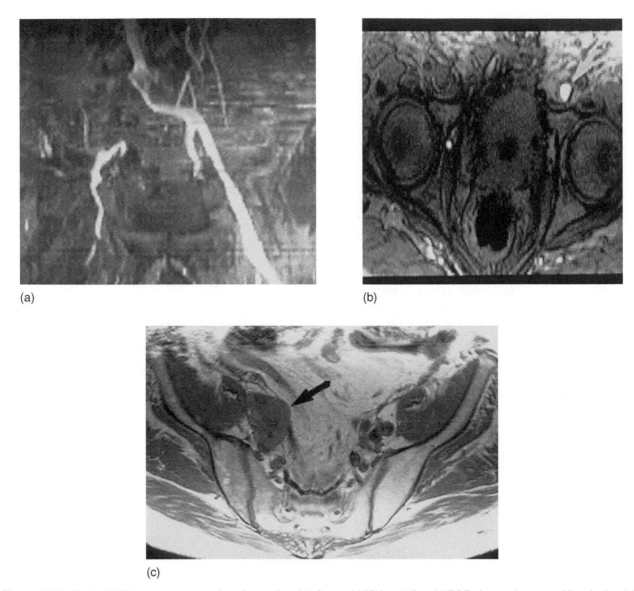

Figure 22.6 Pelvic DVT: nodal mass causing obstruction. (a) Coronal MIP from 2D axial TOF shows absence of flow in the right common iliac vein although there is flow in the femoral vein. The left femoral and iliac veins are patent. (b) Axial 2D TOF source image shows a patent left external iliac vein (arrow) with absence of vascular signal intensity on the right. (c) Axial T2 weighted image at a more superior plane than (b) shows a nodal mass (arrow) obstructing the iliac vein. MRI in combination with MR venography increases the accuracy for not only identifying thrombo-occlusive disease, but also for elucidating the cause.

and late-phase equilibrium fat-saturation T1-weighted sequences. Heavily T2-weighted sequences are highly accurate for detailing the anatomy of the vascular malformation. A T2*-weighted sequence can help detect hemorrhage or thrombus.

Rijswijk et al showed that sensitivity of conventional MRI in differentiating venous and non-venous malformations is 100% with a specificity of 24–33%, increasing to 95% when dynamic contrast-enhanced MR imaging is added. Despite its accuracy and lack of ionizing radiation, MR evaluation of vascular malformations remains inferior to catheter angiography for revealing vascular detail and for intervention planning.

Expanding role of MRV: hemodialysis access and portal venous imaging

The application of MRV continues to grow into vascular territories routinely evaluated by US or catheter angiography/venography. One such arena is the evaluation of hemodialysis arteriovenous fistulas (radio- or brachiocephalic) and synthetic arteriovenous bridge grafts (AVGs) in patients with end-stage renal disease. Diagnosis of hemodynamically significant stenosis (≥50%) is crucial for maintenance of acceptable vascular access and aids in prevention of access failure by stenosis or thrombosis.

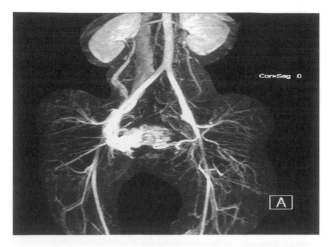

Figure 22.7 32-year-old woman with post-partum vaginal bleeding due to uterine arteriovenous malformation. Coronal MIP from 3D CE-MRV/MRA shows a tangle of vessels in the uterus. Note the preferential venous drainage to the right ovarian and iliac vessels. Image courtesy of Shigeaki Umeoka.

Several surveillance techniques are available to detect access stenosis. Venous pressure measurement performed during dialysis can trace more distally located stenosis in the venous outflow tract, but the development of inflow resistance is not measured. Ultrasound is an appropriate technique to morphologically visualize thrombus or to assess flow changes with clinical suspicion of stenosis or thrombosis. Besides being operator dependent, US is less accurate at venous mapping and poor at evaluating thoracic venous anatomy. It can sometimes overestimate or underestimate stenosis at the arterial anastomosis, and it is inaccurate in the detection of stenosis of the outflow vessels.

Digital subtraction angiography (DSA) is the current method of choice for anatomic hemodialysis access evaluation, but subjects the patient to ionizing radiation and involves nephrotoxic iodinated contrast. DSA performed with gadolinium has also been used, but with inferior contrast-to-noise ratio, and it is limited to only a few injections given the total body limits of gadolinium contrast.

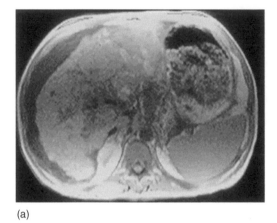

(a)

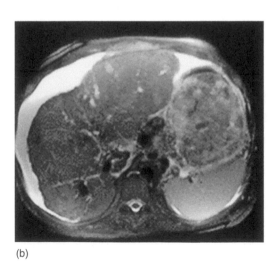

(b)

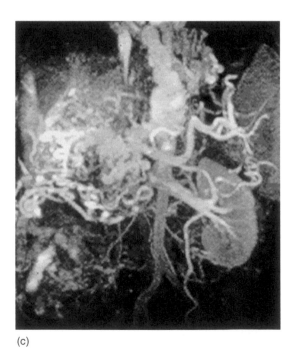

(c)

Figure 22.8 Portal vein thrombosis. (a, b) Axial T1-weighted and T2-weighted images show a cirrhotic liver with ascites. There is a complex tangle of low signal intensity in the gastric and paraesophageal region corresponding to varices. The portal vein is not well seen. (c) 3D CE-MRV confirms gastric and paraesophageal varices. A normal portal vein is not seen due to thrombosis with a resultant cavernous transformation.

Although MR-guided access intervention is not yet widely available, MRV offers an accurate alternative modality for venous mapping prior to creation of hemodialysis access and for evaluation of hemodynamically significant stenosis after placement. Hemodialysis access MRV involves placing the patient in a semi-oblique supine position on the shunt arm with the upper extremities lying next to the body. The antecubital vein contralateral to the fistula or graft limb serves as the site for intravenous contrast injection. Two-dimensional TOF surveys of the inflow–outflow tract and shunt region from the wrist to the subclavian vein are performed with a lipid marker on the dialysis access to accurately plan the contrast-enhanced portion. Indirect 3D CE-MRV is then performed with the aid of a test bolus. In one study by Froger et al, no complications occurred in the evaluation of 282 vascular segments, with excellent correlation to DSA for detection of significant stenosis: sensitivity 97%, specificity 99%, positive predictive value 96%, and negative predictive value 99%.

Another vascular structure successfully evaluated by MRV is the portal venous system. Accurate assessment of portal venous flow in patients with portal hypertension is needed to determine if the cause is pre-, intra-, or posthepatic. The most common prehepatic cause is portal vein thrombosis, usually in the setting of advanced cirrhosis (Figure 22.8). Ultrasound is usually the first imaging modality used in patients with portal hypertension and is accurate in the assessment of the portal venous system. But for patients with variceal bleeding in need of portosystemic shunt procedures, a more exact diagnostic modality that covers the whole portal venous system, such as DSA or CT, is often used for preoperative planning. However, Kreft et al showed that 3D CE-MRV of the portal venous flow is highly accurate compared to DSA with overall sensitivity, specificity, and accuracy for the detection of thrombosis of 100%, 98%, and 99%, respectively. In another study by Boeve et al, 3D CE-MRV in combination with MRI was superior to catheter intra-arterial DSA for detection of malignancy and portal venous occlusion in candidates for liver transplantation and transjugular intrahepatic portosystemic or splenorenal shunt.

CONCLUSIONS

MR venography has been shown to be accurate in evaluating thrombo-occlusive disease of the upper and lower extremities and venous malformations. It is more accurate than either US or CT for evaluating renal vein and IVC tumor thrombosis and can image areas not accessible by US or is limited by catheter venography or CT, for example the pelvis

and ovarian veins. It has shown promise in other clinical applications such as the assessment of hemodynamically significant stenosis in hemodialysis access and evaluation for thrombosis of the portal venous system. As new MR techniques are developed, MRV will continue to serve an expanding role in imaging the peripheral circulation.

FURTHER READING

Aschauer M, Deutschmann HA, Stollberger R et al. Value of a blood pool contrast agent in MR venography of the lower extremities and pelvis: preliminary results in 12 patients. Magnet Reson Med 2003; 50: 993–1002.

Bluemke DA, Wolf RL, Tani I et al. Extremity veins: evaluation with fast-spin-echo MR venography. Radiology 1997; 204: 562–5.

Boeve WJ, Kok T, Haagsma EB et al. Superior diagnostic strength of combined contrast enhanced MR-angiography and MR-imaging compared to intra-arterial DSA in liver transplantation candidates. Magnet Reson Imag 2001; 5: 609–22.

Butty S, Hagspiel KD, Leung DA et al. Body MR venography. Radiol Clin North Am 2002; 40: 899–919.

Cham MD, Yankelevitz DF, Shaham D et al. Deep venous thrombosis: detection by using indirect CT venography. Radiology 2000: 216: 744–51.

Evans AJ, Sostman HD, Knelson MH et al. 1992 ARRS Executive Council Award. Detection of deep venous thrombosis: prospective comparison of MR imaging with contrast venography. AJR 1993; 161: 131–9.

Finn JP, Zisk JH, Edelmann RR et al. Central venous occlusion: MR angiography. Radiology 1993; 187: 245–51.

Fraser DGW, Moody AR, Morgan PS et al. Diagnosis of lower limb deep venous thrombosis: a prospective blinded study of magnetic resonance direct thrombus imaging. Ann Intern Med 2002; 136: 89–98.

Fraser DGW, Moody AR, Davidson IR et al. Deep venous thrombosis: diagnosis by venous enhanced subtracted peak arterial MR venography versus conventional venography. Radiology 2003; 226: 812–20.

Froger CL, Dujim LE, Liem YS et al. Stenosis detection with MR angiography and digital subtraction angiography in dysfunctional hemodialysis access fistulas and grafts. Radiology 2005; 234: 284–91.

Herborn CU, Goyen M, Lauenstein TC et al. Comprehensive time-resolved MRI of peripheral vascular malformations. AJR 2003; 181: 729–35.

Katz DS, Loud PA, Bruce D et al. Combined CT venography and pulmonary angiography: a comprehensive review. Radiographics 2002; 22: S3–S24.

Kreft B, Strunk H, Flacke S et al. Detection of thrombosis in the portal venous system: comparison of contrast-enhanced MR angiography with intraarterial digital substraction angiography. Radiology 2000; 216: 86–92.

Kubik-Hutch RA, Hebisch G, Huch R et al. Role of duplex color Doppler ultrasound, computed tomography, and MR angiography in the diagnosis of septic puerperal ovarian vein thrombosis. Abdom Imag 1999; 24: 85–91.

Laissy JP, Fernandez P, Karila-Cohen P et al. Upper limb vein anatomy before hemodialysis fistula creation: cross-sectional anatomy using MR venography. Eur Radiol 2003; 13: 256–61.

Larsson EM, Sundeh P, Olsson CG et al. MR venography using an intravenous contrast agent: results from a multicenter phase 2 study of dosage. AJR 2003; 180: 227–32.

Li W, David V, Kaplan R, Edelman RR. Three-dimensional low dose gadolinium-enhanced peripheral MR venography. J Magnet Reson Imag 1998; 8: 630–3.

Li W, Salanitri J, Tutton S et al. Ferumoxytol-enhanced MR evaluation of deep venous thrombosis (DVT) using dual contrast mechanism. Radiology 2006 (in press).

Martel AL, Fraser D, Delay GS et al. Separating arterial and venous components from 3D dynamic contrast-enhanced MRI studies using factor analysis. Magnet Reson Med 2003; 49: 928–33.

Quinlan DJ, Alikhan R, Gishen P, Sidhu PS. Variations in lower limb venous anatomy: implications for US diagnosis of deep venous thrombosis. Radiology 2003; 228: 443–8.

Rijswijk CS, van der Linden E, van der Woude HJ et al. Value of dynamic contrast-enhanced MR imaging in diagnosing and classifying peripheral vascular malformations. AJR 2002; 178: 1181–7.

Ruehm SG, Zimny K, Debatin JF. Direct contrast-enhanced 3D MR venography. Eur Radiol 2001; 11: 102–12.

Sharafuddin MJ, Stolpen AH, Dang YM et al. Comparison of MS-325 and gadodiamide-enhanced MR venography of iliocaval veins. J Vasc Interven Radiol 2002; 13: 1021–7.

Spritzer CE, Arata MA, Freed KS. Isolated pelvic deep venous thrombosis: relative frequency as detected with MR imaging. Radiology 2001; 219: 521–5.

Vogt FM, Herborn CU, Goyen M. MR Venography. Magnet Reson Imag Clin North Am 2005; 13: 113–29.

Index

Page numbers in italic refer to figures and tables